ESSENTIAL
CARDIOLOGY

THIRD EDITION
ESSENTIAL CARDIOLOGY

Adam D. Timmis

MD, FRCP, FESC
Consultant Cardiologist
London Chest Hospital

Anthony W. Nathan

MD, FRCP, FACC, FESC
Consultant Cardiologist
St Bartholomew's Hospital
London

With a chapter by
Ian D. Sullivan

Consultant Cardiologist
Great Ormond Street Hospital
for Children

Blackwell
Science

© 1988, 1993, 1997 by
Blackwell Science Ltd
Editorial Offices:
Osney Mead, Oxford OX2 0EL
25 John Street, London WC1N 2BL
23 Ainslie Place, Edinburgh EH3 6AJ
350 Main Street, Malden
  MA 02148 5018, USA
54 University Street, Carlton
  Victoria 3053, Australia

Other Editorial Offices:
Blackwell Wissenschafts-Verlag GmbH
Kurfürstendamm 57
10707 Berlin, Germany

Blackwell Science KK
MG Kodenmacho Building
7–10 Kodenmacho Nihombashi
Chuo-ku, Tokyo 104, Japan

First published 1988
Reprinted 1989
Four Dragons edition 1989
Second edition 1993
Reprinted 1993, 1995
Four Dragons edition 1993
Third edition 1997
International edition 1997

Set by Semantic Graphics, Singapore
Printed and bound in Great Britain
by MPG Books Ltd, Bodmin, Cornwall

The Blackwell Science logo is a
trade mark of Blackwell Science Ltd,
registered at the United Kingdom
Trade Marks Registry

DISTRIBUTORS

Marston Book Services Ltd
PO Box 269
Abingdon, Oxon OX14 4YN
(*Orders*: Tel: 01235 465500
         Fax: 01235 465555)

USA
Blackwell Science, Inc.
Commerce Place
350 Main Street
Malden, MA 02148 5018
(*Orders*: Tel: 800 759 6102
              781 388 8250
         Fax: 781 388 8255)

Canada
Copp Clark Professional
200 Adelaide St West, 3rd Floor
Toronto, Ontario M5H 1W7
(*Orders*: Tel: 416 597-1616
              800 815-9417
         Fax: 416 597-1617)

Australia
Blackwell Science Pty Ltd
54 University Street
Carlton, Victoria 3053
(*Orders*: Tel: 3 9347 0300
         Fax: 3 9347 5001)

A catalogue record for this title
is available from the British Library

ISBN 0-632-04843-3 (BSL)
     0-632-04845-X (IE)

Library of Congress
Cataloging-in-Publication Data

Timmis, Adam D.
    Essential cardiology / Adam D. Timmis,
  Anthony W. Nathan ; with a chapter by
  Ian D. Sullivan. — 3rd ed.
        p.   cm.
    Rev. ed. of: Essentials of cardiology / Adam D.
  Timmis, Anthony W. Nathan. 2nd ed. 1993.
    Includes bibliographical references and index.
    ISBN 0-632-04843-3
    1. Cardiology. 2. Heart—Diseases.
    I. Timmis, Adam D.
  Essentials of cardiology. II. Nathan,
  Anthony W. III. Sullivan, Ian D. IV. Title.
    [DNLM: 1. Heart Diseases—diagnosis.
    2. Heart Diseases—therapy.
  WG 210 T584e 1997]
  RC667.T56   1997
  616.1'2—dc21
  DNLM/DLC
  for Library of Congress   97-14105
                                                  CIP

Contents

CONTENTS

Colour plates fall between pp. 244 and 245.

Preface

It is four years since the second edition of *Essentials of Cardiology*, and in preparing this new edition considerable changes have been necessary in order to keep the reader abreast with the broad range of technological and therapeutic developments which have occurred in the intervening period. The authorship of the book has once again been expanded to include Ian Sullivan from Great Ormond Street Hospital who has completely rewritten the chapter on paediatric cardiology, in order to provide a contemporary, hands-on perspective to this rapidly evolving cardiological subspecialty. Cardiac abnormalities are more common than congenital defects of any other system and in this new chapter the reader will find a detailed account of the current approaches to diagnosis and treatment which have resulted in more and more of these children surviving into adulthood. Despite the expanded authorship every effort has been made to retain the uniformity of style which has contributed to the popularity of the first two editions of the book.

Elsewhere the book has seen other important changes. Indeed, every chapter has been modified, particularly those on heart failure and coronary artery disease where investigative and therapeutic advances have been most dramatic. Thus, the role of ACE inhibition for improving prognosis in all grades of heart failure is now emphasised, while the importance of primary and secondary prevention of coronary heart disease is reflected in new sections devoted to these topics. In addition, the book describes the increasing application of interventional techniques in clinical cardiology, including intravascular ultrasound, coronary angioplasty, coronary stenting, balloon valvuloplasty and ablation therapy. Several illustrations of these new technologies are provided while other illustrations serve to highlight the important roles of transoesophageal echocardiography and magnetic resonance imaging in modern cardiological practice. Finally, acknowledgement is made of the drive towards evidence-based medicine by provision of structured summaries of some landmark clinical trials which have had a major impact on the way cardiological patients are now managed.

Essentials of Cardiology has once again undergone substantial revision in this new edition but it still aims to provide a concise, highly illustrated account of current cardiological practice. We hope that readers of this book will come to share some of our enthusiasm for this fascinating subject which remains one of the most exciting fields in clinical medicine.

Adam D Timmis, Anthony W Nathan, Ian Sullivan

List of Abbreviations

ACE	angiotensin-converting enzyme	IVUS	intravascular ultrasound
AF	atrial fibrillation	JVP	jugular venous pulse
AIDS	acquired immunodeficiency syndrome	LDH	lactic dehydrogenase
		LDL	low-density lipoprotein
APB	atrial premature beat	LGL	Lown–Ganong–Levine
AR	aortic regurgitation	LV	left ventricular
ARDS	adult respiratory distress syndrome	LVF	left ventricular failure
		MI	myocardial infarction
AS	aortic stenosis	MIBI	Methoxy isobutyl nitrile
AST	aspartate transaminase	MR	mitral regurgitation
AV	atrioventricular	MRI	magnetic resonance imaging
AVNRT	atrioventricular nodal re-entrant tachycardia	MS	mitral stenosis
		PA	posteroanterior
AVRT	atrioventricular re-entrant tachycardia	PAT	paroxysmal atrial tachycardia
		PE	pulmonary embolism
CK	creatine kinase	RVF	right ventricular failure
CT	computed tomography	SA	sinoatrial
CVA	cerebrovascular accident	SAM	systolic anterior motion
CXR	chest X-ray	SVT	supraventricular tachycardia
DC	direct current	TAPVC	total anomalous pulmonary venous connection
DVT	deep venous thrombosis		
ECG	electrocardiogram	tPA	tissue-type plasminogen activator
EPS	electrophysiological study	TR	tricuspid regurgitation
ESR	erythrocyte sedimentation rate	TS	tricuspid stenosis
GI	gastrointestinal	VF	ventricular fibrillation
GU	genitourinary	VPB	ventricular premature beat
HDL	high-density lipoprotein	VT	ventricular tachycardia
ICD	implantable cardioverter defibrillator	WPW	Wolff–Parkinson–White

CHAPTER 1

Symptoms and Signs of Heart Disease

SUMMARY

A careful history and examination are potentially diagnostic of most of the common cardiac disorders. Chest pain caused by myocardial ischaemia is called angina and is identified by its location, character and relation to provocative stimuli, particularly exertion. Dyspnoea and fatigue are important symptoms of heart failure and, like angina, are associated with exertion, though dyspnoea may also be provoked by lying flat, when it is called orthopnoea. Palpitation may be symptomatic of cardiac arrhythmia, particularly when its onset and termination are abrupt; description of the rate, rhythm (regular or irregular), duration and relation to provocative stimuli is required for accurate diagnosis. Cardiac syncope is always the result of abrupt cerebral hypoperfusion and, by definition, must be brief if death is to be avoided. Causes range from the trivial (vasovagal or postural attacks) to the serious (Stokes–Adams attacks, aortic stenosis).

During the cardiac examination, the patient should recline at a 45° angle while note is made of body habitus and general appearance. The radial pulse is examined for rate and rhythm but the carotid pulse provides more useful information about volume and waveform, a slow upstroke indicating aortic stenosis and a rapid upstroke aortic regurgitation. Blood pressure is measured by sphygmomanometry, phase V (disappearance of Korotkoff sounds) usually providing the best measure of diastolic pressure. The jugular venous pressure (JVP) reflects right atrial pressure and is elevated in right heart failure. It has a flickering character due to 'a' and 'v' waves, abnormalities of which provide additional diagnostic information. On examination of the chest, the position of the apex beat and the character of the left and right ventricular impulses should be noted. Auscultation of the heart requires identification of the first sound (S1) and both aortic and pulmonary components of the second sound (S2) which should split physiologically during inspiration. Abnormalities of S2 are an important sign of heart disease. Low-frequency rapid filling sounds early (S3) and late (S4) in diastole may be physiological in the young and elderly, respectively, but in other contexts are abnormal, often reflecting advanced ventricular dysfunction. Valve opening is usually silent but causes an early diastolic 'opening snap' in mitral stenosis and may also cause an early systolic 'ejection click' in aortic stenosis, particularly when the valve is bicuspid. Turbulent flow through diseased heart valves produces characteristic murmurs, the loudness, quality, location and timing of which should all be noted.

SYMPTOMS

The extent to which a patient is limited by symptoms of heart disease provides the basis for the New York Heart Association functional classification.

Class 1—asymptomatic (no functional limitation).

Class 2—symptomatic on extra exertion.

Class 3—symptomatic on mild exertion.

Class 4—symptomatic at rest or on minimal exertion (severe functional limitation).

This classification provides a simple means of describing functional capacity but it does not always reflect accurately the severity of disease in individual patients. Nevertheless, in large groups, the classification has been shown to provide a useful indication of disease severity and prognosis.

Chest pain

The common cardiovascular causes of chest pain are myocardial ischaemia, myocardial infarction, pericarditis, aortic dissection and pulmonary embolism.

Myocardial ischaemia results from an imbalance between myocardial oxygen supply and demand which produces pain called angina. Angina is usually a symptom of coronary artery disease (which impedes oxygen supply) but may also occur when left ventricular hypertrophy or rapid tachyarrhythmias cause excessive oxygen demand. Sensory impulses from the myocardium enter the upper cervical spine at the same level as impulses from the anterior chest wall, arm, throat and jaw. Angina is usually experienced in the anterior chest wall as a retrosternal constricting discomfort but it may radiate into any other of these areas. A number of anginal syndromes are recognized (see page 108) but the most common is chronic stable angina in which the pain is provoked by stimuli that increase myocardial oxygen demand, particularly exertion and emotion.

Symptoms are relieved within 2–10 minutes by rest. The location and character of the pain, its relation to provocative stimuli and its duration are essential criteria for the clinical diagnosis of chronic stable angina.

Myocardial infarction produces pain that is similar in location and character to angina. However, the pain is usually more severe, occurring at rest without provocation, and may last for several hours.

In *pericarditis*, chest pain is central or left-sided and is characteristically sharp. It is aggravated by deep inspiration, coughing or changes in posture and often lasts for several days.

Aortic dissection produces intense, tearing pain in either the front or back of the chest. The onset of symptoms is abrupt, unlike the crescendo quality of ischaemic cardiac pain.

Massive *pulmonary embolism* may cause central chest pain difficult to distinguish from myocardial ischaemia. Small pulmonary embolism, however, is often asymptomatic unless it causes a pulmonary infarct when pleuritic pain occurs over the affected area.

Rare cardiovascular causes of chest pain include mitral valve disease associated with massive left atrial dilatation. This causes discomfort in the back which is sometimes associated with dysphagia due to oesophageal compression. Aortic aneurysms can also cause pain in the chest due to local compression.

Dyspnoea

Dyspnoea is an abnormal awareness of breathing, occurring at rest or at an unexpectedly low level of exertion. It is a prominent symptom in a wide variety of cardiac disorders, including coronary, myocardial, valvular and pericardial disease. Nevertheless, *left heart failure* is the major cardiac cause of dyspnoea.

Acute left heart failure. The left atrium is in continuity with the pulmonary capillaries through the pulmonary venous bed. There are no valves in the pulmonary veins and the elevated left atrial pressure that characterizes acute left heart failure produces corresponding elevation of the pulmonary capillary pressure. This increases fluid transudation into the pulmonary interstitium and, as pressure rises, interstitial oedema progresses to alveolar oedema. The oedematous lung is stiff and the extra effort required for ventilation produces the sensation of dyspnoea. In alveolar oedema, impaired gas exchange leads to hypoxaemia which exacerbates dyspnoea by its effect on the respiratory centre. Reduction of left atrial pressure with diuretics and opiates leads to prompt relief of dyspnoea.

Chronic left heart failure. Chronic left heart failure caused by left ventricular or mitral disease is also associated with elevation of the left atrial pressure which rises still further on lying flat (due to gravitational effects), causing *orthopnoea* (Fig. 1.1a). Thus patients with left heart failure prefer to sleep with extra pillows. In advanced cases, frank pulmonary oedema in the supine position causes

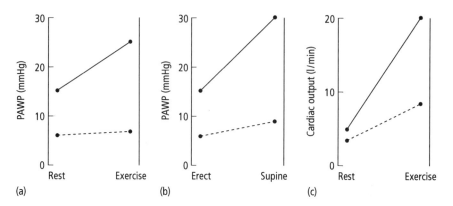

Fig. 1.1 (a) Orthopnoea, (b) exertional dyspnoea and (c) fatigue in left heart failure. Responses of normal individuals (broken line) are compared with those of patients with heart failure (continuous line). Note that in patients with heart failure, lying supine and exercise both cause a sharp increase in the pulmonary artery wedge pressure (PAWP) (an indirect measure of left atrial pressure) in contrast to normal patients in whom the wedge pressure is lower and shows little tendency to change. Despite the sharp rise in wedge pressure with exercise, however, the cardiac output response is markedly attenuated in heart failure compared with normal individuals.

paroxysmal nocturnal dyspnoea. This usually occurs during sleep and wakens the patient with distressing shortness of breath and fear of imminent death. These symptoms are corrected by sitting or standing upright, when gravitational pooling of blood lowers left atrial pressure. *Exertional dyspnoea* (Fig. 1.1b) is the most troublesome symptom in left heart failure. The mechanism is complex because, although left atrial pressure rises abnormally in response to exercise, it correlates poorly with the severity of dyspnoea. Moreover, drugs that lower left atrial pressure do not always improve exercise tolerance. Thus other factors must contribute to exertional dyspnoea in left heart failure. These may include respiratory muscle fatigue, increases in physiological dead space in the lungs and metabolic signals such as exertional acidosis.

Fatigue

Exertional fatigue (Fig. 1.1c) is an important symptom of both left and right heart failure. It is caused by inadequate delivery of oxygen to exercising skeletal muscle and reflects the combined effects of arteriolar vasoconstriction and impaired cardiac output. Drugs that improve the output response to exercise may correct fatigue if regional arteriolar vasodilatation allows the increased output to be distributed to skeletal muscle.

Palpitation

Palpitation is awareness of the heart beat. It is physiological during vigorous exertion or heightened emotion but under other circumstances it is often symptomatic of a cardiac arrhythmia. Occasional awareness of either the pause or the forceful beat that follows an extrasystole is a common complaint but rarely reflects important heart disease. Patients with bradyarrhythmias may be aware of the slow heart beat but tachyarrhythmias are a more common cause of symptoms. The abrupt onset and termination of paroxysmal tachyarrhythmias are particularly noticeable. Irregular palpitation indicates atrial fibrillation or ectopic beats but regular palpitation may be caused by atrial or ventricular arrhythmias. A history of termination of arrhythmia by vagal manoeuvres (Valsalva, rubbing the neck or eyes) suggests a re-entrant tachycardia either within the atrioventricular (AV) node or involving an accessory pathway.

Dizziness and syncope

Cardiac disorders produce dizziness and syncope through abrupt reductions in blood pressure associated with disturbance of cerebral perfusion. Prolonged attacks (> 4 minutes) are inevitably fatal because of the brain's obligatory oxygen requirement. Thus, almost by definition, recovery from cardiac dizziness and syncope occurs within a minute or two, unlike most other common causes of syncope (e.g. stroke, epilepsy, overdose) in which full recovery may be delayed for several hours.

Postural hypotension becomes more troublesome with advancing age. It is due to inadequate baroreceptor-mediated reflex vasoconstriction on standing up from the lying or sitting position. This produces a pronounced fall in blood pressure and cerebral perfusion which may cause the patient to fall to the ground whereupon the condition corrects itself. Vasodilator drugs must be avoided and patients should be encouraged to change posture gradually. If postural symptoms are associated with severe bradycardia, pacemaker therapy may be helpful but in most cases there is no specific treatment.

Vasovagal attacks usually occur in response to emotional or painful stimuli. Autonomic overactivity, manifested by yawning, nausea or sweating, causes vasodilatation in skeletal muscle and inappropriate slowing of the pulse; these combine to reduce blood pressure and cerebral perfusion. Recovery is rapid if the patient lies down. In the large majority of cases specific treatment is unnecessary and simple reassurance suffices. In patients with the very disabling 'malignant vasovagal syndrome', however, pacemaker therapy should be considered to prevent bradycardia although it does not, of course, affect the reflex vasodilatation.

Carotid sinus syncope affects the elderly. It arises when an exaggerated vagal discharge occurs in response to stimulation of the carotid sinus. Reflex vasodilatation and excessive slowing of the pulse lower the blood pressure and lead to dizziness and syncope. Rarely, stimuli such as a tight shirt collar may trigger attacks but more commonly they occur without obvious provocation. Pacemaker therapy is not always effective because, although it prevents slow heart rates, it has less effect on reductions in blood pressure caused by reflex vasodilatation.

Stokes–Adams attacks are caused by self-limiting episodes of asystole or ventricular tachyarrhythmias during which there is no effective cardiac output. Blood pressure becomes unrecordable and the patient loses consciousness.

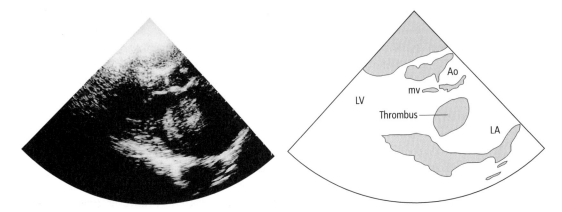

Fig. 1.2 Left atrial ball thrombus. This two-dimensional ECG (parasternal long axis view) shows massive dilatation of the left atrium (LA) in a patient with severe mitral valve disease. A large echogenic thrombus is clearly visible within the left atrium (LA), partially obstructing the mitral valve (mv).

Recovery is rapid following restoration of normal rhythm, when flushing occurs as circulation through the cutaneous bed is restored. Attacks caused by intermittent asystole are readily prevented by pacemaker therapy. Paroxysmal ventricular tachyarrhythmias are more difficult to treat (see page 240).

Valvular obstruction, either fixed or intermittent, is an important cardiac cause of syncope. In aortic stenosis, syncope typically occurs during exertion due to fixed valvular obstruction which prevents a normal increase in cardiac output into the dilated skeletal muscle vascular bed. Reductions in blood pressure and cerebral perfusion lead to syncope. Paroxysmal ventricular arrhythmias (Stokes–Adams attacks) also cause syncope in aortic stenosis. Intermittent valvular obstruction is usually caused by *left atrial myxoma* or ball thrombus (Fig. 1.2). These are mobile tumours which fall into the mitral valve orifice during diastole, thereby obstructing ventricular filling. The abrupt decline in cardiac output and cerebral perfusion causes syncope and if obstruction is unrelieved, death may ensue.

Other symptoms

Other symptoms of heart disease include *cough* and *haemoptysis* in left heart failure due to congestion of the bronchial tree. *Fever* and *flu-like* symptoms accompany infective endocarditis. A variety of other systemic disorders involve the cardiovascular system (see Chapter 16).

SIGNS

General examination

The general examination should first concentrate on the appearance of the patient. Severe obesity may be associated with diabetes, hyperlipidaemia or hypertension, while malnutrition and cachexia occur in advanced heart failure. Other signs of heart failure include tachypnoea, oedema, cyanosis and scleral jaundice. The distinctive features of specific congenital syndromes should be recognized because they are often associated with cardiovascular disorders (see Chapter 15). *Splinter haemorrhages* in the nail beds are a common but non-specific manifestation of infective endocarditis. Other 'classical' manifestations of this condition (clubbing, Osler's nodes, Janeway lesions) are now rarely seen.

Corneal arcus—a white ring around the iris—is common in the elderly, but in younger patients it may indicate hypercholesterolaemia, particularly when the arcus is eccentric. The presence of xanthelasmata—yellowish, fatty deposits in the eyelids—is also a non-specific sign of hypercholesterolaemia. However, *tendon xanthomata* are considerably more specific and are commonly associated with premature coronary artery disease. *Argyll–Robertson pupils* (irregular, unequal, and reacting to accommodation but not to light) are diagnostic of syphilis which was an important cause of coronary and aortic disease in the past. Fundoscopy may reveal signs of hypertensive or diabetic vascular disease, both of which are commonly associated with coronary artery disease.

Inspiratory crackles at the lung base occur commonly in left heart failure. *Hepatic* and splenic enlargement reflect visceral engorgement in right heart failure. In advanced heart failure, signs of *ascites* may also be present. Abdominal *aortic aneurysms* can usually be located by deep palpation and may be the cause of bruits heard during auscultation of the abdomen. Carotid and femoral bruits provide additional evidence of vascular disease.

Oedema

Oedema that pits in response to digital pressure is an important sign of congestive heart failure. The salt and water retention that characterizes heart failure expands plasma volume and increases capillary hydrostatic pressure. As pressure rises, the equilibrium between hydrostatic forces driving fluid out of the capillary and osmotic forces reabsorbing it cannot be maintained and oedema fluid accumulates in the interstitial space. The effect of gravity on capillary hydrostatic pressure ensures that dependent parts of the body are worst affected. Thus oedema is most prominent in the ankles in the ambulant patient, and over the sacrum in the bedridden patient.

Worsening salt and water overload leads to oedema of the legs, genitalia and trunk with engorgement of the abdominal viscera. Hepatic engorgement produces abdominal discomfort and nausea; jaundice may develop if hepatic dysfunction is severe. In advanced cases ascites occurs, particularly when disordered protein synthesis in the liver lowers plasma osmotic pressure. Effusion into the pleural and pericardial spaces may also occur.

Cyanosis

Cyanosis is a blue discoloration of the skin and mucous membranes caused by an increased concentration of reduced haemoglobin (greater than 5 g/100 ml) in the superficial blood vessels.

Peripheral cyanosis

Peripheral cyanosis affects the skin and the lips but spares the mucous membranes of the palate. It is caused by cutaneous vasoconstriction which slows blood flow in the skin and increases oxygen extraction. Peripheral cyanosis is physiological during exposure to cold but is also an important manifestation of heart failure, when sympathetically mediated cutaneous vasoconstriction occurs in response to reduced cardiac output. In severe mitral stenosis, cyanosis is often prominent over the cheeks producing the characteristic mitral facies.

Central cyanosis

Central cyanosis is caused by reduced arterial oxygen saturation and affects the skin and the mucous membranes of the mouth. Important cardiac causes of central cyanosis are acute pulmonary oedema and congenital heart disease. In acute pulmonary oedema, oxygenation of the blood is inadequate due to alveolar flooding. In congenital heart disease, central cyanosis is usually the result of right-to-left ('reversed') shunting of blood through a septal defect or a patent ductus arteriosus. Desaturated venous blood bypasses the lungs and enters the arterial circulation. Cyanosis caused by reversed shunting through a patent ductus arteriosus may be more prominent in the lower part of the body (differential cyanosis) because desaturated venous blood enters the aorta below the origins of the carotid and subclavian arteries. In adults, cyanotic congenital heart disease is usually associated with digital clubbing.

Skin temperature

Skin temperature provides a useful indication of cutaneous flow. In high-output states, such as pregnancy, the skin is vasodilated and warm, while in low-output states, such as heart failure or haemorrhage, reflex vasoconstriction causes cooling of the skin. Measurements of skin temperature are widely used in intensive care units for monitoring changes in cardiac output in response to treatment.

Clubbing of the fingers and toes

Congenital cyanotic heart disease is almost invariably associated with the development of clubbing during infancy; it is not present at birth. Clubbing may also be seen in pulmonary heart disease, but it is now a rare manifestation of infective endocarditis.

Arterial pulse and blood pressure

The arterial pulse is generated by the systolic contractions of the left ventricle. At the onset of ejection, the aortic valve is forced open and arterial pressure rises rapidly to a peak. The early decline in arterial pressure is checked by the dicrotic notch which marks aortic valve closure. There follows a more gradual decline in pressure as blood runs off into the peripheral circulation. Peak systolic pressure rises progressively as distance from the heart increases, because reflected pressure waves from the branch arteries summate with the main wave (Fig. 1.3). Pressure in the legs may be 20 mmHg higher than in the thoracic aorta. A small decline in peak systolic pressure occurs during inspiration, due to the increased vascular capacity of the inflated lung which reduces pulmonary venous return to the left atrium. Full examination of the pulse requires documentation of rate, rhythm and character. Finally, the symmetry of the peripheral pulses should be assessed and the blood pressure measured.

Rate and rhythm

Both are traditionally assessed by palpation of the right radial artery. Pulse rate, expressed in beats per minute, is measured by counting over a timed period of at

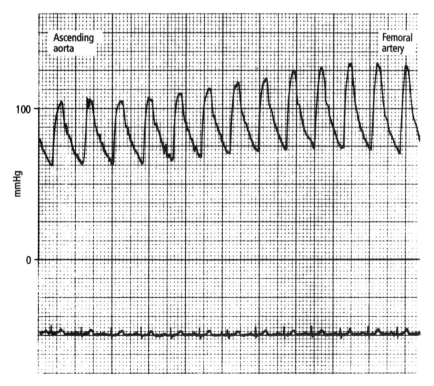

Fig. 1.3 Arterial pressure recording during catheter withdrawal from the ascending thoracic aorta to the femoral artery. Note the progressive rise in pressure as distance from the heart increases.

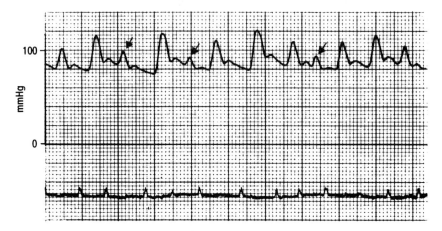

Fig. 1.4 Arterial pressure recording in atrial fibrillation. The ECG shows the irregularly irregular rhythm of atrial fibrillation. There is beat-to-beat variation of arterial pressure. The pulse pressure is lowest in those beats which follow very short diastolic intervals.

least 15 seconds. If the rhythm is irregular, the rate should be measured by auscultation at the cardiac apex, because beats that follow very short diastolic intervals may not generate sufficient pressure to be palpable at the radial artery. In rapid atrial fibrillation the apex–radial pulse deficit may be greater than 20 beats per minute (Fig. 1.4).

The rhythm is described as regular or irregular. Normal sinus rhythm is regular but may show phasic variation in rate during respiration (sinus arrhythmia), particularly in young patients. Frequent ectopic beats cause an irregular rhythm which may be difficult to distinguish from atrial fibrillation unless they occur predictably in bigeminal or trigeminal sequence. The irregularly irregular rhythm that characterizes atrial fibrillation is shown in Fig. 1.4.

Character

The character of the pulse, defined by its volume and waveform, should be evaluated at the (right) carotid artery. This is closest to the heart and is least subject to damping and distortion during passage through the arterial tree. A small, *low-volume* pulse reflects reduced stroke volume and occurs in advanced heart failure. Conversely, a *large-volume* pulse reflects increased stroke volume which characterizes aortic regurgitation and conditions associated with a hyperkinetic circulation (such as anaemia, pregnancy, fever or thyrotoxicosis).

Of greater diagnostic importance is the *waveform* of the pulse (Fig. 1.5). A slow upstroke pulse with a delayed peak characterizes aortic stenosis and reflects left ventricular outflow obstruction. In aortic regurgitation, backflow through the valve volume-loads the left ventricle in diastole, stimulating vigorous systolic ejection (Starling's law) with a rapid upstroke pulse and an exaggerated systolic peak; backflow also causes abrupt collapse of the pulse in early diastole with an

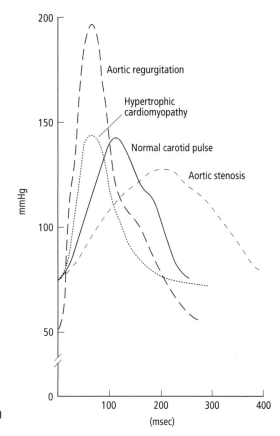

Fig. 1.5 The normal carotid arterial pulse recording compared with recordings in hypertrophic cardiomyopathy, aortic regurgitation and aortic stenosis. Note the very rapid upstroke of the pulse in hypertrophic cardiomyopathy and aortic regurgitation compared with the slow upstroke in aortic stenosis. The pulse pressure in aortic regurgitation is widened because of the exaggerated systolic peak and the diastolic collapse.

exaggerated diastolic nadir. Thus the pulse pressure (systolic minus diastolic pressure) is widened and prominent pulsations in the neck (Corrigan's pulse) are clearly visible. A *bisferiens* pulse, in which two systolic peaks can be felt, is characteristic but not diagnostic of mixed aortic stenosis and regurgitation. In hypertrophic cardiomyopathy, left ventricular contraction is vigorous and ejection is near complete by mid-systole. The pulse has a jerky quality with a rapid upstroke and a very early peak.

An alternating pulse always indicates severe left ventricular failure. The alternating high and low systolic peaks are particularly prominent in the beats that follow an extrasystole and can usually be detected by palpating the carotid pulse (Fig. 1.6). The mechanism is unknown.

A paradoxical pulse is an exaggeration of the normal inspiratory decline in systolic pressure. A decline greater than 10 mmHg (measured by sphygmomanometry) is usually pathological (Fig. 1.7). It is always present in cardiac tamponade because the normal inspiratory increase in right ventricular output is prevented. This exacerbates the inspiratory reduction in pulmonary venous return to the left atrium. A paradoxical pulse also occurs, albeit less frequently, in constrictive pericarditis and obstructive pulmonary disease.

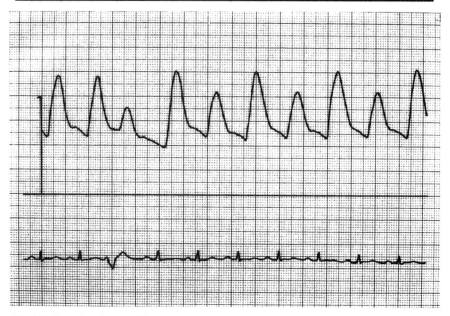

Fig. 1.6 Alternating pulse—arterial pressure recording in severe left ventricular failure. After the second beat a ventricular premature beat triggers an episode of alternating pulse.

Symmetry

The presence and symmetry of the following pulses should always be confirmed: radial, brachial, carotid, femoral, popliteal, posterior tibial and dorsalis pedis. A pulse that is absent or reduced in volume indicates an obstructive lesion more proximally in the arterial tree which is usually due to atherosclerosis or thromboembolism. Auscultation over the abdomen, or the carotid or femoral pulses, may reveal arterial bruits due to turbulent flow within the diseased vessels. Coarctation of the aorta is an important cause of symmetrical reduction of the femoral pulses which are 'delayed' compared with the radial pulses (radio-femoral delay).

Measurement of blood pressure

Blood pressure is measured indirectly using a sphygmomanometer. Supine and erect measurements should be recorded to provide an assessment of baroreceptor function. A cuff attached to a mercury or aneroid manometer is placed around the arm above the elbow. The width of the cuff should be at least 40% of the circumference of the arm, in order to avoid over-estimation of blood pressure, and in obese patients a large 'thigh cuff' may be required. The cuff is inflated until the brachial pulse disappears, then gradually deflated during auscultation over the brachial artery which should be held at the same level as the heart. Five phases of Korotkoff sounds can be distinguished during deflation of the cuff.

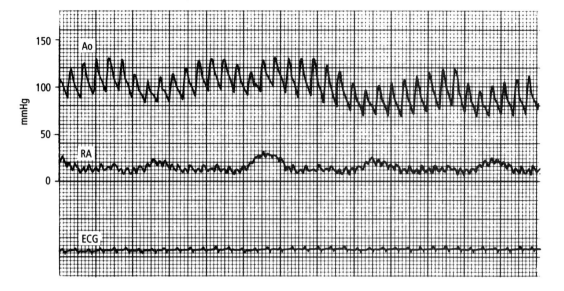

Fig. 1.7 Paradoxical pulse and Kussmaul's sign. Pericardial effusion (evidenced by the small voltage deflexions on the ECG) has caused tamponade. Respiratory fluctuations in the aortic (Ao) and right atrial (RA) pressure signals are seen. During inspiration aortic pressure falls markedly (paradoxical pulse) and right atrial pressure rises (Kussmaul's sign).

Phase I—the first appearance of an audible Korotkoff sound, marking systolic blood pressure.

Phase II/III—increasingly loud turbulence as blood flows through the constricted artery.

Phase IV—abrupt muffling of the Korotkoff sounds.

Phase V—disappearance of the Korotkoff sounds. This is usually within 10 mmHg of Phase IV.

In pregnancy, aortic regurgitation or patients with large arteriovenous fistulae, phase V may be difficult to identify and phase IV should be used as the measure of diastolic pressure. In all other situations, phase V should be used, not only because it corresponds more closely with directly measured diastolic pressure but also because its identification is less subjective.

Jugular venous pulse

Fluctuations in right atrial pressure during the cardiac cycle generate a pulse which is transmitted backwards into the internal jugular vein. Although the JVP is rarely palpable it may be visualized using a tangential light source while the patient reclines at a 45° angle. A more horizontal position may be required to visualize the pulse if right atrial pressure is low, or manual pressure applied to the upper abdomen may be used to produce a transient increase in venous return to the heart which elevates the JVP. The (vertical) level of the pulse above the sternal angle provides a measure of right atrial pressure while analysis of the waveform provides more specific diagnostic information.

Level of JVP

The upper limit of normal is 4 cm vertically above the sternal angle corresponding to a right atrial pressure of 6 mmHg. Elevation indicates increase of right atrial pressure, unless the superior vena cava is obstructed, producing engorgement of the neck veins.

During inspiration, pressure within the chest falls and there is a corresponding fall in the level of the JVP, despite an increase in venous return to the heart. In constrictive pericarditis, however, and less commonly in tamponade, the increased venous return during inspiration cannot be accommodated within the constricted right ventricle. This produces a paradoxical inspiratory rise in the level of the JVP—Kussmaul's sign (Fig. 1.7).

Waveform of JVP

The JVP has a flickering character due to 'a' and 'v' waves separated by 'x' and 'y' descents (Fig. 1.8). The 'a' wave produced by atrial systole precedes tricuspid valve closure, and is followed by the 'x' descent, marking the descent of the tricuspid valve ring. The 'x' descent is interrupted by the diminutive 'c' wave, marking tricuspid closure. Atrial pressure then rises again ('v' wave) as the chamber fills passively during ventricular systole. The decline in atrial pressure, as the tricuspid valve opens to allow ventricular filling, produces the 'y' descent. These events are difficult to distinguish on inspection, although they are clear on pressure recordings. The 'a' wave, however, is usually the most prominent deflexion and precedes ventricular systole which can be identified by simultaneous palpation of the carotid pulse on the opposite side of the neck.

Giant 'a' wave

Forceful atrial contraction against a stenosed tricuspid valve or a non-compliant hypertrophied right ventricle produces an unusually prominent (giant) 'a' wave.

Cannon 'a' wave (see Fig. 10.6)

Atrial systole against a closed tricuspid valve also produces prominent 'a' waves called cannon waves, which occur irregularly when atrial and ventricular rhythms are dissociated in complete heart block or ventricular tachycardia. They mark the random coincidence of atrial and ventricular systole. In junctional tachycardias, atrial and ventricular systole are simultaneous; cannon 'a' waves are therefore regular. Note that, because cannon 'a' waves occur during ventricular systole, their timing is coincident with the normal 'v' wave.

Giant 'v' wave (see Fig. 9.12)

This is an important sign of tricuspid regurgitation. The regurgitant jet produces

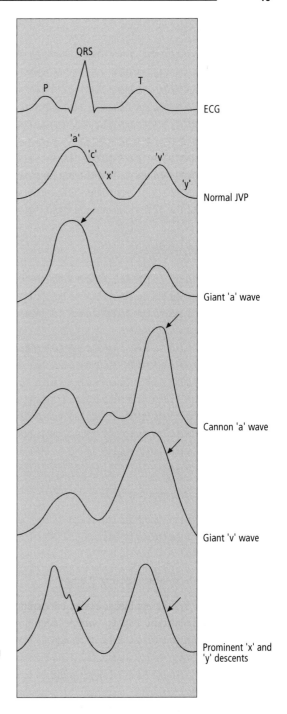

Fig. 1.8 The jugular venous pulse (JVP). Electrical events always precede mechanical events. Thus the P wave of the ECG (representing atrial depolarization) and the QRS complex (representing ventricular depolarization) precede the 'a' wave and the 'v' wave of the JVP, respectively.

pulsatile systolic waves in the jugular veins, which coincide with the period normally associated with passive atrial filling. They are therefore called giant 'v' waves, even though they are generated by an entirely different mechanism from the normal 'v' wave.

Prominent 'x' and 'y' descents (see Fig. 7.7)

Prominence of either the 'x' or the 'y' descent produces an unusually dynamic JVP although clinical distinction between these two negative waves is difficult. Tamponade produces a prominent 'x' descent because the vigorous right ventricular contraction causes exaggerated descent of the tricuspid valve ring. In constrictive pericarditis, ventricular contraction often shows variable impairment and the 'x' descent may not be so marked. The 'y' descent, however, is always prominent because ventricular filling is unusually rapid following the opening of the tricuspid valve due to the elevated right atrial pressure.

Examination of the heart

Inspection of the chest

Common chest-wall deformities include *pectus excavatum* (depressed sternum) and *straight back syndrome* (loss of dorsal curvature of thoracic spine), either of which may compress the heart and displace the apex beat laterally, giving a spurious impression of cardiac enlargement. Cardiac compression may also cause turbulence in the ventricular outflow tracts and produce 'innocent' ejection murmurs without affecting cardiac function. *Pectus carinatum* (pigeon chest) is sometimes associated with Marfan's syndrome but does not itself affect the heart. Large ventricular or aortic aneurysms may produce visible pulsations on the chest wall. Obstructions of the superior or inferior vena cava produce prominent venous collaterals on the anterior chest wall with caudal or cranial flow, respectively.

Palpation of the chest

The *apex beat* is the lowest and most lateral point on the chest wall at which the cardiac impulse is palpable while the patient sits upright. Location of the beat inferior or lateral to the intersection of the mid-clavicular line and the fifth intercostal space usually indicates cardiac enlargement.

The quality of the apex beat (as opposed to its location) is best appreciated with the patient lying on the left side. A *thrusting* impulse occurs in patients with left ventricular enlargement (dilatation or hypertrophy), particularly if stroke volume is increased, such as in aortic regurgitation. A *double* apical impulse may occur in patients with third or fourth heart sounds (see below). Indeed, these low-frequency added heart sounds are often more easy to feel than to hear.

Ventricular aneurysms and non-aneurysmal dyskinetic segments, following myocardial infarction, can be palpated as a more diffuse impulse medial to the apex beat. Right ventricular enlargement produces a systolic thrust in the left parasternal area.

The turbulent flow responsible for heart murmurs may produce palpable vibrations called 'thrills' on the chest wall. The location of thrills and their timing in the cardiac cycle match the location and timing of the murmur with which they are associated. Thrills are most commonly associated with aortic stenosis, but the murmurs of aortic regurgitation, mitral regurgitation, ventricular septal defect and patent ductus arteriosus may also be palpable if turbulence is sufficiently vigorous.

Percussion of the heart

Percussion plays no useful role in the cardiac examination. Although the area of cardiac dullness provides a crude measure of heart size, the location of the apex beat and the chest X-ray provide more accurate information.

Auscultation of the heart

A stethoscope with a diaphragm and bell must be used for appreciation of high-pitched and low-pitched auscultatory events, respectively. The apex and lower left, upper left and upper right sternal edges should be auscultated in turn. These correspond to the mitral, tricuspid, pulmonary and aortic areas, respectively, and loosely identify the sites at which murmurs from the four heart valves are best heard.

The *diaphragm* must be used at each of these sites but the *bell* is only used at the apex and lower left sternal edge where the important low-frequency sounds and murmurs occur. During auscultation the patient should recline at 45°; the sitting forward and lateral decubitus positions accentuate sounds and murmurs from the base (aortic and pulmonary areas) and apex of the heart, respectively.

To ensure identification of all auscultatory events in the cardiac cycle, a systematic approach should be adopted, listening to the first and second heart sounds and the systolic and diastolic intervals in sequence. Simultaneous palpation of the carotid pulse distinguishes systole from diastole when there is doubt about timing.

Heart sounds

First sound (S1)

This coincides with mitral and tricuspid valve closure at the onset of ventricular systole. The valve leaflets themselves do not produce S1, the precise cause of which is unknown. Electromechanical events on the right side of the heart are slightly delayed with respect to the left side, and narrow splitting of S1 into mitral followed by tricuspid components can occasionally be appreciated. Mitral closure makes the major contribution to S1. The normal mitral valve leaflets fall together following atrial systole, such that at the onset of ventricular systole the valve is already partially closed. In *mitral stenosis*, however, diastolic filling of the ventricle through the restricted mitral orifice is prolonged and the valve leaflets remain widely separated at the onset of ventricular systole. Valve closure therefore generates unusually vigorous vibrations and S1 is accentuated. In very advanced mitral stenosis, the valve is rigid and immobile and S1 becomes soft again.

Second sound (S2)

This coincides with aortic and pulmonary valve closure and marks the end of ventricular ejection (Fig. 1.9). S2 may be heard as a single sound during expiration, but during inspiration the increased venous return to the right side of the heart delays pulmonary valve closure, to produce physiological splitting into aortic followed by pulmonary components. *Right bundle branch block* delays right ventricular activation and exaggerates the normal splitting of S2. Conditions

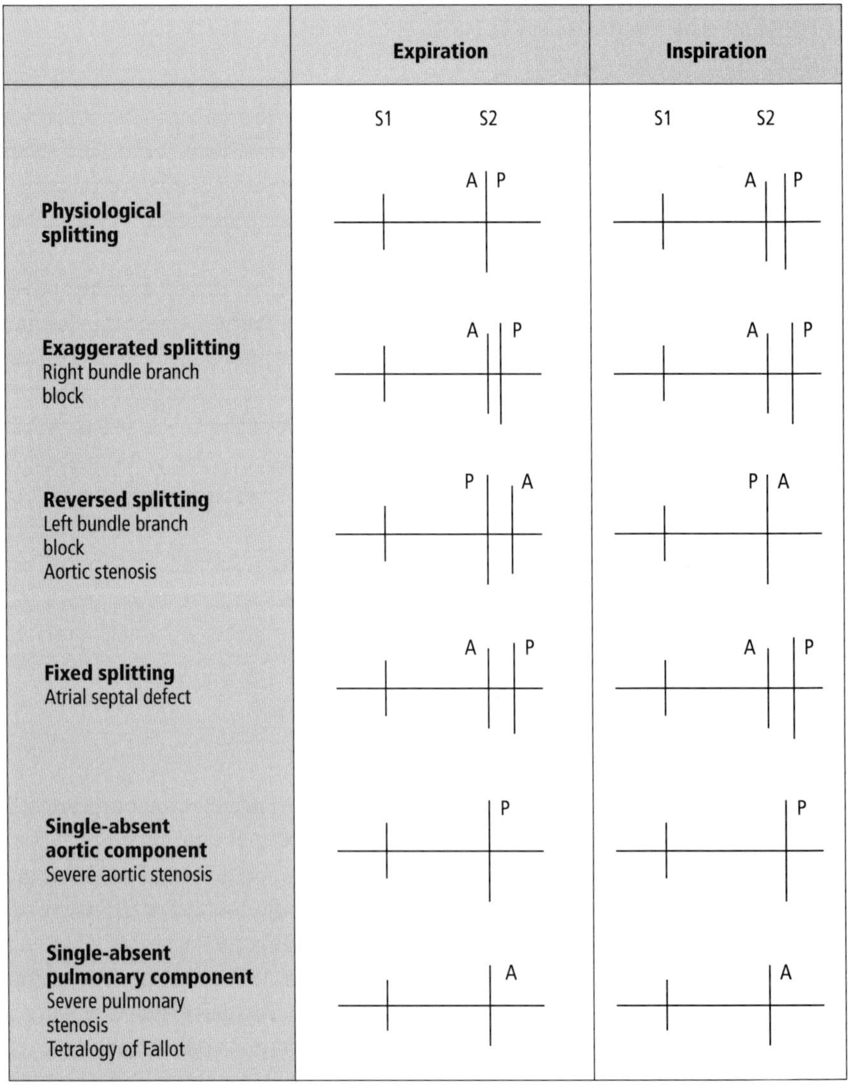

	Expiration	Inspiration
	S1 S2	S1 S2
Physiological splitting	A | P	A | P
Exaggerated splitting Right bundle branch block	A | P	A | P
Reversed splitting Left bundle branch block Aortic stenosis	P | A	P | A
Fixed splitting Atrial septal defect	A | P	A | P
Single-absent aortic component Severe aortic stenosis	P	P
Single-absent pulmonary component Severe pulmonary stenosis Tetralogy of Fallot	A	A

Fig. 1.9 Splitting of the second heart sound.

associated with delayed aortic valve closure (*left bundle branch block, aortic stenosis*) produce reversed splitting of S2; pulmonary followed by aortic components are heard separately during expiration, but during inspiration the physiological delay in the pulmonary component produces a single sound. In *atrial septal defect*, fixed splitting of S2 occurs throughout the respiratory cycle. The left-to-right shunt increases right ventricular stroke volume and delays pulmonary valve closure resulting in a split S2; during inspiration, increased venous return to the right atrium reduces the shunt such that the split remains fixed. S2 is single throughout the respiratory cycle when either the aortic or pulmonary component is absent. This occurs in severe *aortic* or *pulmonary stenosis*, and also in *tetralogy of Fallot* (absent pulmonary component). The aortic and pulmonary components of S2 are loud in *systemic* and *pulmonary hypertension*, respectively.

Third and fourth heart sounds (S3, S4)

These low-frequency diastolic sounds are associated with rapid ventricular filling, which occurs early in diastole (S3) following atrioventricular valve opening, and again later in diastole (S4) due to atrial contraction. When present, they give a characteristic gallop to the cardiac rhythm—best heard at the apex with the bell of the stethoscope.

In children and young adults the left ventricle is relatively thin and relaxes rapidly, permitting rapid filling in early diastole. S3 is therefore physiological in this age group, but tends to disappear beyond the age of 40, as increase in ventricular mass reduces the velocity of relaxation. S3 may also be present in high-output states caused by anaemia, fever, pregnancy or thyrotoxicosis. After the age of 40, S3 is nearly always pathological, usually indicating left ventricular failure or, less commonly, mitral regurgitation or constrictive pericarditis (see Fig. 4.6).

S4 is nearly always pathological, and occurs when vigorous atrial contraction late in diastole is required to augment filling of a hypertrophied non-compliant left ventricle, such as in hypertension, aortic stenosis or hypertrophic cardiomyopathy.

Systolic clicks and opening snaps

In the normal heart, valve opening is silent (unlike valve closure) and cannot be detected during auscultation. Under certain circumstances, however, aortic or pulmonary valve opening produces an *ejection click* in early systole, while mitral valve opening produces an *opening snap* in early diastole (tricuspid opening is only rarely audible). An *aortic ejection click is* heard in aortic stenosis if the valve leaflets are mobile. The click precedes the ejection murmur and is particularly prominent in patients with a congenitally bicuspid valve (see Fig. 9.8). In advanced calcific disease, the aortic leaflets are rigid and do not generate an ejection click. A *pulmonary ejection click* occurs in conditions associated with dilatation of the main pulmonary artery, including pulmonary hypertension and valvular pulmonary stenosis. A click later in systole (*mid-systolic click*) usually signifies mitral valve prolapse. It may be followed by a murmur if mitral regurgitation is present (see Fig. 9.6).

The *mitral opening snap* is best heard at the cardiac apex and is pathognomonic of mitral stenosis. It is related to forceful opening of the valve due to elevated left atrial pressure (see Fig. 9.4). As mitral stenosis worsens, left atrial pressure rises and leaflet rigidity increases; these cause the opening snap to occur progressively earlier in diastole and to become progressively quieter, respectively. The timing of the opening snap is unaffected by respiration, helping to distinguish it from the pulmonary component of the second heart sound.

Heart murmurs

Heart murmurs detected during auscultation are vibrations caused by turbulent flow within the heart (Fig. 1.10). The turbulence is usually the result of one of the following:

1 Valve disease.

2 Increased flow through a normal valve—usually aortic or pulmonary—causing an 'innocent' flow murmur (see below).

3 Abnormal communications between the left and right sides of the heart (e.g. septal defects, sinus of Valsalva aneurysms).

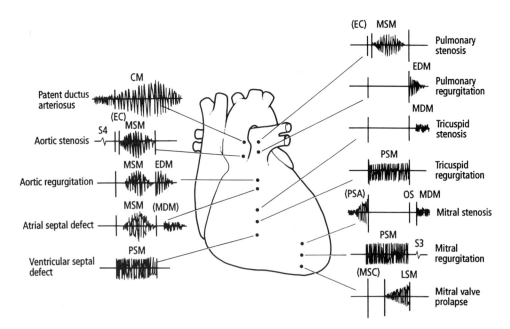

Fig. 1.10 Heart murmurs: CM, continuous murmur; MSM, mid-systolic murmur; PSM, pansystolic murmur; LSM, late systolic murmur; EDM, early diastolic murmur; MDM, mid-diastolic murmur; PSA, presystolic accentuation of murmur; EC, ejection click; MSC, mid-systolic click; OS, opening snap; S3, third heart sound; S4, fourth heart sound. Parentheses indicate those auscultatory findings which are not constant.

Table 1.1 Grading system for describing the loudness of heart murmurs.

Grade	Description
1	The faintest detectable murmur
2	Faint murmur, readily detectable
3	Moderately loud murmur
4	Loud murmur
5	Very loud murmur
6	Extra loud murmur, detectable with stethoscope raised off the chest wall

Murmurs are defined by four characteristics: loudness, quality, location and timing.

The *loudness* of a murmur is graded from 1 to 6 (Table 1.1) and is determined principally by the degree of turbulence, which in turn relates to volume and velocity of flow rather than to the severity of the cardiac lesion. Indeed, although turbulent flow often reflects valvular disease or an intracardiac shunt, it may also occur when the volume or velocity of flow through a normal valve is exaggerated. Thus, the hyperdynamic circulation in anaemia or pregnancy may cause turbulence in the ventricular outflow tracts and produce murmurs that are difficult to distinguish from those associated with aortic or pulmonary stenosis.

A variety of adjectives have been used to describe the *quality* of heart murmurs (blowing, musical, honking, rumbling) but their interpretation is very subjective. The quality of a murmur relates to its frequency (or pitch) and is therefore best described as low, medium or high pitched. The mid-diastolic murmurs of mitral and tricuspid stenosis are low pitched, the systolic murmurs of aortic and pulmonary stenosis and mitral and tricuspid regurgitation are medium pitched, and the early diastolic murmurs of aortic and pulmonary regurgitation are high pitched. The *location* of a murmur on the chest wall is determined by its origin, while its *radiation* is determined by the direction of the blood flow. The locations of the aortic, pulmonary, tricuspid and mitral areas have already been described (page 17) and murmurs from the respective valves are usually best heard in these areas. Localization is not always specific, and aortic systolic murmurs, for example, are often clearly audible all over the left precordium. Significant radiation of murmurs occurs only when flow velocity is rapid. The high-velocity systolic flow in *mitral regurgitation* and *aortic stenosis* is directed towards the left axilla and the neck, respectively. Thus murmurs related to these lesions radiate to the same area. The high-velocity diastolic flow in *aortic regurgitation* is directed towards the left sternal edge, where the murmur is often more clearly audible than at the aortic area.

It is not adequate to describe the *timing* of a murmur as systolic or diastolic without referring more specifically to the length of the murmur and the phase of systole or diastole during which it is heard: *systolic* murmurs are either mid-systolic, pansystolic or late systolic; *diastolic* murmurs are either early diastolic, mid-diastolic or presystolic in timing. Continuous murmurs are audible in both phases of the cardiac cycle.

A *mid-systolic* ('*ejection*') murmur is caused by turbulence in the left or right ventricular outflow tracts during ejection. It starts following opening of the aortic or pulmonary valve, reaches a crescendo in mid-systole, and disappears before the second heart sound. The murmur is loudest in the aortic area (with radiation to the neck) when it arises from the left ventricular outflow tract, and in the pulmonary area when it arises from the right ventricular outflow tract. It is best heard with the diaphragm of the stethoscope while the patient sits forward. Important causes of *aortic ejection murmurs* are aortic stenosis and hypertrophic cardiomyopathy. Aortic regurgitation also produces an ejection murmur due to increased stroke volume and velocity of ejection. *Pulmonary ejection murmurs* may be caused by pulmonary stenosis or infundibular stenosis (Fallot's tetralogy). In atrial septal defect the pulmonary ejection murmur results from right ventricular volume loading and does not indicate organic valvular disease. *'Innocent' murmurs* unrelated to heart disease are always mid-systolic in timing and are caused by turbulent flow in the left (sometimes right) ventricular outflow tract. In most cases there is no clear cause but they may reflect a hyperkinetic circulation in conditions such as anaemia, pregnancy, thyrotoxicosis or fever. They are rarely louder than grade 3, often vary with posture, may disappear on exertion, and are not associated with other signs of organic heart disease.

Pansystolic murmurs are audible throughout systole from the first to the second heart sounds. They are caused by regurgitation through incompetent atrioventricular valves and by ventricular septal defects. The pansystolic murmur of *mitral regurgitation* is loudest at the cardiac apex and radiates into the left axilla. It is best heard with the diaphragm of the stethoscope with the patient lying on the left side. The murmurs of *tricuspid regurgitation* and *ventricular septal defect* are loudest at the lower left sternal edge. Inspiration accentuates the murmur of tricuspid regurgitation because the increased venous return to the right side of the heart increases the regurgitant volume. *Mitral valve prolapse* may also produce a pansystolic murmur but, more commonly, prolapse occurs in mid-systole producing a click followed by a late-systolic murmur (see Fig. 9.6).

Early diastolic murmurs are high pitched and start immediately after the second heart sound, fading away in mid-diastole. They are caused by regurgitation through incompetent aortic and pulmonary valves and are best heard using the diaphragm of the stethoscope while the patient leans forward. The early diastolic murmur of *aortic regurgitation* radiates from the aortic area to the left sternal edge where it is usually easier to hear. *Pulmonary regurgitation* is loudest in the pulmonary area.

Mid-diastolic murmurs are caused by turbulent flow through the atrioventricular valves. They start following valve opening, relatively late after the second sound, and continue for a variable period during mid-diastole. *Mitral stenosis* is the principal cause of a mid-diastolic murmur which is best heard at the cardiac apex using the bell of the stethoscope while the patient lies on the left side. Increased flow across a non-stenotic mitral valve occurs in *ventricular septal defect* and *mitral regurgitation* and may produce a mid-diastolic murmur. In severe *aortic regurgitation*, preclosure of the anterior leaflet of the mitral valve by the regurgitant jet may produce mitral turbulence associated with a mid-diastolic murmur

(Austin–Flint murmur). A mid-diastolic murmur at the lower left sternal edge, accentuated by inspiration, is caused by *tricuspid stenosis* and also by conditions that increase tricuspid flow, e.g. atrial septal defect, tricuspid regurgitation.

In *mitral* or *tricuspid stenosis*, atrial systole produces a presystolic murmur immediately before the first heart sound when the patient is in sinus rhythm. The murmur is perceived as an accentuation of the mid-diastolic murmur associated with these conditions. Because presystolic murmurs are generated by atrial systole they do not occur in patients with atrial fibrillation.

Continuous murmurs are heard during systole and diastole and are uninterrupted by valve closure. The commonest cardiac cause is *patent ductus arteriosus* in which flow from the high-pressure aorta to the low-pressure pulmonary artery continues throughout the cardiac cycle, producing a murmur over the base of the heart which, though continuously audible, is loudest at end-systole and diminishes during diastole. Ruptured sinus of Valsalva aneurysm also produces a continuous murmur (see Fig. 13.2).

In patients with a hyperkinetic circulation flow in the jugular veins is sometimes audible as a continuous hum over the base of the heart, abolished by lying the patient supine.

Pericardial friction rub

In *pericarditis*, the movement of the visceral layer of the pericardium against the parietal layer produces a high-pitched, scratching noise called a friction rub. This may be audible during any part of the cardiac cycle and over any part of the left precordium depending on the extent of pericardial involvement. It is best heard using the diaphragm of the stethoscope while the patient sits forward.

FURTHER READING

Anonymous. Clinical signs in heart failure. *Lancet* 1989; ii: 309.

Constant J. *Bedside Cardiology*, 4th edn. Edinburgh: Churchill Livingstone, 1993.

Craige E. Should auscultation be rehabilitated? *N Engl J Med* 1988; 318: 1611.

Henkind SJ, Benis AM, Teichholz LE. The paradox of pulsus paradoxus. *Am Heart J* 1987; 114: 198.

Leatham A. Auscultation and phonocardiography: a personal view of the past 40 years. *Br Heart J* 1987; 57: 397.

CHAPTER 2

The Electrocardiogram and Arrhythmia Detection

CONTENTS

SUMMARY

The electrocardiogram (ECG) records the electrical activity of the heart at the skin surface and consists of three bipolar leads (I, II, III) and nine unipolar leads (aVR, aVL, aVF and V1–V6). The orientation of each lead with respect to the heart is different and consequently the positive and negative depolarization changes recorded by each lead are also different. However, in normal sinus rhythm, the sequence of changes is always the same, each sinus impulse initiating atrial depolarization (P wave) followed by ventricular depolarization (QRS complex) and ventricular repolarization (T wave). In analysing the ECG, the rate, rhythm and frontal plane QRS axis should first be noted. Examination of P wave and QRS morphology provides evidence not only of myocardial disease involving the atria and ventricles but also of conducting tissue disease as it affects the PR interval, the duration of the QRS complex and P wave–QRS association. ST segment analysis is important for diagnosis of acute ischaemia, myocardial infarction and pericarditis.

The ECG is the most useful tool for arrhythmia detection, and if a 12-lead recording can be obtained during symptoms it is usually diagnostic. For patients with intermittent arrhythmias, a recording may be obtained by ambulatory ECG monitoring, either in hospital using a central monitoring station or on an outpatient basis using a small portable recording device. When the history suggests arrhythmias in association with specific activities, the ECG recorded during provocative testing may be helpful, using stress testing for exercise-induced symptoms or tilt testing for postural symptoms. In some cases electrophysiological study (EPS) is required in which one or more electrode catheters are positioned within the cardiac chambers to record the intracardiac electrogram and to deliver electrical impulses for stimulating and terminating arrhythmias. More recently EPS has also been used for delivering therapy in patients requiring catheter ablation of conducting tissue and arrhythmogenic foci.

THE ELECTROCARDIOGRAM

The ECG is a record of the electrical activity of the heart recorded at the skin surface. A good-quality 12-lead ECG is essential for the proper evaluation of the cardiac patient.

Generation of electrical activity

The interior of the resting cardiac cell is electrically negative relative to the exterior, due to active extrusion of sodium ions which maintain a transmembrane voltage difference of approximately -90 mV. Reduction of the voltage difference to a threshold of -60 mV triggers a self-perpetuating action potential.

In the Purkinje cell (Fig. 2.1a) this occurs in response to electrical stimulation which reduces the voltage difference to threshold by increasing membrane permeability to sodium ions. The action potential has five parts:

0 rapid depolarization caused by rapid influx of sodium ions;

1 early repolarization caused by efflux of sodium ions;

2 plateau during which depolarization is temporarily arrested by slow influx of calcium ions;

3 rapid repolarization due to completion of cation efflux; and

4 diastole during which the resting transmembrane voltage difference remains at -90 mV until the cell is once again stimulated.

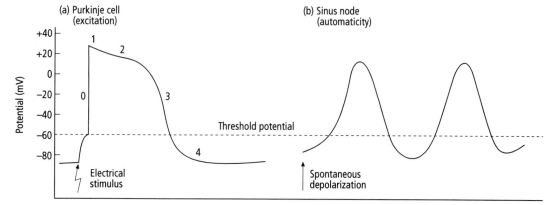

Fig. 2.1 Action potential recordings from (a) a Purkinje cell and (b) a pacemaker cell of the sinus node. Depolarization of the Purkinje cell occurs in response to excitation but in the sinus node depolarization is spontaneous.

In the sinus and atrioventricular nodes (Fig. 2.1b) depolarization to threshold occurs spontaneously and is not dependent upon electrical stimulation. All the specialized conduction tissues are capable of spontaneous depolarization (*automaticity*) but because the sinus node has the fastest intrinsic rate, it provides the pacemaker for the normal heart. The action potential of the sinus node pacemaker cells is principally dependent on the influx of calcium ions, and exhibits a different contour from that of the His–Purkinje cells.

In the normal heart, the impulse generated by the sinus node spreads first through the atria, producing atrial systole, and then through the atrioventricular (AV) node and His–Purkinje tissue, producing ventricular systole (Fig. 2.2). The AV node and bundle of His provide the only pathway connecting atria and ventricles; the remainder of the AV ring tissue is electrically inert. Moreover, impulse conduction through the AV node is slow and cannot proceed above a certain rate. These anatomical and physiological properties of AV conduction ensure that:

1 ventricular filling is complete before the onset of systole; and
2 the ventricles will not respond to excessively rapid atrial rates.

Within the ventricles, the impulse is conducted rapidly through the bundle of His into the upper part of the interventricular septum and thence through the left and right bundle branches to the free walls of the ventricles. The wave of depolarization that spreads through the heart during each cardiac cycle has vector properties defined by its direction and magnitude. At any instant depolarization occurs in multiple directions as the activation wave is propagated. Thus the instantaneous direction of the wave recorded at the skin surface is the

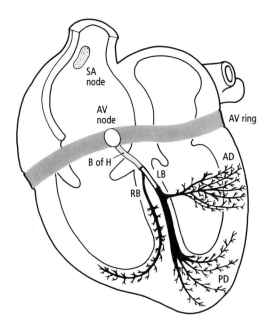

Fig. 2.2 Normal conduction pathways. SA, sinoatrial; AV, atrioventricular; B of H, bundle of His; LB, left bundle; RB, right bundle. Note that the left bundle branch divides into anterior and posterior divisions (AD and PD). The electrically inert atrioventricular ring tissue is indicated by the shaded band.

resultant of multiple 'minivectors' throughout the heart. Since the sinus node is in the high right atrium, the predominant direction of the activation wave is downwards and to the left. This produces the P wave on the ECG. Ventricular depolarization is initiated in the upper part of the septum following passage of the impulse through the AV node into the bundle of His. The predominant direction of the activation wave is downwards and slightly leftwards due to the greater thickness of the wall of the left ventricle compared with the right ventricle. This produces the QRS complex on the ECG.

An activation wave approaching the recording electrode produces, by convention, a *positive* deflexion on the ECG, whilst a wave moving in the opposite direction produces a *negative* deflexion. Importantly, if the direction of the wave is at right angles to the recording electrode it produces no deflexion at all. Thus every gradation of deflexion (positive and negative) can be produced by the same activation wave depending on the precise orientation of the recording electrode (Fig. 2.3). During the normal depolarization process, the (resultant) direction of the activation wave is continuously changing as it spreads throughout the heart. The ECG deflexions change accordingly during each cardiac cycle, being positive at one moment and negative at another.

The magnitude of the activation wave is a function of muscle mass and therefore the ECG deflexion produced by depolarization of the atrium (the P wave) is smaller than that produced by depolarization of the more muscular ventricles (QRS complex). Consequently, patients with *ventricular hypertrophy* tend to have exaggerated QRS voltage deflexions on the ECG. As previously stated, the magnitude of the activation wave perceived by a recording electrode is also influenced by its direction; the deflexions, regardless of muscle mass, become progressively smaller as the orientation of the recording electrode to the activation wave approaches right angles.

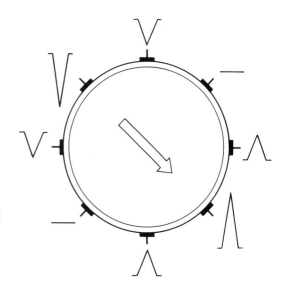

Fig. 2.3 A unidirectional activation wave (large arrow) and the voltage deflections recorded by eight electrodes. As the activation wave approaches an electrode it records a positive deflexion and as it moves away it records a negative deflexion. The greatest deflexions (both positive and negative) are recorded by electrodes orientated along the long axis of the activation wave. Electrodes at right angles record no deflexion at all.

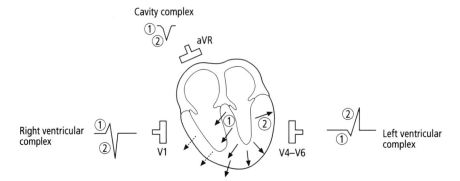

Fig. 2.4 Inscription of the QRS complex. The first (1) and second (2) ventricular depolarization vectors as perceived by recording electrodes orientated towards the right ventricle (V1) and the left ventricle (V4–V6). Note that lead aVR is orientated towards the ventricular cavities and therefore records an entirely negative deflexion.

Inscription of the QRS complex

The shape of the QRS complex is determined by the ventricular depolarization vector and the orientation of the recording electrode with respect to the heart. The ventricular depolarization vector can, for convenience, be resolved into two components (Fig. 2.4). The first, septal depolarization, spreads from left to right while the second, ventricular free wall depolarization, spreads from endocardium to epicardium.

Because the left ventricular depolarization vector dominates that of the thin-walled right ventricle, the net direction of the second vector component is from right to left. Therefore, leads orientated to the *left ventricle* record a small negative deflexion (Q wave) as the septal depolarization vector moves away, followed by a large positive deflexion (R wave) as the ventricular depolarization vector moves towards the recording electrode. The sequence of deflexions in leads orientated towards the *right ventricle* is in the opposite direction, to give an RS complex (Fig. 2.4).

Mean frontal QRS axis

This is the mean direction of the ventricular depolarization vector in those leads (1–aVF) that lie in the frontal plane of the heart. Although the direction of the depolarization vector is continuously changing, its mean direction can be determined by identifying the limb lead in which the net QRS deflexion (positive and negative) is least pronounced, i.e. the lead where positive and negative deflexions are most equal. The mean frontal QRS axis is at right angles to this lead and is quantified using a hexaxial reference system (Fig. 2.5).

The principal importance of the mean frontal QRS axis relates to its wide range of normality from −30° to +90°. This explains the wide variation of limb-lead QRS patterns that are consistent with a normal ECG. Correct inter-

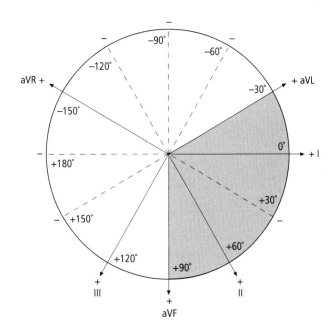

Fig. 2.5 Hexaxial reference system. When the mean frontal QRS is directed towards lead I it is arbitrarily defined as 0°; the dominant positive deflexion is in lead I and the equiphasic deflexion is in aVF. Axis shifts are ascribed a negative sign if directed leftwards (towards aVL) and a positive sign if directed rightwards (towards aVF). Axes between −30° and + 90° are normal (shaded area). Axes less than − 30° (left axis deviation) or greater than + 90° (right axis deviation) are abnormal.

pretation of the ECG must therefore take account of the mean frontal QRS axis. An abnormal axis often indicates heart disease but does not itself identify the nature of the disorder. Nevertheless, *left axis deviation* is usually associated with conduction block in the anterior fascicle of the left bundle branch ('left anterior hemiblock'—see Fig. 5.23) while *right axis deviation* may indicate right ventricular strain or a block in the posterior fascicle of the left bundle branch (left posterior hemiblock, see Figs 14.4 and 14.6).

The normal ECG

Figure 2.6 shows a standard 12-lead ECG. The recording is normal. Note the following features.

1 There are six limb leads. Leads I–III are the bipolar limb leads. Leads aVR–aVF are the augmented unipolar limb leads.

2 There are six unipolar chest leads, V1–V6.

3 The orientation of each lead to the wave of depolarization is different. Consequently the perceived direction and magnitude of the wave shows considerable variation, as reflected by the difference in the shapes of the complexes.

4 Despite this variation the sequence of deflexions is identical in each lead. The small P wave (atrial depolarization) is followed by the larger QRS complex (ventricular depolarization) and the T wave (ventricular repolarization).

5 The paper speed is 25 mm/second so that each small square (1 mm) represents 0.04 seconds and each large square (5 mm) represents 0.20 seconds.

6 The square wave is a calibration signal: 1 cm vertical deflexion = 1 mV.

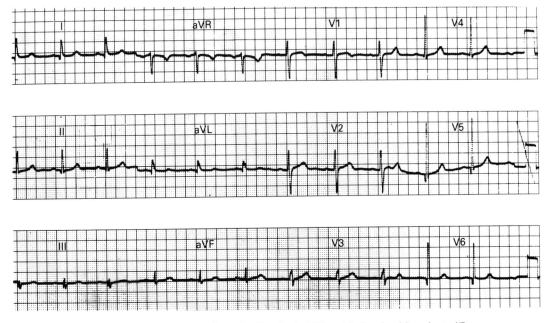

Fig. 2.6 Standard 12-lead ECG. Normal recording. Note that lead III is equiphasic and at right angles to aVR which is dominantly negative. Thus the mean frontal QRS axis is +30°.

The limb leads

The standard bipolar leads (I–III) each measure the potential difference between two limbs:

lead I: left arm–right arm;

lead II: left leg–right arm;

lead III: left leg–right arm.

An earth electrode is attached to the right leg to minimize electrical interference.

The heart may be considered as the centre of an equilateral triangle (Einthoven's triangle) formed by the two arms and the left leg (Fig. 2.7). By simple subtraction of vectors, the orientation of each standard lead with reference to the heart may be calculated.

The augmented unipolar limb leads (aVR–aVF) each consist of an exploring electrode connected to a limb: an indifferent electrode is connected to the other two limbs through high electrical resistance. The potential of the indifferent electrode is thus reduced to a very low level. This has two important effects.

1 The voltage deflexion on the ECG is augmented.

2 The orientation of the augmented lead with reference to the heart is very close to that of the limb to which the exploring electrode is attached. Thus in Fig. 2.7 the orientation of the limbs (RA, LA, F) is essentially the same as the orientation of aVR, aVL and aVF with reference to the heart.

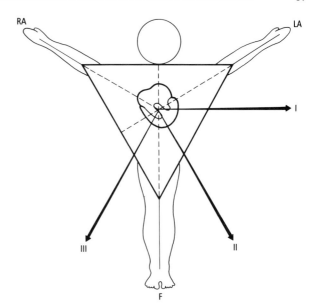

Fig. 2.7 Einthoven's triangle. Lead I measures the potential difference between the left and right arms. Since the right arm carries the negative electrode the resultant direction of the lead I vector is obtained by bisecting the angle between the left arm and a point directly opposite the right arm. The resultant directions of leads II and III are obtained in a similar way. RA, right arm; LA, left arm; F, foot.

The chest leads

Each of the unipolar leads V1–V6 consists of an exploring electrode on the chest wall (Fig. 2.8) and an indifferent electrode connected to the three limbs through high electrical resistance. The very low (effectively zero) potential of the indifferent electrode ensures that the orientation of each chest lead with respect to the heart is defined almost exactly by the position of the exploring electrode on the chest wall.

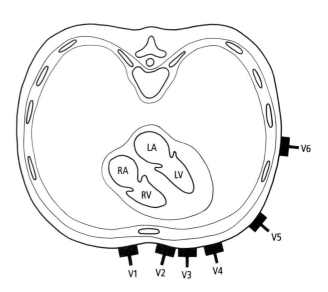

Fig. 2.8 The chest leads. This horizontal section through the chest shows the orientation of the chest leads with respect to the chambers of the heart. V1 is orientated towards the right ventricle, V2 and V3 face the interventricular septum, and V4–V6 extend around the free wall of the left ventricle.

Analysis of the ECG

Figure 2.9 illustrates the normal ECG complex.

Heart rate

The ECG is usually recorded at a paper speed of 25 mm/second such that each large square (5 mm) represents 0.20 seconds. Heart rate is conveniently calculated by counting the number of large squares between consecutive R waves and dividing this into 300.

Rhythm

In normal sinus rhythm, P waves precede each QRS complex. The rhythm is regular or shows phasic variations in rate with respiration (sinus arrhythmia). Absence of P waves and an irregular rhythm indicate atrial fibrillation. Other arrhythmias are discussed in Chapters 10 and 11.

Electrical axis

Evaluation of the mean frontal plane QRS axis is described on page 28.

P-wave morphology

The P wave is a small deflexion caused by atrial depolarization. Upper limits of normal for height and duration are 3.0 mm and 0.1 seconds, respectively. The

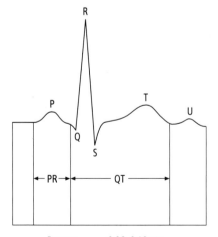

P wave:	0.06–0.10 sec
PR interval:	0.12–0.20 sec
QRS complex:	0.08–0.12 sec
QT interval:	0.35–0.45 sec

Fig. 2.9 The normal ECG complex.

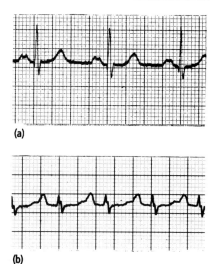

Fig. 2.10 P-wave abnormalities. (a) P mitrale. (b) P pulmonale.

deflexion is negative in aVR and often biphasic in III and VI; in all other leads the P wave is positive.

Atrial depolarization is initiated by the sinus node in the high right atrium and proceeds downwards and to the left. *Right atrial enlargement* in pulmonary hypertension accentuates the early depolarization vector, producing a tall, peaked P wave (P pulmonale). *Left atrial enlargement* in left heart failure accentuates the late depolarization vector, producing a broad notched P wave (P mitrale, Fig. 2.10). If an ectopic atrial focus assumes pacemaker function, atrial depolarization proceeds by abnormal pathways resulting in altered P-wave morphology. This is particularly obvious for foci in the low right atrium around the coronary sinus, when atrial depolarization occurs from below upwards resulting in an inverted P wave (coronary sinus rhythm).

Failure of atrial depolarization results in absence of the P wave. This occurs in sinus arrest with junctional or ventricular escape. In atrial fibrillation or atrial flutter, P waves are replaced by fibrillation or flutter waves, respectively.

PR interval

The PR interval is measured from the onset of the P wave to the first deflexion of the QRS complex, and represents the time taken for the sinus node impulse to reach the ventricular myocardium. The normal duration is 0.12–0.20 seconds *Prolongation* of the PR interval occurs when conduction through the AV node is delayed by disease or drugs (first-degree AV block). If AV conduction fails, either intermittently (second-degree AV block) or completely (third-degree AV block), the normal 1 : 1 relation between the P wave and the QRS complex is lost.

A *short PR interval* (< 0.12 seconds) occurs when a rapidly conducting tract bypasses the AV node permitting early ventricular activation, e.g. in Wolff–Parkinson–White or Lown–Ganong–Levine syndromes. Shortening of the PR interval also occurs in low atrial or coronary sinus escape rhythms because of the proximity of the escape focus to the AV node.

QRS morphology

The QRS complex (caused by ventricular depolarization) is the most prominent deflexion in the ECG. Its duration should not exceed 0.12 seconds. Prolongation indicates slow ventricular depolarization caused sometimes by pre-excitation (Wolff–Parkinson–White syndrome) or hyperkalaemia but most commonly by bundle branch block (Fig. 2.11). In *right bundle branch block* depolarization of the right ventricle is delayed, resulting in a late positive deflexion in leads facing the right ventricle (V1) and a late negative deflexion in leads facing the left ventricle (I, V6). In *left bundle branch block* the entire sequence of ventricular depolarization is disorganized and the QRS complex is broad and bizarre. Septal depolarization no longer occurs from left to right and the small septal Q waves in leads V4–V6 are therefore lost.

Exaggerated QRS deflexions indicate ventricular hypertrophy (Fig. 2.12). Voltage criteria for *left ventricular hypertrophy* are fulfilled when the sum of the S and R wave deflexions in leads V1 and V6 respectively exceeds 35 mm (3.5 mV). However, these criteria may be normal in narrow-chested individuals. Other ECG manifestations of left ventricular hypertrophy include T-wave inversion in left ventricular leads (strain pattern). *Right ventricular hypertrophy* causes tall R waves in right ventricular leads (V1 and V2), often associated with T-wave inversion.

Diminished QRS deflexions occur when pericardial effusion, hyperinflated lungs (emphysema) or severe obesity partially insulate the heart from the skin surface. Myxoedema may also be associated with diminished QRS deflexions.

Pathological Q waves (duration > 0.04 seconds), associated with variable loss of height of the ensuing R wave, usually indicate myocardial infarction. Note, however, that in leads orientated towards the cavity of the left ventricle (aVR, sometimes V1, rarely V2) a deep Q wave is normal and simply reflects the

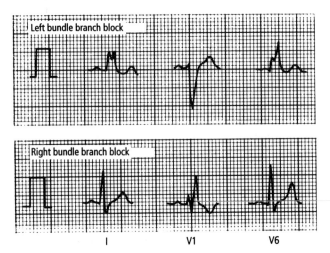

Fig. 2.11 Bundle branch block with widening of the QRS complex.

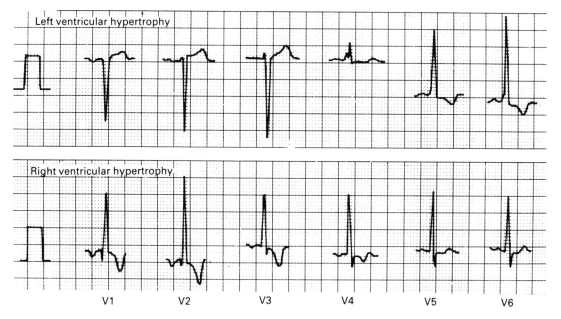

Fig. 2.12 Left and right ventricular hypertrophy causing exaggerated voltage deflexions in leads V1–V6, often associated with T-wave inversion in leads V5–V6 and V1–V3, respectively ('strain' pattern).

endocardial-to-epicardial depolarization vector directed away from the lead on the opposite side of the ventricle (see Fig. 2.4).

ST segment

The ST segment is the isoelectric segment between the end of the QRS complex and the start of the T wave. Deviation of the ST segment above or below the isoelectric line may indicate heart disease (Fig. 2.13). However, minor degrees of ST elevation (early repolarization) occur as a normal variant, particularly in patients of African origin. *Pathological ST elevation* is caused by acute myocardial infarction, variant angina and pericarditis. In acute infarction and variant angina, the ST elevation is typically convex upwards ('coved'), affecting leads orientated towards the threatened myocardium. In pericarditis, the changes are more widespread and the ST elevation is concave upwards. Elevation of the early part of the ST segment occurs in severe hypothermia and is caused by a J wave at the junction of the QRS complex and the ST segment.

Depression of the junction between the QRS complex and the ST segment (J point) with an upwards sloping ST segment is physiological during exertion, unlike the horizontal ('planar') ST depression that indicates myocardial ischaemia. In acute myocardial infarction, however, ST depression affecting leads opposite the infarct zone occurs as a 'reciprocal' phenomenon and does not necessarily indicate remote ischaemia. Other important causes of ST depression include digoxin therapy and hypokalaemia, both of which cause sagging of the ST segment which may be difficult to distinguish from ischaemia.

ST elevation

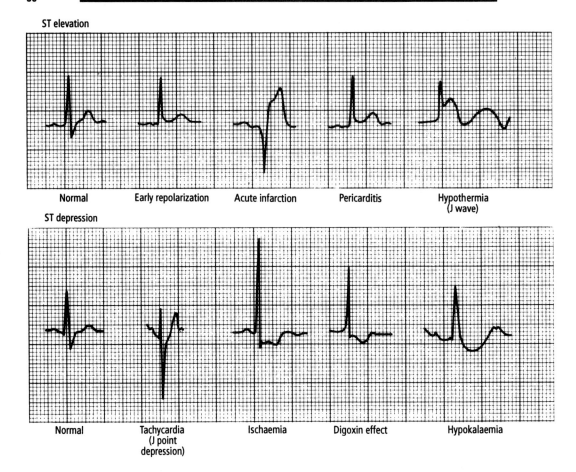

Normal   Early repolarization   Acute infarction   Pericarditis   Hypothermia (J wave)

ST depression

Normal   Tachycardia (J point depression)   Ischaemia   Digoxin effect   Hypokalaemia

Fig. 2.13 Abnormalities of the ST segment.

T wave

The T wave represents ventricular repolarization, and its orientation (positive or negative) is usually the same as the QRS complex. Thus T-wave *inversion* is normal in leads aVR and V1. Widespread T-wave inversion is common in cardiomyopathy and occurs as a non-specific response to viral infection, hypothermia and hyperventilation. More important causes of T-wave inversion include left ventricular hypertrophy and myocardial ischaemia and infarction; in small non-Q-wave infarcts this may be the only abnormality.

Exaggerated *peaking* of the T wave is seen as a hyperacute phenomenon in the early hours of acute myocardial infarction and also occurs in hyperkalaemia.

QT interval

This is measured from the onset of the QRS complex to the end of the T wave and represents the duration of *electrical* systole (*mechanical* systole starts between the QRS complex and the T wave). The QT interval (0.35–0.45 seconds) is very rate sensitive, shortening as heart rate increases. *Abnormal prolongation* of the QT interval predisposes to ventricular arrhythmias and may be congenital or occur in response to hypokalaemia, rheumatic fever or drugs (e.g. quinidine, amiodarone, tricyclic antidepressants). *Shortening* of the QT interval is caused by hyperkalaemia and digoxin therapy.

U wave

The cause of the U wave is unknown. It is a small, often invisible, deflexion following the T wave and orientated in the same direction. Although U-wave abnormalities are rarely of diagnostic importance, inversion may occur in ischaemic disease while peaking is seen in hypokalaemia.

ARRHYTHMIA DETECTION

The effective management of cardiac arrhythmias depends upon accurate diagnosis. Although the history and examination are sometimes useful, special investigations are required in most cases in order to obtain electrocardiographic documentation of the arrhythmia.

Electrocardiogram

The ECG is the basic tool for arrhythmia diagnosis. A single lead or monitor strip is sometimes adequate but accurate diagnosis often requires a full 12-lead ECG. If a patient has an arrhythmia at the time of presentation all efforts should be made to get a 12-lead recording, even if the patient is hypotensive. Appropriate future management may depend on the ECG obtained at that time. Occasionally special ECG leads are required, particularly when atrial activity is not clearly visible. The electrocardiographic diagnosis of arrhythmias will be discussed in Chapter 11.

Ambulatory ECG monitoring

Many patients present with symptoms suggesting an intermittent arrhythmia or conduction disturbance. Although an ECG obtained during symptoms may be diagnostic, this is often not practical and some form of ambulatory monitoring must be performed.

In-hospital ECG monitoring

Patients who have severe arrhythmias, thought to be life-threatening, should be managed in hospital with continuous ECG monitoring. Unless the patient is being individually nursed, a central monitoring system is required, ideally with a computerized alarm triggered by abrupt alterations in rate or QRS morphology. Patients may be connected directly to the system or monitored at a distance using radiotelemetry. Either way, continuous surveillance by trained staff is essential.

Continuous ambulatory ECG monitoring (24-hour or Holter monitors)

This utilizes a small recording device (either magnetic tape or solid state) called a 24-hour or Holter monitor which records at least two ECG channels. It is worn during normal activities while the patient keeps a diary of symptoms; activities known to trigger symptoms should be encouraged during the monitoring period. Tape analysis is computer assisted and rhythm abnormalities are usually displayed at standard paper speed. Alternatively, a full disclosure of the entire ECG can be displayed at very slow speed (Fig. 2.14). If an arrhythmia is documented it is usually diagnostic, particularly when it coincides with symptoms entered into the diary.

An advantage of continuous ambulatory monitoring is that not only symptomatic and asymptomatic arrhythmias, but also the start and end of attacks may be recorded (Fig. 2.14). Events leading up to a sustained arrhythmia can be examined in detail. Unfortunately, however, in patients with paroxysmal arrhythmias who do not experience attacks each day, the chances of recording an abnormality by this technique may be small.

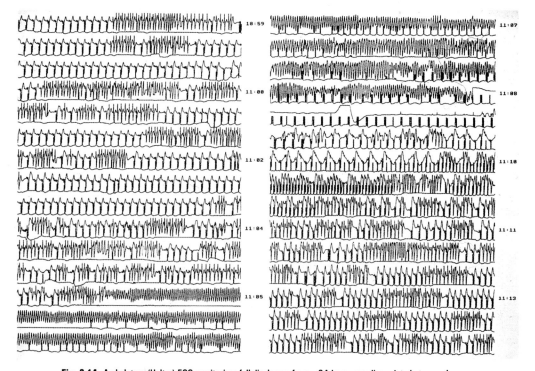

Fig. 2.14 Ambulatory (Holter) ECG monitoring: full disclosure from a 24-hour recording printed at very slow paper speed showing recurrent paroxysms of ventricular tachycardia.

Event recorders

These are useful for patients with infrequent symptoms and often have a facility for transtelephonic transmission of rhythm recordings which may then be examined by the cardiologist. The recorder is patient activated and is applied to the chest wall in the event of symptoms in order to obtain an ECG which is then stored for later analysis. Some units are capable of storing only one arrhythmic episode, while others can store several. More sophisticated devices are available; these are continuously connected to the patient, recording events that fulfil certain trigger criteria (automatic mode) and also events that provoke symptoms (manual mode). These devices have a loop facility so that when they are triggered manually by the patient during symptoms, a record of the ECG in the seconds leading up to the episode is obtained. The most sophisticated of these devices will also alert the patient if a dangerously abnormal rhythm occurs.

Provocative testing

This is helpful when the history suggests cardiac rhythm disturbance in association with specific activities, e.g. exercise or swallowing (Fig. 2.15). In certain patients, an ECG obtained during the activity will be diagnostic if the arrhythmia is recorded.

The *exercise ECG* is frequently used for provocation of arrhythmias caused by ischaemia or increased sympathetic activity. However, it must be emphasized that although ventricular tachycardia in particular is usually associated with coronary artery disease, it is not usually triggered by an acute ischaemic episode and for this reason exercise testing is often unhelpful as a provocative test.

Tilt testing is another provocative test, particularly useful in the diagnosis of malignant vasovagal syndrome, an autonomic disorder causing bradycardias and syncope. The patient is placed on a tilt table at 60°, with adequate restraint, and the blood pressure and ECG are monitored for up to 40 minutes. Most patients with malignant vasovagal syndrome become suddenly bradycardic and/or hypotensive, and lose consciousness unless the table is tilted back to the horizontal.

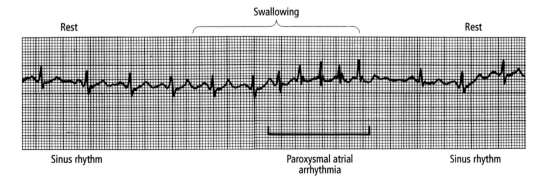

Fig. 2.15 Atrial tachycardia induced by swallowing.

Assessing risk (e.g. Wolff–Parkinson–White syndrome, ventricular arrhythmias)
Elucidating difficult ECGs
Investigating palpitations or syncope when non-invasive techniques have failed
Assessing therapy (especially after drugs, ablation, surgery or special devices)
Delivering therapy (catheter ablation)

Table 2.1 Indications for electrophysiological study.

Carotid sinus massage (after excluding carotid bruits) during simultaneous ECG recording is useful for provoking symptomatic bradycardia in the carotid sinus syndrome. The test is positive if it provokes a bradycardia (pauses longer than 3 seconds) and reproduces symptoms, usually dizziness or syncope.

Electrophysiological study

Indications for electrophysiological study (EPS) are shown in Table 2.1. It is used to investigate usually tachyarrhythmias, less commonly bradyarrhythmias. Depending on the type of study being performed, one or more multipolar electrode catheters are positioned in the right atrium and right ventricle, across the tricuspid valve (to record the His bundle deflection), in the coronary sinus (to record left atrial and ventricular activity), in the left ventricle and occasionally in the left atrium (Fig. 2.16). The catheters are used to record the intracardiac

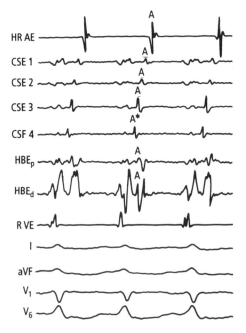 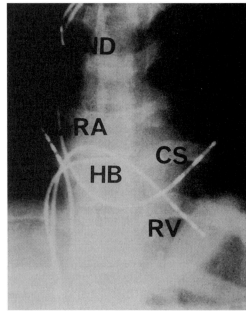

Fig. 2.16 Electrophysiological study. Surface ECG and intracardiac recordings (left panel) obtained from electrodes positioned strategically within the heart (right panel) in a patient with Wolff–Parkinson–White syndrome. The paper speed is accelerated (100 mm/second) in order to permit accurate timing of the abnormal atrial activation that characterizes this syndrome. A* = earliest atrial activation; CSE = coronary sinus electrodes; HBE = His bundle electrodes; HRAE = high right atrial electrode; RVE = right ventricular electrode.

electrogram and to deliver electrical impulses for stimulating and terminating arrhythmias. Although the original application of EPS was in arrhythmia diagnosis and monitoring therapy, more recently it has been used for delivering therapy in patients requiring catheter ablation of conduction tissue and arrhythmogenic foci (see page 248). The EPS is a powerful tool and, though invasive, is usually safe. However, because it may involve deliberate induction of ventricular tachycardia or fibrillation, considerable expertise is required and resuscitation equipment must always be available.

SPECIAL TECHNIQUES TO IDENTIFY PATIENTS AT RISK OF ARRHYTHMIAS

In patients recovering from acute myocardial infarction, special techniques may be employed to identify those at greatest risk of developing lethal arrhythmias early after discharge from hospital, so that specific treatment can be given to protect them from sudden death. Electrophysiological studies (see above) to test susceptibility to arrhythmia induction by ventricular stimulation are often used for this purpose. Recently, however, a number of non-invasive methods have been developed to identify patients at risk of arrhythmias.

The signal-averaged ECG

This technique permits identification of low-voltage signals by means of high-gain amplification of the ECG. A large number of cycles are recorded; these are superimposed and filtered so that electrical noise is averaged out while the low-voltage signal remains amplified. The technique was originally used to record His bundle potentials non-invasively but now finds greater application in the identification of ventricular late potentials (Fig. 2.17). These are low-amplitude deflections at the end of the QRS complex which indicate a heightened risk of ventricular tachyarrhythmias. Their presence has been used for prognostic assessment after myocardial infarction.

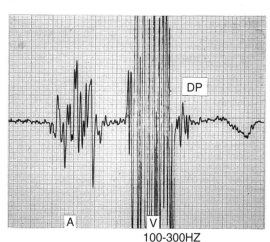

Fig. 2.17 Signal-averaged ECG showing atrial (A) and ventricular (V) potentials. Delayed potentials (DP) late after ventricular activation are clearly visible.

100-300HZ

Heart-rate variability

The heart rate varies during the respiratory cycle, autonomic influences causing it to increase during inspiration and decrease during expiration. This may be quantified by 24-hour ECG recording while the patient breathes normally. Loss of heart-rate variability is seen in autonomic neuropathy and may also occur early after acute myocardial infarction when it is a poor prognostic sign.

FURTHER READING

Ayres SM. The electrocardiogram in acute coronary syndromes. *J Am Coll Cardiol* 1990; 16: 1026.

Zipes DP. Sympathetic stimulation and arrhythmias. *N Engl J Med* 1991; 325: 656–7.

Jaffe AS, Atkins JM, Mentzer RM *et al.* Recommended guidelines for in-hospital cardiac monitoring of adults for detection of arrhythmias. *J Am Coll Cardiol* 1991; 18: 1431.

Knoebel SB, Crawford MN, Dunn MI *et al.* Guidelines for ambulatory electrocardiography. *J Am Coll Cardiol* 1989; 13: 249.

Ward DE. Can the technicalities of electrophysiological testing for ventricular tachycardia be simplified? *Br Heart J* 1987; 58: 437.

Cardiac Imaging and Catheterization

SUMMARY

The chest X-ray permits assessment of heart size, which should not exceed 50% of the transverse diameter of the chest. Enlargement is usually caused by dilatation (as opposed to hypertrophy) of one or more cardiac chambers, although only the left atrium can be accurately identified on the posteroanterior film. The lateral chest X-ray permits assessment of left and right ventricular size and diseased intracardiac structures may be visible if they are calcified. Lung-field abnormalities in cardiovascular disease are caused by alterations of pulmonary flow or increased left atrial pressure. Increased pulmonary flow (e.g. in atrial septal defect) causes prominent vascular markings while reduced flow causes oligaemia which may be regional (e.g. in pulmonary embolism) or global (e.g. in Eisenmenger's syndrome). Increased left atrial pressure in left heart failure produces corresponding increments in pulmonary venous and pulmonary capillary pressures. Prominence of the upper lobe veins is an early sign but, as pressure rises, interstitial and alveolar oedema develop, evidenced by Kerley B lines and perihilar air-space consolidation, respectively.

The echocardiogram utilizes ultrasound to provide unidimensional (M-mode) and two-dimensional images of the heart, of particular value for diagnosis of myocardial, pericardial, valvular and congenital defects. Transthoracic imaging is usually satisfactory, but better quality information is obtained by the transoesophageal approach which is particularly useful for imaging the left atrium, aorta and prosthetic heart valves. The role of echocardiography has been extended by Doppler ultrasound which identifies the direction and velocity of flow within the heart, permitting evaluation of the severity of stenotic and regurgitant valve lesions and localization of intracardiac shunts through septal defects.

Radionuclide imaging with a gamma camera provides an alternative diagnostic method, the application of which depends on the isotope used and its uptake within the cardiopulmonary system. Scintigraphic analysis of ventricular function and myocardial perfusion are widely used in the investigation of patients with heart failure and coronary artery disease, while ventilation-perfusion imaging of the lungs is one of the most reliable methods for diagnosing pulmonary embolism.

Computed tomography and, more recently, *magnetic resonance imaging* represent a quantum leap forwards in terms of image quality (and cost). Already, these technologies are widely used for diagnosis of aortic dissection and intracardiac masses, and other applications are expected to emerge.

Cardiac catheterization is an invasive method for delivery of radiographic contrast material into the area of interest. This permits angiographic assessment of ventricular function, valvular competence and pulmonary perfusion and is the only reliable technique for imaging the coronary arteries. Cardiac catheterization is also used for intracardiac pressure measurement and for haemodynamic evaluation of valvular stenosis, intracardiac shunts and cardiac output. In addition to its important diagnostic role, catheter technology is now being used increasingly for the interventional management of cardiovascular disease where procedures such as valvuloplasty, angioplasty and coronary stenting are extending the therapeutic role of the cardiologist into areas that were once exclusively surgical.

NON-INVASIVE IMAGING

The chest X-ray

Good quality posteroanterior (PA) and lateral chest X-rays make an important contribution to the cardiac assessment.

Cardiac silhouette

Because the radiodensity of cardiac tissue is similar to that of blood, intracardiac structures can rarely be identified unless they are calcified (Fig. 3.1). However, the cardiac silhouette contrasts strongly with the adjacent radiolucent lung fields, permitting accurate appreciation of the heart size. The heart is long and thin in ectomorphic individuals but is more bulky in endomorphic individuals. Nevertheless, the maximum transverse measurement should not exceed 50% that of the chest. Cardiac enlargement is caused either by pericardial effusion or by dilatation of the cardiac chambers and great vessels. Myocardial hypertrophy without chamber dilatation rarely causes radiographic cardiac enlargement.

Pericardial effusion

Pericardial effusion separates the parietal layer of the pericardial sac from the wall of the heart. The cardiac silhouette enlarges, but differential diagnosis from other causes of cardiac enlargement cannot be made with confidence. Typically, however, the effusion gives the cardiac silhouette a 'globular' appearance with an unusually crisp ('stencilled') appearance because the parietal pericardium is immobilized by the effusion, eliminating movement artefact at the interface with the lung.

Atrial dilatation

Right atrial dilatation is usually due to right ventricular failure and tricuspid regurgitation but occurs as an isolated finding in tricuspid stenosis and Ebstein's anomaly. It produces cardiac enlargement without specific radiographic signs.

The left atrium is the only cardiac chamber than can be accurately identified on the PA chest X-ray. Dilatation occurs in left ventricular failure and mitral valve disease. This causes the following features (Fig. 3.2).
• Flattening and later bulging of the left heart border below the main pulmonary artery due to leftwards displacement of the atrial appendage.
• Elevation of the left main bronchus with widening of the carena.
• Appearance of the medial border of the left atrium behind the right side of the heart (double density sign).

Ventricular dilatation

Ventricular dilatation commonly accompanies heart failure, particularly when this is caused by myocardial disease or regurgitant valvular disease. Although the PA chest X-ray does not reliably distinguish left from right ventricular dilatation, the lateral view may be more helpful. Thus, dilatation of the posteriorly located left ventricle encroaches on the retrocardiac space, while dilatation of the anteriorly located right ventricle encroaches on the retrosternal space (see Fig. 9.3).

Vascular dilatation

Dilatation and lengthening of the thoracic aorta is common in the elderly and produces an 'unfolded' appearance. Aortic dilatation caused by aneurysm or dissection may be focal, but more commonly produces widening of the entire upper mediastinum. Localized dilatation of the proximal aorta occurs in aortic valve disease and produces a prominence in the right upper mediastinum. Dilatation of the main pulmonary artery occurs in pulmonary hypertension and pulmonary stenosis and produces a prominence below the aortic knuckle (Fig. 3.3).

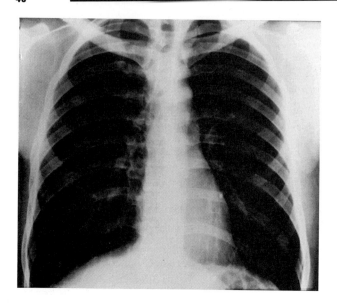

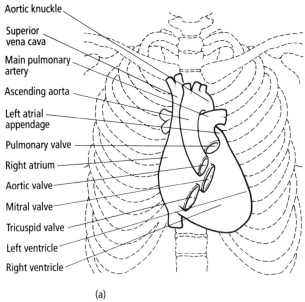

Aortic knuckle

Superior vena cava

Main pulmonary artery

Ascending aorta

Left atrial appendage

Pulmonary valve

Right atrium

Aortic valve

Mitral valve

Tricuspid valve

Left ventricle

Right ventricle

(a)

Fig. 3.1 (a) Normal chest X-ray—posteroanterior projection.

Intracardiac calcification

Disease of any of the cardiac tissues may result in calcification. This may be visible on the penetrated chest X-ray, but is better visualized using fluoroscopy in the catheter laboratory. Pericardial calcification is characteristic of tuberculous disease but is less common in other causes of constrictive pericarditis (Fig. 3.4). Myocardial calcification may occur in the walls of a ventricular aneurysm and sometimes in the left atrial wall in advanced mitral disease (see Fig. 9.3). Valvular calcification occurs most commonly in aortic and mitral disease and may involve

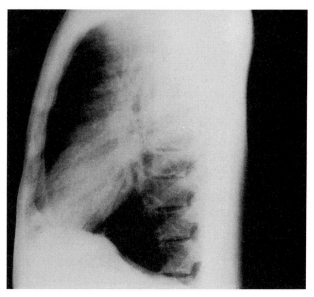

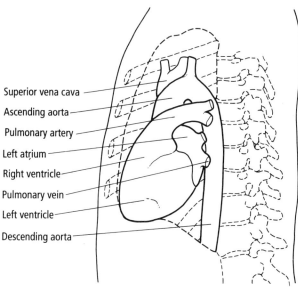

Superior vena cava
Ascending aorta
Pulmonary artery
Left atrium
Right ventricle
Pulmonary vein
Left ventricle
Descending aorta

Fig. 3.1 (*Continued*) (b) Normal chest X-ray—left lateral projection.

(b)

the leaflets—causing stenosis, the ring tissue—when valve function is often unaffected, or both. Identification of the calcified valve usually requires a lateral chest X-ray in which the aortic valve lies anterior and the mitral valve posterior to the long axis of the heart. Vascular calcification may affect the coronary arteries in atheromatous disease, the wall of the ascending aorta in syphilitic aortitis, or the main pulmonary artery in pulmonary hypertension (Fig. 3.3). Most commonly, however, vascular calcification is seen in the aortic arch and represents a benign degenerative process in the elderly.

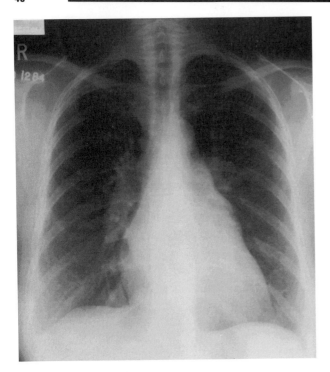

Fig. 3.2 Left atrial enlargement in a patient with mitral valve disease. Note the bulging of the left heart border below the main pulmonary artery with elevation of the left main bronchus and the 'double density' at the right heart border.

Lung fields

In cardiovascular disease the common lung-field abnormalities are caused either by alterations in pulmonary flow or by increased left atrial pressure.

Pulmonary flow

Increased pulmonary flow, sufficient to cause radiographic abnormalities, is usually caused by a left-to-right intracardiac shunt, e.g. atrial septal defect, ventricular septal defect. Prominence of the vascular markings gives the lung fields a 'plethoric' appearance.

Reduced pulmonary flow may be regional or global. *Regional oligaemia* occurs in emphysema and pulmonary embolism; vascular markings in the affected area are diminished and contrast with the normal vascularity elsewhere in the lung. *Global reductions* occur in obliterative pulmonary vascular disease (e.g. primary pulmonary hypertension, Eisenmenger's syndrome) and are most marked in the peripheral lung field—'peripheral pruning'. The main pulmonary artery is always dilated due to long-standing pulmonary hypertension.

Increased left atrial pressure. Increased left atrial pressure occurs in mitral valve disease and left ventricular failure and produces a corresponding rise in pulmonary venous and pulmonary capillary pressures. Prominence of the pulmonary

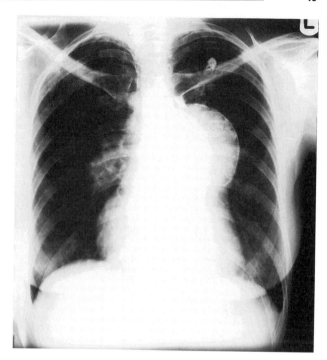

Fig. 3.3 Pulmonary arterial calcification. The main pulmonary artery is very dilated due to longstanding pulmonary hypertension. Calcification of the artery is clearly visible.

veins—most marked in the upper lobes—is an early radiographic sign. As left atrial and pulmonary capillary pressures rise above 18 mmHg, transudation into the lung produces interstitial pulmonary oedema (see Fig. 4.5) characterized by prominence of the interlobular septa, particularly at the lung bases (Kerley B lines). Further rises in pressure lead to alveolar pulmonary oedema with air-space consolidation in a perihilar ('bat's-wing') distribution (Fig. 3.5).

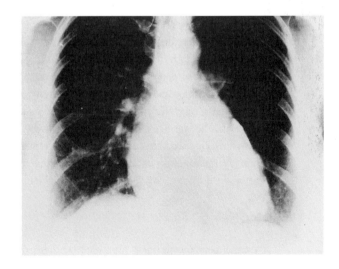

Fig. 3.4 Pericardial calcification. In this patient with constrictive pericarditis the pericardial calcification is clearly visible on the posteroanterior chest X-ray. In most cases, however, pericardial calcification is better appreciated on the lateral chest X-ray.

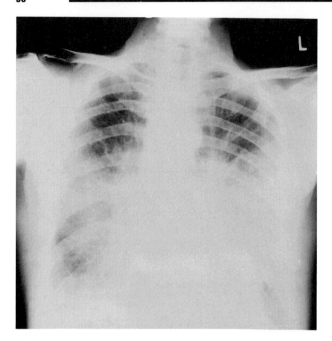

Fig. 3.5 Alveolar pulmonary oedema. The perihilar 'bat's-wing' distribution of the pulmonary oedema is clearly visible. Small bilateral pleural effusions are also present.

Bony abnormalities

Bony abnormalities are unusual in cardiovascular disease, apart from coarctation of the aorta and thoracic outlet syndromes. In coarctation, dilated bronchial collateral vessels erode the inferior aspect of the ribs to produce notches although they are rarely present before adolescence.

Cervical ribs may compress the neurovascular bundle in the thoracic outlet, and special thoracic outlet views are necessary for radiographic diagnosis.

Echocardiography

Echocardiography is one of the most versatile non-invasive imaging techniques in clinical cardiology. Because it does not utilize ionizing radiation, it is free of known risk and can be used safely throughout pregnancy. Transthoracic imaging with the transducer applied to the chest wall is usually satisfactory, but better quality information is obtained by the transoesophageal approach in which the transducer is mounted on a probe and positioned in the oesophagus, directly behind the heart. This provides better-quality images because there are no intervening ribs and the probe is closely applied to the posterior aspect of the heart. It is particularly useful for imaging the left atrium, the aorta and prosthetic heart valves.

Principles

A transducer containing a piezoelectric element converts electrical energy into an ultrasound beam which can be directed towards the heart. The beam is reflected when it strikes an interface between tissues of different density. The reflected ultrasound, or *echo*, is converted back to electrical energy by the piezoelectric element, which permits construction of an image using two basic units of information:

1 the *intensity* of the echoes, which defines the density difference at tissue interfaces within the heart; and

2 the *time* taken for echoes to arrive back at the transducer, which defines the distance of the cardiac structures from the transducer.

Density differences within the heart are greatest between the blood-filled chambers and the myocardial and valvular tissues, all of which are clearly visible on the echocardiogram. Because the depth of the myocardial and valvular tissues with respect to the transducer changes constantly throughout the cardiac cycle, the time taken for echo reflection changes accordingly. Thus, real-time imaging throughout the cardiac cycle provides a dynamic record of cardiac function.

M-mode echocardiogram

M-mode echocardiography (Fig. 3.6) provides a unidimensional 'ice-pick' view through the heart. Continuous recording on photographic paper supplies an additional time dimension, thereby permitting appreciation of the dynamic component of the cardiac image. By convention, cardiac structures closest to the transducer are displayed at the top of the record and more distant structures are displayed below. Thus, on the transthoracic M-mode echocardiogram, anteriorly located ('right-sided') structures lie above the posteriorly located ('left-sided') structures, but on the transoesophageal echocardiogram the display is reversed.

Two-dimensional echocardiogram

The two-dimensional echocardiogram (Fig. 3.6) provides more detailed informa-tion about morphology than the M-mode recording. By projecting a fan of echoes in an arc of up to 80°, a two-dimensional 'slice' through the heart can be obtained, the precise view depending on the location and angulation of the transducer. The most widely used transthoracic views are shown in Figs 3.6 and 3.7; transoesophageal views are shown in Figs 3.8 and 3.9.

Clinical applications

Congenital heart disease

Echocardiography, particularly the two-dimensional technique, has revolution-ized the diagnosis of congenital heart disease, obviating the need for invasive investigation by cardiac catheterization in the majority of cases. The relationships of the cardiac chambers and their connections with the great vessels are readily determined. Valvular abnormalities and septal defects can also be recognized.

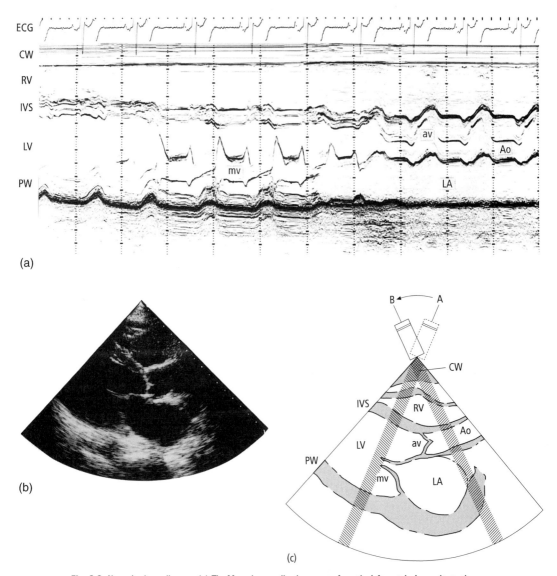

(a)

(b)

(c)

Fig. 3.6 Normal echocardiogram. (a) The M-mode recording is a sweep from the left ventricular cavity to the ascending aorta and was obtained by angling the transducer through an arc from A to B (c). (b) The two-dimensional recording obtained from the left parasternal area is a long axis view of the left ventricle as illustrated in (c). CW, chest wall; RV, right ventricle; IVS, interventricular septum; LV, left ventricle; LA, left atrium; PW, posterior wall; mv, mitral valve; av, aortic valve; Ao, aorta.

Recent technology has permitted *in utero* fetal imaging for the antenatal diagnosis of cardiac defects (see page 302).

Myocardial disease

Echocardiography permits accurate assessment of cardiac dilatation, hypertrophy and contractile function. Congestive cardiomyopathy produces ventricular

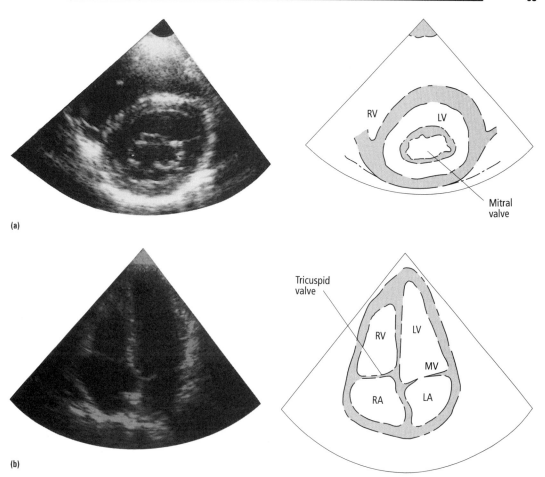

Fig. 3.7 Normal two-dimensional echocardiogram. (a) A short axis view through the left ventricle at mitral valve level, obtained from the left parasternal area. (b) A four-chamber view of the heart obtained from the cardiac apex.

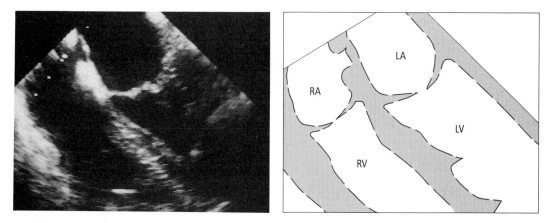

Fig. 3.8 Normal transoesophageal echocardiogram: four-chamber view (horizontal plane). This view provides a clear image of the interatrial septum, particularly useful for identifying septal defects.

Horizontal plane views

Vertical plane views

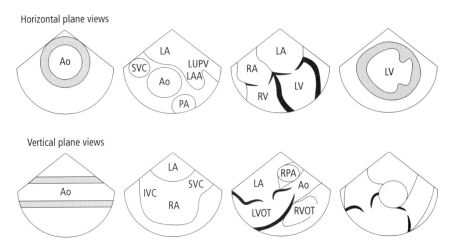

Fig. 3.9 Standard horizontal and vertical plane views obtained during transoesophageal echocardiography. Ao, aorta; SVC, superior vena cava; IVC, inferior vena cava; PA, pulmonary artery; RPA, right pulmonary artery; LAA, left atrial appendage; LVOT, left ventricular outflow tract; LUPV, left upper pulmonary vein; RVOT, right ventricular outflow tract.

dilatation with *global* contractile impairment. This must be distinguished from the *regional* contractile impairment that follows myocardial infarction in patients with coronary artery disease. Hypertrophic cardiomyopathy is characterized by thickening (hypertrophy) of the left ventricular myocardium, usually with disproportionate involvement of the interventricular septum (asymmetrical septal hypertrophy). In aortic and hypertensive heart disease, on the other hand, left ventricular hypertrophy is usually symmetrical.

Valvular disease

Echocardiography is of particular value in identifying both structural and dynamic valvular abnormalities and any associated chamber dilatation or hypertrophy. The severity of valvular involvement in congenital, rheumatic, degenerative and infective disease may thus be defined; the technique is diagnostic of bicuspid aortic valve and mitral valve prolapse, and readily identifies valve thickening and calcification in rheumatic and calcific disease. Vegetations in infective endocarditis can usually be visualized if they are large enough (> 3 mm). The transoesophageal approach is usually necessary for endocarditis involving prosthetic heart valves.

Pericardial disease

Although the echocardiogram is of little value in constrictive pericarditis, it is the most sensitive technique available for the diagnosis of pericardial effusion. The effusion appears as an echo-free space distributed around the ventricles but usually avoiding the potential space behind the left atrium.

Other clinical applications

Intracardiac tumours, particularly myxomas and thrombi, are readily visualized by echocardiography, and the oesophageal technique has found an important application in the identification of thrombus in the left atrial appendage. The oesophageal technique is also helpful for diagnosing aortic disease such as aneurysm and dissection because it provides better views of the thoracic aorta than are obtained with conventional two-dimensional echocardiography. The application of stress echocardiography for diagnosis of coronary artery disease is currently investigational (see page 112).

Doppler echocardiography

Doppler echocardiography permits evaluation of the direction and velocity of blood flow within the heart and great vessels. It is widely used for measuring the severity of valvular stenosis and for identifying valvular regurgitation and intracardiac shunts through septal defects.

Principles

According to the Doppler principle, when an ultrasound beam is directed towards the bloodstream the frequency of the ultrasound reflected from the blood cells is altered. The frequency shift or Doppler effect is related to the direction and velocity of flow. If continuous-wave Doppler is used, blood flow at any point along the path of the ultrasound beam is detected, such that a 'clean' Doppler signal from the area of interest may be difficult to obtain. Pulsed Doppler, however, has a range-gating facility that permits frequency sampling from any specific point within the heart, preselected on the echocardiogram. This lends greater precision to the technique. Nevertheless, pulsed Doppler is less able than continuous-wave Doppler to quantify very high velocity jets, such as those that occur in aortic stenosis.

Colour-flow mapping has been a major technological advance. Instead of the unidirectional ultrasound beam used in continuous-wave and pulsed Doppler imaging, the beam is rotated through an arc. Frequency sampling throughout the arc permits construction of a colour-coded map, red indicating flow towards, and blue away from, the transducer. Colour-flow data can be superimposed on the standard two-dimensional echocardiogram to identify precisely the patterns of flow within the four chambers of the heart. This simplifies the interpretation of Doppler imaging and provides more useful qualitative data, although it is less useful for quantitative assessment of valve gradients which requires the precision of conventional Doppler technique.

Clinical applications (Fig. 3.10)

In paediatric cardiology, the combination of two-dimensional echocardiography

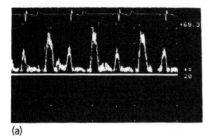

(a)

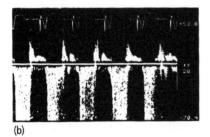

(b)

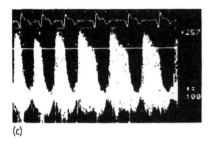

(c)

Fig. 3.10 Doppler studies of mitral flow. Flow velocity (cm/second) is represented by the vertical dots according to the scale shown on the right side of each recording. (a) Normal mitral flow shows a biphasic pattern peaking in early diastole immediately after the valve opens and again late in diastole as the left atrium contracts. (b) In mitral regurgitation the normal diastolic flow pattern is preserved, but during systole a high-velocity regurgitant jet is recorded. (c) Mitral stenosis produces a high-velocity jet during diastole. Atrial fibrillation eliminates atrial contraction and ensures complete loss of the normal biphasic flow pattern.

and colour-flow Doppler mapping has made possible the 'non-invasive' diagnosis of the large majority of congenital defects, often without the need for cardiac catheterization. These techniques have also revolutionized the diagnosis of valvular disease in all age groups. In valvular regurgitation, the retrograde flow that occurs after valve closure is readily detected by Doppler echocardiography, although only an approximate estimate of its severity is possible. In valvular stenosis, peak velocity (as opposed to volume) of flow across the valve is directly related to the degree of stenosis. Thus measurement of Doppler flow velocity (ideally by continuous wave) permits quantification of stenosis by the application of the Bernoulli equation: pressure gradient = $4 \times \text{velocity}^2$.

Cardiovascular radionuclide imaging

Principles

All radionuclide techniques require the internal administration of a radioisotope; the distribution of radioactivity in the area of interest is then imaged with a gamma camera. Ideally, the isotope should be distributed homogeneously in that part of the cardiovascular system under investigation; thus, isotopes that remain in the intravascular space during imaging are used for radionuclide angiography. In myocardial perfusion scintigraphy, however, isotopes taken up by the myocardium are required. Because of their potential toxicity, isotopes with a short half-life are usually used.

Clinical applications

Radionuclide angiography

Radionuclide angiography is used for assessment of ventricular function. Red cells labelled with technetium-99m are allowed to equilibrate in the blood pool and the heart is then imaged under the gamma camera (Fig. 3.11). The waxing and waning of radioactivity within the ventricular chambers during diastole and systole, respectively, permits construction of a dynamic ventriculogram. Left ventricular contractile function can be evaluated quantitatively—by calculation of ejection fraction, or qualitatively—by observation of wall movement. Global left ventricular impairment is characteristic of cardiomyopathy, while regional defects are seen following myocardial infarction. Stress radionuclide angiography using exercise or peripheral cold stimulation (cold pressor test) is used for detection of myocardial ischaemia: provocation of reversible regional wall-motion abnormalities is strongly suggestive of coronary artery disease.

Myocardial perfusion scintigraphy

Myocardial perfusion scintigraphy is used for diagnosis of coronary artery disease (Fig. 3.12). The investigation requires a standardized exercise stress test with

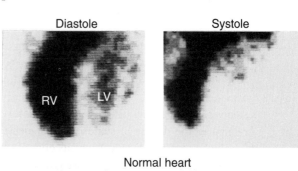

Diastole   Systole

RV   LV

Normal heart

RV

LV

Cardiomyopathy

Fig. 3.11 Radionuclide angiography. The right and left ventricles separated by the interventricular septum are clearly visible. Note that in the normal heart the left ventricular cavity is small and during systole contracts vigorously. In cardiomyopathy the left ventricle is considerably dilated and there is global impairment of contractile function.

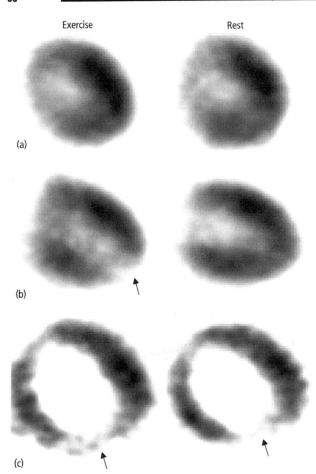

(a)

Exercise

Rest

(b)

(c)

Fig. 3.12 Myocardial perfusion scintigraphy. (a) In the normal LV scintigram there is homogeneous distribution of radioisotope both at peak exercise and at rest (4 hours later). (b) Exercise-induced myocardial ischaemia has produced a reversible perfusion defect (arrowed) towards the apex of the left ventricle which normalizes during rest. (c) In the patient with myocardial infarction, on the other hand, the perfusion defect of the inferoapical area (arrowed) seen at peak exercise is irreversible and persists during the resting study.

continuous ECG monitoring in order to provoke myocardial ischaemia in susceptible subjects. Thallium-201 is used most commonly but the more recently introduced technetium-99m-labelled MIBI (methoxy isobutyl nitrile) provides better image quality. Isotope is injected intravenously at peak exercise and the heart is imaged under a gamma camera. Isotope is distributed homogeneously in normally perfused myocardium, ischaemic or infarcted areas appearing as scintigraphic defects. If thallium-201 is used, repeat imaging after 2–4 hours' rest permits reassessment of scintigraphic defects, those that disappear (reversible defects) indicating areas of exercise-induced ischaemia, those that persist (fixed defects) indicating infarcted myocardium. If technetium-99m-labelled MIBI is used, resting images for assessment of reversibility require a separate injection of isotope 24 hours after (or before) the exercise images.

Hot-spot scintigraphy

Hot-spot scintigraphy permits diagnosis of acute myocardial infarction but in practice is rarely used (Fig. 3.13). Technetium-99m pyrophosphate is taken up by

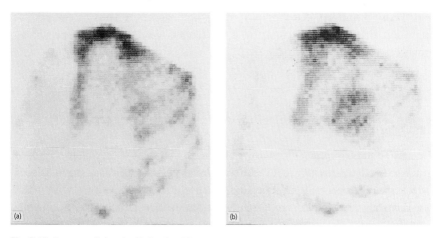

Fig. 3.13 Hot-spot scintigraphy. Technetium-99m pyrophosphate is taken up by normal bone and in the normal study (a) the ribs are clearly visible. Following myocardial infarction (b) the isotope has localized in the infarcted area of the left ventricle producing a large 'hot spot' which is clearly visible on the scintigram.

recently infarcted myocardium, producing a localized 'hot spot' of radioactivity on the scintigram. Diagnostic sensitivity is greatest during the first week following infarction.

Pulmonary scintigraphy

Pulmonary scintigraphy is used for the diagnosis of pulmonary embolism (Fig. 3.14). Technetium-99m-labelled microspheres, injected intravenously, become trapped within the pulmonary capillaries. The normal pulmonary perfusion scintigram shows homogeneous distribution of radioactivity throughout both lung fields. Pulmonary embolism causes regional impairment of pulmonary flow, which results in a perfusion defect on the scintigram; however, the appearance is non-specific and occurs in many other pulmonary disorders, particularly chronic obstructive pulmonary disease. Specificity is enhanced by simultaneous ventilation scintigraphy. Inhaled xenon-133 is distributed homogeneously throughout the normal lung and, in pulmonary embolism (unlike other

Fig. 3.14 Pulmonary ventilation perfusion scintigraphy. In this patient with pulmonary emboli there are multiple defects visible on the perfusion scan (a). The ventilation scan (b) is entirely normal. Ventilation–perfusion mismatch is highly specific for pulmonary embolism.

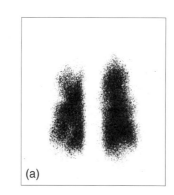

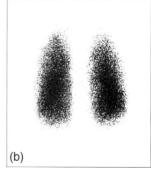

pulmonary disorders), distribution remains homogeneous. Thus a scintigraphic perfusion defect not 'matched' by a ventilation defect is highly specific for pulmonary embolism.

Computed tomography

Principles

Computed tomography (CT) measures the attenuation of X-rays after they have traversed body tissues (Fig. 3.15). Attenuation is greatest for tissues such as bone which are relatively radio-opaque, and least for tissues such as lung or fat which are relatively radiotranslucent. From X-ray attenuation measurements, taken as

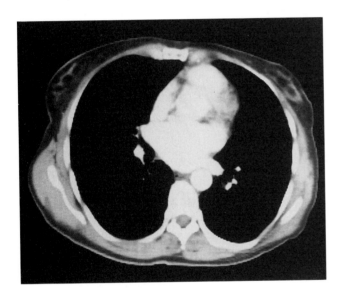

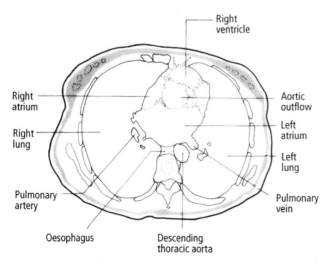

Fig. 3.15 Computed tomography. A normal thoracic tomogram at left atrial level is shown. The vascular spaces have been enhanced by the injection of contrast medium into the bloodstream.

a sensor rotates around the chest, cross-sectional images are constructed. Image resolution is excellent and contrast injection into a peripheral vein provides adequate opacification of the blood pool for identification of intracardiac structures. In the past, the clinical application of CT in cardiology was limited by image acquisition times of up to 5 seconds, during which the constant motion of the heart degraded the image. The current generation of ultrafast CT scanners (with image acquisition times of less than 1 second) provide high-resolution cardiac images in both static and video mode; measurements of blood flow can also be obtained by the application of indicator dilution principles.

Clinical applications

CT (with contrast enhancement) is widely used for the non-invasive diagnosis of aortic dissection, when two contrast columns separated by an intimal flap can be clearly seen. It is also used for accurate assessment of pericardial thickness in constrictive disease and diagnosis of cardiac tumours. Additional applications of ultrafast CT include the evaluation of graft patency following coronary bypass surgery, analysis of ventricular wall motion, and blood-flow quantification in congenital heart disease permitting dynamic assessment of shunts and other defects.

Magnetic resonance imaging

Principles

Magnetic resonance imaging (MRI) utilizes the fact that certain nuclei with an intrinsic spin generate magnetic fields and behave like tiny bar magnets. Placed in a magnetic field, these nuclei align and adopt a resonant frequency that is unique to that nucleus and the strength of the magnetic field. If the nuclei are exposed to pulsed radiowaves of that frequency, they resonate and release energy which allows the location of the nucleus to be determined.

For imaging purposes, the patient lies in a strong magnetic field which is artificially graded. The hydrogen protons of fat and water are imaged and, on exposure to pulsed radiowaves, they resonate at different frequencies in different parts of the imaging zone. Analysis of the emitted frequencies permits construction of tomographic and three-dimensional images of the heart. If data acquisition is gated to a specific part of the cardiac cycle, motion artefact is eliminated and excellent image resolution can be obtained.

Clinical applications

MRI is already being used in the diagnosis of aortic dissection (Fig. 3.16) and for imaging cardiac tumours. Potential applications may include coronary artery imaging without the need for contrast material, identification of histological and metabolic disorders of the myocardium, and assessment of myocardial perfusion

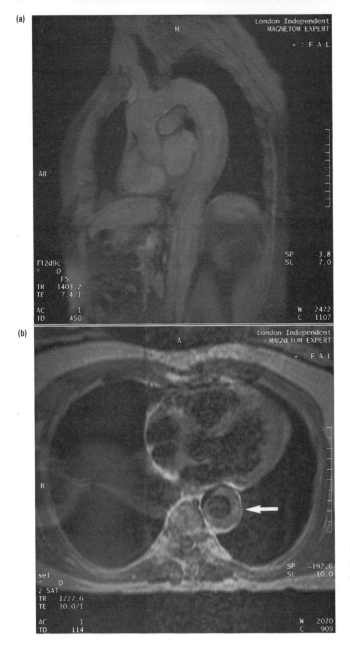

Fig. 3.16 Magnetic resonance imaging: aortic dissection. (a) Coronal section showing extensive dissection extending from the aortic root through the arch and into the abdominal aorta. (b) Transverse section through the heart and descending aorta. Note the circumferential false lumen filled with clot in the descending thoracic aorta (arrowed).

using paramagnetic contrast agents. The realization of this exciting potential will ensure an important role for MRI in clinical cardiology.

CARDIAC CATHETERIZATION

Catheters introduced into an artery or vein may be directed into the left or right sides of the heart, respectively. Vascular access is usually percutaneous, using the femoral vessels, or by surgical cut-down, using the antecubital vessels. Originally developed for diagnostic purposes, catheter techniques are now being used increasingly for the interventional management of cardiovascular disease.

Diagnostic catheterization

Catheters introduced into the heart or great vessels are used both for the delivery of radiographic contrast medium (angiography) and for the measurement of pressure within the chambers of the heart and cardiac output.

Cardiac angiography

Four diagnostic investigations account for the majority of angiographic procedures:
* aortic root angiography;
* left ventricular angiography;
* coronary arteriography; and
* pulmonary arteriography.

For coronary arteriography, relatively small volumes of contrast (5–8 ml) injected manually are used, but for other angiographic procedures much larger amounts (up to 50 ml), introduced by power injection, are required. Digital subtraction techniques permit reductions in contrast volume but have, at present, only a limited role in cardiovascular angiographic diagnosis (see below). Until recently, images have been recorded on high-speed cine film or video, to provide a dynamic record of ventricular wall movement, blood flow and intravascular anatomy. The current generation of angiographic laboratories, however, utilize digital technology and provide better-quality images which may be stored electronically.

Aortic root angiography

Contrast injection into the aortic root demonstrates the vascular anatomy in suspected aneurysm or dissection, and also permits evaluation of aortic valve function (Fig. 3.17). The normal aortic valve prevents diastolic backflow of contrast, but in aortic regurgitation variable opacification of the left ventricle occurs, depending on the severity of the valve lesion.

Left ventricular angiography

Contrast injection into the left ventricle defines ventricular anatomy and wall motion, and also permits evaluation of mitral valve function (Fig. 3.18). Dilatation of the ventricle and contractile dysfunction occurs in left ventricular failure. Exaggerated contractile function with systolic obliteration of the cavity occurs in hypertrophic cardiomyopathy. Filling defects within the ventricular lumen may indicate thrombus or, less commonly, neoplasm. The normal mitral valve prevents systolic backflow of contrast into the left atrium, but in mitral regurgi-

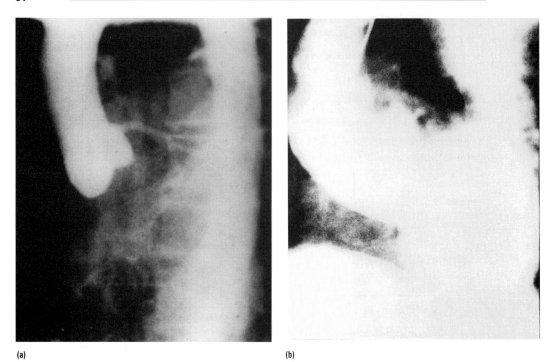

(a)   (b)

Fig. 3.17 Aortic root angiography. Contrast medium has been injected into the ascending aorta. (a) A normal study. (b) Aortic regurgitation causes dilatation of the ascending aorta and opacification of the left ventricle due to diastolic backflow through the diseased aortic valve.

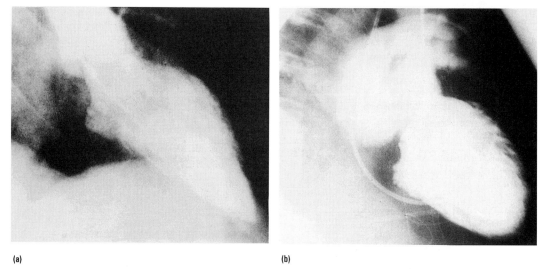

(a)   (b)

Fig. 3.18 Left ventricular angiography. Contrast medium has been injected into the left ventricle. (a) A normal study. (b) Mitral regurgitation causes left ventricular dilatation and opacification of the left atrium due to systolic backflow through the diseased valve.

tation variable atrial opacification occurs, depending on the severity of the valve lesion.

Coronary arteriography

Coronary arteriography is the only reliable technique for diagnostic imaging of the coronary arteries. It requires selective injection of contrast into the left and right coronary arteries (Fig. 3.19) and multiple views in different projections are necessary for a complete study. Intraluminal filling defects or occlusions indicate coronary artery disease, which is nearly always caused by atherosclerosis.

Pulmonary arteriography

Injection of contrast medium into the main pulmonary artery opacifies the arterial branches throughout both lung fields. The normal flow distribution is homogeneous. Vascular occlusions with regional perfusion defects usually indi-

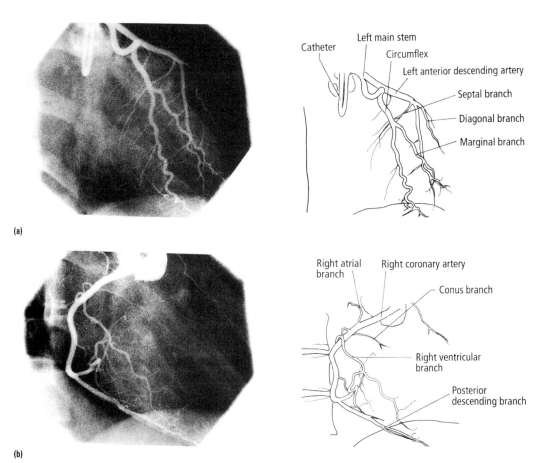

(a)

(b)

Fig. 3.19 Contrast medium has been injected into (a) the left and (b) the right coronary arteries. These are normal coronary arteriograms.

cate pulmonary thromboembolism (particularly when intraluminal filling defects are present) but may also occur in advanced emphysema.

Digital subtraction angiography

Digital subtraction angiography employs computerized subtraction of the background image so that only the contrast medium in the heart and great vessels stands out. Its most enthusiastic proponents hoped this would permit high-resolution imaging with injection of contrast into a peripheral vein without the need for cardiac catheterization. However, this has proved unrealistic because although contrast resolution is increased, contrast delivery to the area of interest is severely diminished and spatial resolution is poor. At present, therefore, the intravenous digital subtraction technique is useful only for imaging large and relatively static arteries such as the aortic arch (for diagnosis of coarctation) and the carotid arteries. It also has a limited role in determining the patency of coronary bypass grafts since these are not subject to the motion artefact of the native coronary system.

Intravascular ultrasound

An ultrasound transducer mounted at the tip of a coronary catheter can now be used to provide cross-sectional images of an artery. The technique permits visualization of coronary plaques and provides information about plaque composition and structure that cannot be obtained from angiographic images (Fig. 3.20). Indeed, it is already apparent from ultrasound studies that coronary arteries which appear angiographically 'normal' may in reality be extensively diseased. Intravascular ultrasound has already found a clinical role in coronary

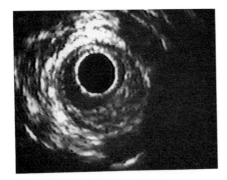

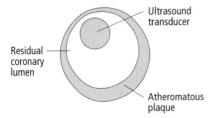

Fig. 3.20 Intravascular ultrasound (IVUS): coronary artery disease. A large crescentic coronary plaque extending from the 1 o'clock to the 7 o'clock positions is shown, severely reducing the coronary arterial lumen.

angioplasty and stenting when 'before' and 'after' images can be used to document satisfactory patency of the vessel.

Interventional catheterization

Interventional catheterization represents one of the most exciting fields in the treatment of cardiovascular disease and has found important application in both paediatric and adult practice, often extending the role of the cardiologist into areas that were once exclusively surgical. The earliest example was the insertion of electrode-tipped catheters into the heart for pacing patients with bradyarrhythmias (see page 219). Pacing technology has now reached a high level of sophistication and the interventional management of arrhythmias has expanded to include treatment of resistant tachyarrhythmias by overdrive pacing and, more recently, by the electrical ablation of conduction tissue with catheters placed strategically within the heart (see page 248). Balloon angioplasty is a catheter technique used widely for the treatment of coronary artery disease (see page 118), particularly when medical treatment fails to control symptoms. Intracoronary stents mounted on balloon catheters are also widely used for maintaining patency after angioplasty (see page 118). Balloon valvuloplasty is finding increasing application in the treatment of mitral stenosis, and in paediatric practice is the treatment of choice for congenital pulmonary stenosis (see page 323). The insertion of obstructors for closure of patent ductus arteriosus using specially adapted catheters represents a recent advance that is reducing the requirement for surgery in young children (see page 321) while in neonates with transposition of the great arteries emergency balloon atrial septostomy is potentially life saving (see page 330).

Intracardiac pressure measurement

Cardiac catheterization for measurement of blood flow and pressure within the heart and great vessels is widely used both for diagnostic purposes and to guide treatment (Fig. 3.21). The fluid-filled catheter is attached to a pressure transducer which converts the pressure waves into electrical signals. For measurement of right-sided pressures, the catheter is directed by the venous route into the right atrium and then advanced through the right ventricle into the pulmonary artery. For measurement of left-sided pressures, the catheter is directed by the arterial route into the ascending aorta and guided retrogradely through the aortic valve into the left ventricle. Because access to the left atrium is technically difficult, left atrial pressure is usually measured indirectly using the pulmonary artery wedge pressure.

The pulmonary artery wedge pressure is obtained during the right heart catheterization by advancing the catheter distally into the pulmonary arterial tree until the tip wedges in a small branch. Alternatively, a catheter with a preterminal balloon (Swan–Ganz catheter) may be used. Inflation of the balloon in the pulmonary artery causes the catheter tip to be carried with blood flow into a more distal branch which becomes occluded by the balloon. Regardless of

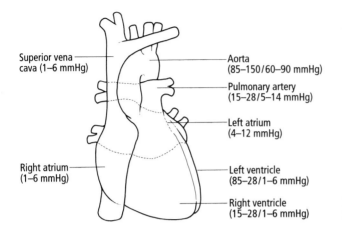

Superior vena cava (1–6 mmHg)

Aorta (85–150/60–90 mmHg)

Pulmonary artery (15–28/5–14 mmHg)

Left atrium (4–12 mmHg)

Right atrium (1–6 mmHg)

Left ventricle (85–28/1–6 mmHg)

Right ventricle (15–28/1–6 mmHg)

Fig. 3.21 Normal pressure measurements within the heart and great vessels.

which method is used, the wedge pressure recorded at the catheter tip is a more-or-less accurate measure of the left atrial pressure transmitted retrogradely through the pulmonary veins and capillaries.

Haemodynamic evaluation of valvular stenosis

In the normal heart there is no pressure gradient across an open valve. Such a gradient usually indicates valvular stenosis (Fig. 3.22) and, as stenosis worsens, the pressure gradient increases. This provides, therefore, a useful index of the severity of stenosis. However, it must be recognized that the pressure gradient is

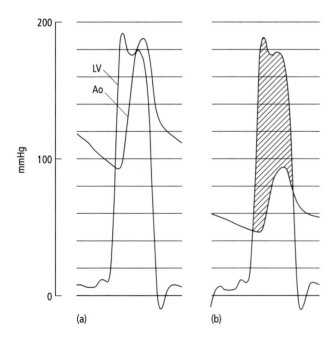

mmHg

200

100

0

LV

Ao

(a)

(b)

Fig. 3.22 Valvular stenosis. Simultaneous measurements of the aortic (Ao) and left ventricular (LV) pressure signals are shown. Note that during systole there is no pressure gradient across the normal aortic valve (a) and the pressure signals are superimposed. Aortic stenosis (b) causes a pressure gradient (shaded area) across the aortic valve throughout systole.

itself influenced by the flow through the valve. For example, if output is very low, the gradient may be small despite the presence of severe stenosis. This applies particularly to the aortic valve because flow velocity is normally high.

Haemodynamic evaluation of intracardiac shunts

Left-to-right intracardiac shunts through atrial or ventricular septal defects introduce 'arterialized' blood into the right side of the heart. This results in an abrupt increase or 'step-up' in the oxygen saturation of venous blood at the level of the shunt, which can be detected by right heart catheterization. Thus, by drawing serial blood samples for oxygen saturation from the pulmonary artery, right ventricle, right atrium and vena cava, the shunt may be localized to the site at which the step-up in oxygen saturation occurs (Table 3.1). The magnitude of the step-up is related to the size of the shunt but precise quantification of the shunt requires measurement of pulmonary and systemic blood flow. The extent to which the pulmonary-systemic flow ratio exceeds 1 is a measure of the size of the shunt.

Measurement of cardiac output

Cardiac output is usually measured by application of the Fick principle. A Swan–Ganz catheter with a right atrial portal and a terminal thermistor is positioned in the pulmonary artery. A known volume of cold saline (usually 10 ml) is injected into the right atrium and the temperature reduction in the pulmonary artery is recorded at the thermistor. The contour of the cooling curve is dependent upon cardiac output, which is calculated by measurement of the area under the curve using a bedside computer.

A relatively simple non-invasive measure of cardiac output can be obtained by Doppler echocardiography using the 'area–length' method. Thus, the length of the column of blood ejected by the left ventricle during a single beat is obtained by multiplying the Doppler aortic flow velocity (cm/second) by the ejection time (seconds). The length of the column of blood is then multiplied by

Table 3.1 Oxygen saturation within the heart and great vessels. Representative values for the normal heart and for patients with a left-to-right shunt are shown.

Region	Normal (%)	Sinus venosus defect (%)	Secundum atrial septal defect (%)	Ventricular septal defect (%)	Patent ductus arteriosus (%)
Superior vena cava	75	85	75	75	75
Right atrium	75	85	85	75	75
Inferior vena cava	75	75	75	75	75
Right ventricle	75	85	85	85	75
Pulmonary artery	75	85	85	85	85
Left ventricle	95	95	95	95	95

the echocardiographic cross-sectional area of the aorta to yield stroke volume (ml/beat). Cardiac output is the product of stroke volume and heart rate.

FURTHER READING

Anonymous. Thallium scintigraphy for diagnosis and risk assessment in coronary artery disease. *Lancet* 1991; 338: 1424.

Daniel WG, Mugge A. Transoesophageal echocardiography. *N Engl J Med* 1995; 332: 1268.

Haire WD, Lieberman RP. Defining the risks of subclavian-vein catheterisation. *N Engl J Med* 1994; 331: 1770.

Higgins CB. The potential role of magnetic resonance imaging in ischemic vascular disease. *N Engl J Med* 1992; 326: 1624.

Matsuzaki M, Toma Y, Kusukawa R. Clinical applications of transesophageal echocardiography. *Circulation* 1990; 82: 709.

Pearlman AS. Transesophageal echocardiography: sound diagnostic technique or two-edged sword? *N Engl J Med* 1991; 324: 841.

Pohost GM, Henzlova MJ. The value of thallium-201 imaging. *N Engl J Med* 1990; 323: 190.

Popp RL. Medical progress: echocardiography. *N Engl J Med* 1990; 323: 101–9 and 179.

Sandham JD, Hull RD, Brant RF. Pulmonary artery flow directed catheter: the evidence. *Lancet* 1996; 348: 1324.

Simpson IA, Camm AJ. Colour Doppler flow mapping. *Br Med J* 1990; 300: 1.

Soni N. Swan song for the Swan Ganz catheter? *Br Med J* 1996; 313: 763.

Steinberg EP. Magnetic resonance coronary angiography—assessing an emerging technology. *N Engl J Med* 1993; 328: 879.

Van der Wall EE, de Roos A, van Voorthuisen AE, Bruschke AVG. Magnetic resonance imaging: a new approach for evaluating coronary artery disease? *Am Heart J* 1991; 121: 1203.

Zaret BL, Wackers FJ. Nuclear cardiology—parts 1 and 2. *N Engl J Med* 1993; 329: 775 (part 1), 855 (part 2).

Heart Failure

SUMMARY

Heart failure, in which cardiac output is inadequate for the perfusion requirements of metabolizing tissues, is usually caused by ischaemic or hypertensive left ventricular disease. Compensatory physiological responses directed at maintaining cardiac output and blood pressure include activation of the sympathoadrenal and renin–angiotensin systems and left ventricular dilatation and hypertrophy. In acute heart failure only sympathoadrenal mechanisms are available to support the circulation, and sharp increments in atrial pressures and reductions in output commonly lead to pulmonary oedema and peripheral hypoperfusion. Chronic heart failure advances more slowly, providing time for compensatory ventricular dilatation and hypertrophy. It is characterized by fluid retention and peripheral hypoperfusion expressed clinically as oedema, exertional dyspnoea and fatigue. Diagnosis is usually clear on clinical grounds but identification of the underlying cause often requires additional tests of which the echocardiogram is most useful. Treatment is aimed at reversing the underlying cause, correcting symptoms and improving prognosis. Although general measures, including arrhythmia and blood-pressure control, are important, most patients require treatment with a diuretic and an ACE inhibitor. Not only does this help to correct symptoms but the ACE inhibitor may also improve prognosis. In intractable heart failure, the addition of digoxin may be helpful but, at this stage, prognosis is poor and heart transplantation becomes the only treatment likely to correct symptoms and prolong survival.

HEART FAILURE

Definition

Heart failure is a syndrome in which a cardiac disorder prevents the delivery of sufficient output to meet the perfusion requirements of metabolizing tissues. This definition is not all-embracing, but it serves to emphasize that the role of the heart is to drive the circulation. Any disturbance of ventricular function that undermines this role may result in heart failure.

Epidemiology

Heart failure is common, with an estimated prevalence in this country of at least 0.4%, rising to nearly 3% in those aged over 65. The incidence (new cases per 1000) doubles with each decade between the ages of 40 and 80, and at any age is more common in men than in women. It is an important cause of morbidity and mortality, accounting for 5% of all adult hospital admissions and carrying a 2-year mortality of between 20 and 75%, depending on its severity. The major causes are coronary artery disease, hypertension, cardiomyopathy and valvular heart disease.

Determinants of ventricular function

Cardiac output is the product of heart rate and stroke volume. Heart rate is under autonomic control and reflects the balance of sympathetic and parasympathetic influences on the sinus node. Stroke volume is determined by the interaction of preload, afterload and contractility (Fig. 4.1).

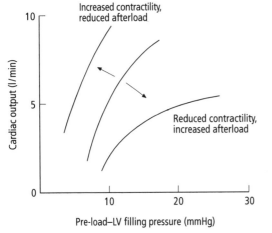

Fig. 4.1 Ventricular function curves. These are Starling curves which define the relation between preload and cardiac output. Because changes in contractility and afterload have an independent influence on ventricular function, a 'family' of Starling curves may be constructed as shown in this figure. Note that as ventricular function improves in response to increments in contractility or reductions in afterload, the contour of the function curve becomes steeper. Deteriorating ventricular function, on the other hand, is associated with a flatter ventricular function curve such that changes in preload have a relatively small effect on cardiac output.

Preload

Changes in ventricular preload produce directionally similar changes in stroke volume. Preload refers to the passive stretch (or tension) of the ventricular myocardium at end-diastole and is equivalent to end-diastolic volume. Because end-diastolic volume is largely pressure dependent, ventricular end-diastolic pressure and atrial pressure (collectively termed ventricular filling pressures) are widely used as measures of preload. The curvilinear relation between preload and stroke volume (as described by Starling) provides a useful means of evaluating ventricular function (Fig. 4.1).

Although ventricular filling pressures provide a convenient measure of preload, the effect of *compliance* (the reciprocal of stiffness) must not be overlooked. Thus the non-compliant (stiff) ventricle which characterizes hypertrophic disease, restrictive cardiomyopathy and constrictive pericarditis requires a higher filling pressure to produce the same end-diastolic volume (or preload) as the normally compliant ventricle (Fig. 4.2).

Afterload

Changes in ventricular afterload produce directionally opposite changes in stroke volume (Fig. 4.1). Afterload is the systolic wall tension developed by the ventricle to expel blood against vascular resistance. It is a function of ventricular pressure and volume and is defined by the law of Laplace:

ventricular wall tension = ventricular pressure × ventricular radius.

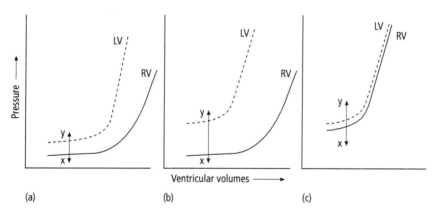

Fig. 4.2 Ventricular pressure–volume ('compliance') curves. (a) The normal heart. The right ventricular (RV) curve lies below the left ventricular (LV) curve because the pressure x required to fill the thin-walled right ventricle in diastole is considerably lower than the pressure y required to fill the thick-walled left ventricle to the same volume. (b) Reduced LV compliance. This is usually caused by LV hypertrophy in patients with hypertension, aortic stenosis or hypertrophic cardiomyopathy. The LV diastolic pressure y must rise considerably to maintain adequate filling. RV diastolic pressure is unaffected. (c) Reduced LV and RV compliance. Tamponade, constrictive pericarditis or restrictive cardiomyopathy usually impede the diastolic filling of both ventricles equally. Thus diastolic pressures of both ventricles (x and y) rise and equilibrate to maintain adequate filling.

Clinically, afterload is equated with systolic pressure, but the contribution of ventricular radius should not be overlooked. Thus, as the failing heart dilates, afterload (as well as preload) increases.

Contractility

Changes in ventricular contractility produce directionally similar changes in stroke volume (Fig. 4.1). Contractility is not easily measured and the term is usually used qualitatively to describe the inherent force and velocity of ventricular contraction, independent of preload and afterload.

Measurement of ventricular function

Ejection fraction

Left ventricular function is usually assessed qualitatively by observation of wall motion and cavity size during dynamic imaging. Any of the major imaging techniques, e.g. echocardiography, radionuclide angiography, contrast ventriculography, are suitable for this purpose. These techniques may also be used for the quantitative assessment of left ventricular function by measurement of the ejection fraction, the fraction of left ventricular blood volume expelled per beat.

$$\text{Ejection fraction} = \frac{\text{end-diastolic volume} - \text{end-systolic volume}}{\text{end-diastolic volume}}$$

At rest, the lower limit of normal for left ventricular ejection fraction is 55%, but during exercise it increases considerably and may exceed 90%. Failure of ejection fraction to increase normally during exercise indicates left ventricular impairment, usually caused by ischaemia or by an intrinsic defect of contractile function. Thus, exercise stress may be used as a provocative test to unmask left ventricular impairment in the patient with a normal resting ejection fraction. Exercise stress is usually applied during radionuclide angiography which allows sequential measurements of the ejection fraction following a single injection of isotope.

Starling relation

Measurement of left atrial pressure (as reflected by pulmonary artery wedge pressure) and cardiac output provides a simple means of evaluating left ventricular function, and is widely used in the intensive care unit. Abnormal elevation of the wedge pressure with a normal or low cardiac output indicates downward displacement of the Starling curve and left ventricular dysfunction. However, these measurements do not define the cause of left ventricular dysfunction, which may result from restricted filling, excessive afterload or myocardial contractile impairment.

Mechanisms of heart failure

Cardiac disorders produce heart failure by one or more of the following mechanisms (Table 4.1).

- Restriction of ventricular filling.
- Imposition of excessive load on the ventricle (volume or pressure).
- Impairment of myocardial contractile function.

Restriction of ventricular filling is the principal cause of heart failure in mitral stenosis where the left ventricle itself is entirely normal. It is also important in hypertrophic and restrictive cardiomyopathy and constrictive pericarditis, where there may be no intrinsic impairment of systolic function, but diastolic filling (or preload) is impaired by the stiff *non-compliant* ventricle (cardiomyopathy) or the diseased pericardium (constriction), resulting in depressed cardiac output (Fig. 4.2).

Excessive loading may be caused by pressure or volume which have their major effects on afterload and preload, respectively. It is important to distinguish between the effects of acute and chronic loading. In acute pressure loading (e.g. pulmonary embolism), heart failure is a direct result of the sudden increase in

Table 4.1 Causes of heart failure.

Ventricular pathophysiology	Clinical examples	Ventricle predominantly affected		
		Left	Right	Both
Restricted filling	Mitral stenosis	•		
	Tricuspid stenosis		•	
	Constrictive pericarditis		•	
	Tamponade		•	
	Restrictive cardiomyopathy			•
	Hypertrophic cardiomyopathy	•		
Pressure loading	Hypertension	•		
	Aortic stenosis	•		
	Coarctation of the aorta	•		
	Pulmonary vascular disease		•	
	Pulmonary embolism		•	
	Pulmonary stenosis		•	
Volume loading	Mitral regurgitation	•		
	Aortic regurgitation	•		
	Pulmonary regurgitation		•	
	Tricuspid regurgitation		•	
	Ventricular septal defect	•		
	Patent ductus arteriosus	•		
Contractile impairment	Coronary artery disease	•		
	Dilated cardiomyopathy			•
	Myocarditis			•
Arrhythmia	Severe bradycardia			•
	Severe tachycardia			•

afterload which depresses stroke volume. Similarly, acute volume loading (e.g. valvular regurgitation in endocarditis) produces heart failure by overwhelming the Starling reserve of the ventricle. However, in chronic pressure or volume loading, compensatory mechanisms may protect against heart failure for prolonged periods (see below). Finally myocardial contractile function deteriorates to the point that the ventricle can no longer tolerate the extra load.

Ventricular contractile dysfunction is the primary cause of heart failure in dilated cardiomyopathy. The Starling curve is displaced downwards and is flattened in contour, such that changes in filling pressure produce relatively small changes in cardiac output (see Fig. 4.1). In myocardial infarction, regional loss of contractile tissue reduces effective muscle mass which has a similar effect on the Starling curve and the dyskinetic ventricular contraction pattern further reduces pump efficiency. Chronic pressure and volume loading ultimately lead to ventricular contractile dysfunction as compensatory mechanisms fail to preserve cardiac output.

Classification of heart failure

Heart failure may be caused by a wide variety of disorders affecting the coronary circulation, myocardium, pericardium or valvular tissue. It is a complex disorder and a number of classifications have been suggested.

Low-output versus high-output heart failure

This classification is physiologically based but has very little practical application because nearly all cases of heart failure encountered clinically are associated with low cardiac output. Rarely, the perfusion requirements of tissue metabolism cannot be met despite considerable increments in cardiac output above the normal range. This is termed high-output heart failure. There are three major causes.
- Chronic elevation of metabolic rate, e.g. in thyrotoxicosis.
- Reduced oxygen-carrying capacity of the blood, e.g. in anaemia.
- Arteriovenous shunting which reduces the fraction of cardiac output delivered to the tissues, e.g. in arteriovenous fistula, beriberi, Paget's disease.

Heart failure is a rare consequence of these disorders and, when it occurs, the mechanisms are often complex. Nevertheless, chronic volume overload is an important factor because of the long-term requirement for increased output.

Systolic versus diastolic heart failure

This classification is also physiologically based but is more helpful because it recognizes that abnormalities of systolic and diastolic function may act independently in the pathogenesis of heart failure. Systolic dysfunction (reduced contractility) is the principal mechanism of heart failure in coronary heart disease and dilated cardiomyopathy, although there may be an additional diastolic component in coronary heart disease related to the reduced compliance of the ischaemic ventricle. In mitral stenosis and restrictive cardiomyopathy, however, diastolic dysfunction is the principal mechanism of heart failure due to obstructed ventricular filling and reduced ventricular compliance, respectively. In hypertrophic left ventricular disease (caused by hypertension, aortic stenosis or hypertrophic cardiomyopathy) diastolic dysfunction due to reduced ventricular compliance is also the major mechanism of heart failure, although systolic dysfunction makes a variable contribution to the haemodynamic derangement.

The value of this classification is undermined by the fact that many patients with heart failure have abnormalities of both systolic and diastolic function. Nevertheless, therapeutic implications may be important because drugs like beta-blockers which slow the heart rate and increase diastolic filling time are often helpful in diastolic heart failure but tend to make systolic heart failure worse. Conversely, vasodilators, including ACE inhibitors, play a major role in the treatment of systolic heart failure but are less helpful in diastolic heart failure.

Left-sided versus right-sided heart failure

This classification is clinically based and probably for this reason is the most widely used. It recognizes that many causes of heart failure have their major impact on either the left- or right-sided cardiac chambers (see Table 4.1), producing a characteristic cluster of symptoms and signs. Coronary artery disease and hypertension, for example, typically damage the left ventricle, causing left-sided heart failure. The patient complains of fatigue and shortness of breath due to reduced cardiac output and increased left ventricular filling pressure (see page 83). Similar complaints characterize mitral stenosis which causes left-sided heart failure by obstructing diastolic filling of the left ventricle. Pulmonary vascular disease in patients with longstanding bronchitis and emphysema, on the other hand, causes right-sided heart failure. The patient complains of fatigue, abdominal discomfort and peripheral oedema due to reduced cardiac output and increased right ventricular filling pressure (see page 83).

This classification has a time-honoured role in clinical cardiology, but its flaws must be recognized. The left and right sides of the heart do not operate independently of each other but as an integrated unit, and this renders the classification rather meaningless in physiological terms. Moreover, in chronic heart failure, almost regardless of cause, fluid retention associated with variable reductions in cardiac output dominates the clinical picture ensuring that most patients present with symptoms of *chronic congestive heart failure* (dyspnoea, oedema, fatigue) defying classification into left- or right-sided failure.

Despite these reservations, the classification into left and right-sided heart failure remains helpful in so far as it encourages the clinician to relate symptoms to aetiological factors and to pathological effects on the cardiac chambers. For this reason, it continues to be used in this chapter although the term 'chronic congestive heart failure' is retained for the syndrome of dyspnoea, oedema and fatigue when no left- or right-sided attribution is intended.

Pathophysiology

Compensatory mechanisms

Compensatory mechanisms in heart failure attempt to maintain cardiac output and blood pressure in the face of abnormal loading and contractile impairment. There are three major mechanisms (Fig. 4.3):
- neurohormonal activation;
- ventricular dilatation; and
- ventricular hypertrophy.

   The principal neurohormonal response is sympathoadrenal activation. This is immediately available when ventricular pump function is threatened, but ventricular dilatation and hypertrophy take longer to develop. Thus, an acute cardiac lesion is less well tolerated than a lesion of similar severity that has developed slowly. Nevertheless, even in chronic disease, the mechanisms that protect against heart failure are of limited potential and do not always prevent decompensation occurring.

Neurohormonal activation (Table 4.2)

There are many neurohormonal changes in heart failure, and the picture is confused by their variation with the severity of heart failure and by differences between untreated and treated patients. Both vasoconstrictor and vasodilator hormones are released, but it is the vasoconstrictor response which predominates.

(a) Sympathoadrenal system. Sympathetic stimulation of cardiac beta-1-adrenoceptors improves ventricular function by increasing heart rate and contractility. In addition, constriction of venous capacitance vessels by adrenergic pathways redistributes flow centrally, and the increased venous return to the heart further

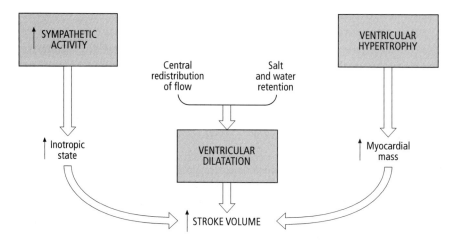

Fig. 4.3 Compensatory physiology in heart failure.

Table 4.2 Summary of neurohormonal changes.

	Hormone	Effects
Vasoconstrictor group		
Catecholamines		
	Noradrenaline ↑↑	Increased contractility
	Adrenaline (↑)	Increased heart rate
	Dopamine (↑)	Vasoconstriction
Renin–angiotensin–aldosterone system	Plasma renin activity	Vasoconstriction
	Angiotensin II ↑↑	Salt retention
	Aldosterone ↑↑	Vascular remodelling?
Antidiuretic hormone (vasopressin)	ADH ↑	Vasoconstriction
		Water retention
Vasodilator group		
Atrial natriuretic peptide	ANP ↑	Salt excretion
		Vasodilation
Others		
Prostaglandins	PGE$_2$, PGI$_2$ ↑	Vasodilation
Bradykinins	Kallikrein ↓	Kinins are mostly
		natriuretic and vasodilation
Endorphins	Beta-endorphin (↑)	Vasodilation?

ADH, antidiuretic hormone; ANP, atrial natriuretic peptide; PGE, prostaglandin; PGI, prostacyclin.

augments ventricular function by the Starling mechanism. To some extent, these beneficial effects are modified by arteriolar constriction in the skin, gut and kidneys, the vascular beds that respond most vigorously to sympathetic stimulation. Although this helps to maintain blood pressure, the increase in afterload tends to depress ventricular function. Moreover, the responsiveness of the heart to chronic adrenergic stimulation becomes attenuated due to reduction in both the density of cardiac adrenoceptors and their sensitivity to catecholamines *(receptor down-regulation)*. Depletion of cardiac noradrenaline stores contributes to this process.

(b) Renin–angiotensin system. Reduced renal perfusion and heightened sympathetic activity are the major stimuli for renin release from the juxtaglomerular apparatus of the kidney, although additional stimulus is provided by some of the drugs commonly used to treat heart failure, particularly diuretics and vasodilators. Renin is the rate-limiting enzyme in the synthesis of angiotensin II, a potent vasoconstrictor which also stimulates aldosterone secretion from the adrenal gland. Angiotensin II-mediated vasoconstriction helps to support the blood pressure, while the action of aldosterone on the distal nephron stimulates salt and water retention which further increases ventricular filling and maintains cardiac output by the Starling mechanism. However, the compensatory potential of the renin–angiotensin system is limited. Vasoconstriction adds significantly to left ventricular afterload exacerbating contractile dysfunction. This further reduces renal perfusion thereby establishing a 'vicious cycle' of increasing renin–

angiotensin II production and deteriorating ventricular function (Fig. 4.4). Moreover, as salt and water retention increases, peripheral and pulmonary congestion
cause oedema and contribute to dyspnoea.

(c) Antidiuretic hormone (vasopressin). Circulating levels of this vasoconstrictor are
also increased in heart failure. Compensatory benefits of blood-pressure support
and increased ventricular filling must be set against the long-term adverse effects
of increased afterload, renal hypoperfusion and fluid retention.

(d) Atrial natiuretic peptide. Circulating levels of this peptide are increased in heart
failure although its precise role remains uncertain. Nevertheless, it has potentially useful properties, including vasodilatation, salt and water diuresis and
inhibition of renin and aldosterone secretion. Thus it has the potential to modify
the adverse consequences of renin–angiotensin activation.

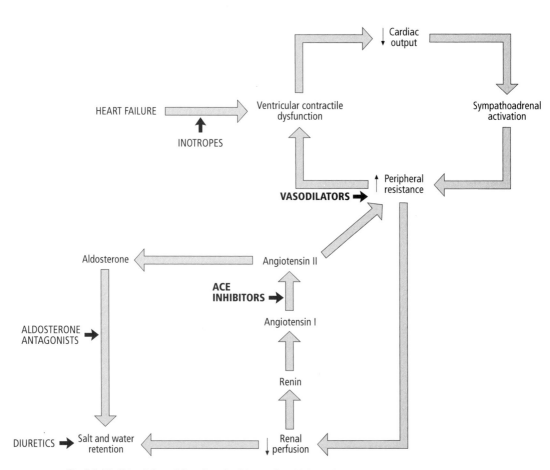

Fig. 4.4 The kidney in heart failure. Note the vicious cycles of falling cardiac output, increasing peripheral
resistance and stimulation of angiotensin secretion. The effects of specific antifailure treatment are shown. Only
ACE inhibitors and vasodilators, however, have the potential to break the vicious cycles.

Ventricular dilatation

When the heart is volume loaded it dilates, and ventricular contraction increases by the Starling mechanism. Thus the dilatation that occurs in valvular incompetence allows 'forward' output to be maintained, despite the regurgitant volume of blood. Dilatation also occurs in myocardial disease due to central redistribution of venous blood and expansion of plasma volume. The increase in preload helps to maintain stroke volume. Once heart failure is established, the compensatory effects of cardiac dilatation become limited by associated increments in afterload (law of Laplace) and by the flattened contour of the Starling curve which diminishes the responsiveness of the ventricle to increasing preload. Ultimately, rising left ventricular filling pressure may lead to pulmonary oedema, further destabilizing the circulation.

Ventricular hypertrophy

Excessive ventricular loading stimulates myocardial hypertrophy which augments the mass of contractile tissue and enables the heart to sustain the extra burden. Hypertrophy is most marked in the pressure-loaded ventricle (e.g. in hypertension, aortic stenosis) when additional sarcomeres are laid down in parallel, producing significant increments in wall thickness. Nevertheless, hypertrophy also occurs in the volume-loaded ventricle (e.g. in valvular regurgitation) but additional sarcomeres are laid down in series as the ventricle dilates, so that wall thickness remains close to normal despite an overall increase in myocardial mass. Hypertrophy takes time to develop and acute overloading is not well tolerated. Moreover, in established myocardial hypertrophy, there is an intrinsic defect in ventricular function affecting both systole and diastole, and, as loading increases, pump function deteriorates. Thus, like all the major compensatory mechanisms, hypertrophy has only limited potential to protect against the development of heart failure.

The kidney in heart failure

The kidney plays a central role in the salt and water retention characterizing chronic congestive heart failure (Fig. 4.4). A significant reduction in glomerular filtration occurs early during heart failure, often before symptoms develop. This is caused by constriction of the preglomerular arterioles in response to increased sympathetic activity and angiotensin II production. The reduction in glomerular filtration inevitably reduces sodium delivery to the nephron but this provides only a partial explanation for salt and water retention in heart failure. Increased sodium reabsorption from the nephron is the more important factor. This occurs particularly in the proximal tubule in the early stages of heart failure but, as the failure worsens, the effects of aldosterone on sodium reabsorption in the distal nephron predominate. Ultimately, feedback regulation of salt and water balance breaks down completely, due to suppression of atrial natriuretic peptide and inappropriate antidiuretic hormone secretion. This produces intractable plasma volume overload and dilutional hyponatraemia.

Oedema in heart failure

In heart failure, oedema is the result of increased capillary hydrostatic pressure. This drives fluid into the interstitial space at a rate which exceeds the combined effects of osmotic reabsorption and the clearing capacity of the lymphatic system.

Pulmonary oedema

Pulmonary oedema occurs in acute left heart failure due to sympathetically mediated central redistribution of flow. It may also occur in chronic congestive heart failure, when plasma volume overload secondary to salt and water retention is the major mechanism. The pulmonary veins and capillaries are in continuity with the left atrium and therefore increments in left atrial pressure produce a similar increase in pulmonary capillary pressure. As left atrial pressure rises above 18–20 mmHg, pulmonary oedema develops.

Systemic oedema

Systemic oedema occurs in chronic congestive heart failure and always reflects plasma volume overload secondary to salt and water retention. The effect of gravity on capillary hydrostatic pressure ensures that dependent parts of the body are particularly prone to oedema formation. With worsening plasma volume overload, oedema of the abdominal viscera and ascites develops. Hepatic engorgement may lead to impaired synthesis of plasma proteins which exacerbates oedema formation by reducing capillary osmotic pressure.

Clinical manifestations

Minor impairment of cardiac function may remain asymptomatic but, as compensatory mechanisms become overwhelmed, the clinical manifestations of heart failure emerge. These relate principally to the consequences of elevated atrial pressures and reduced cardiac output, expressed clinically as congestion and peripheral hypoperfusion, respectively. Increased sympathetic activity also plays an important role. Manifestations of left- and right-sided heart failure are conveniently considered separately although, as discussed previously (page 77), the syndrome of dyspnoea, oedema and fatigue which characterizes most cases of chronic heart failure defies this simple classification and is termed 'chronic congestive heart failure' in this chapter.

Acute left heart failure

This is a medical emergency and is usually caused by myocardial infarction, although other causes include acute aortic and mitral regurgitation, fulminant myocarditis and mitral stenosis. Pulmonary oedema and systemic hypoperfusion are invariable; the patient becomes abruptly dyspnoeic and may expectorate pink, frothy oedema fluid. Central cyanosis, hypotension and oliguria occur and in severe cases cardiogenic shock develops (see page 96).

Chronic left heart failure

This is usually the result of left ventricular failure caused by ischaemic, hypertensive, cardiomyopathic or valvular disease. In mitral stenosis, however, left ventricular contractile function is normal and heart failure is due to impaired left ventricular filling. Elevated left atrial pressure produces orthopnoea and, in advanced cases, paroxysmal nocturnal dyspnoea (see page 3). More troublesome is exertional dyspnoea, causes of which are complex but include exertional elevations of left atrial pressure, respiratory muscle fatigue and metabolic factors such as acidosis. Muscular fatigue due to impaired cardiac output also occurs during exercise.

The physical examination reveals signs of low cardiac output and reflex sympathetic stimulation, which include tachycardia, cool skin and peripheral cyanosis. Auscultation at the lung bases reveals inspiratory crackles reflecting pulmonary congestion; signs of pleural effusion may also be present. Of greater diagnostic significance is the third heart sound which produces a characteristic gallop rhythm. It is associated with rapid ventricular filling in early diastole and therefore never occurs when filling is impeded by mitral stenosis. The cardiac apex is displaced laterally and in severe failure, left ventricular dilatation may stretch the mitral valve ring, producing 'functional' regurgitation manifested by a pansystolic apical murmur. An alternating pulse also occurs in severe failure (see Fig. 1.6).

Acute right heart failure

This is a medical emergency seen in pulmonary embolism and less commonly in right ventricular infarction. Signs are those of critically reduced cardiac output and include cool skin, systemic hypotension and peripheral cyanosis. The jugular venous pulse (JVP) is usually elevated (see also page 141).

Chronic right heart failure

This is usually the result of chronically elevated pulmonary artery pressure in patients with left heart failure or pulmonary disease. In these cases dyspnoea is always prominent but the effects of low cardiac output, elevated right atrial pressure and salt and water retention are also important. Fatigue is invariable, and congestion of the liver and gastrointestinal tract causes abdominal discomfort and loss of appetite. The JVP is elevated and in severe cases a giant 'v' wave indicates 'functional' tricuspid regurgitation due to right ventricular dilatation.

Peripheral oedema may be severe and visceral congestion produces enlargement of the liver and spleen; in longstanding disease, hepatic dysfunction results in jaundice and impaired protein synthesis. Auscultation at the lower left sternal edge may reveal a pansystolic murmur if tricuspid regurgitation is present.

Chronic congestive heart failure

This is the most common mode of presentation and combines clinical features of left- and right-sided failure. Principal complaints are fatigue, dyspnoea and peripheral oedema caused by reduced cardiac output and salt and water retention. In advanced cases orthopnea, abdominal discomfort and loss of appetite develop. Physical signs include tachycardia, peripheral cyanosis, elevation of the JVP, lateral displacement of the cardiac apex, a gallop rhythm, murmurs of mitral and tricuspid regurgitation, inspiratory crackles at the lung bases, and dependent oedema, sometimes associated with ascites and pleural effusions.

Complications

Cardiac arrhythmias occur commonly in heart failure, particularly atrial fibrillation which produces variable haemodynamic deterioration; ventricular arrhythmias are more sinister and an important cause of sudden death. Deep venous thrombosis (the result of sluggish flow in the veins of the legs and pelvis) may lead to pulmonary embolism which may also cause sudden death; thrombosis within the dilated cardiac chambers may cause both systemic and pulmonary embolism. Chronic pulmonary congestion in left heart failure predisposes to chest infection.

Major organ failure is an inevitable consequence of advanced heart failure. Hypoperfusion in the kidney may lead to worsening renal failure. Liver failure with jaundice and elevation of liver enzymes is usually reversible following correction of visceral congestion, but in longstanding right heart failure cardiac cirrhosis develops, characterized by centrilobular necrosis and fibrosis ('nutmeg liver').

Diagnosis

Heart failure can usually be recognized on clinical grounds, but full diagnosis demands identification of its cause.

ECG

This is usually abnormal in heart failure but the changes are often non-specific. Most common are T-wave inversion, bundle branch block and atrial fibrillation. ECG abnormalities pointing to an aetiology include pathological Q waves in ischaemic disease, and left ventricular hypertrophy in hypertensive and aortic valve disease.

Chest X-ray

Cardiac enlargement is the most consistent finding and, in left-sided failure, this may be associated with pulmonary venous dilatation or pulmonary oedema (Fig. 4.5). In mitral stenosis, pulmonary congestion may occur without cardiac enlargement, though signs of left atrial dilatation are usually present. Cardiac enlargement without pulmonary congestion is seen in tamponade and primary right-sided failure.

Non-invasive imaging

The echocardiogram is potentially diagnostic of many of the cardiac defects that lead to heart failure. The presence of left ventricular dilatation and *regional* contractile impairment indicates ischaemic disease (Fig. 4.6), whilst the presence of four-chamber dilatation and *global* contractile impairment indicates dilated cardiomyopathy (see Fig. 6.1). Heart failure due to valvular disease and tamponade is readily apparent (see Figs 7.5, 9.10 and 9.11). Simultaneous Doppler studies permit identification of regurgitant jets through incompetent valves and shunting through septal defects.

Radionuclide ventriculography provides an alternative way of examining left ventricular cavity size and wall-motion abnormalities. It is particularly useful for quantitating ejection fraction and for identifying early ventricular impairment by application of provocative tests.

Cardiac catheterization

Right heart catheterization is occasionally of diagnostic value in acute myocardial infarction, particularly for identification of relative hypovolaemia when low

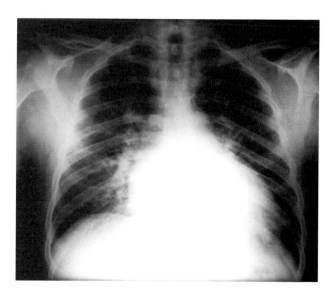

Fig. 4.5 Left ventricular failure. The chest X-ray shows cardiac enlargement, dilatation of the upper lobe veins and interstitial pulmonary oedema. Kerley B lines are seen in the right costophrenic angle.

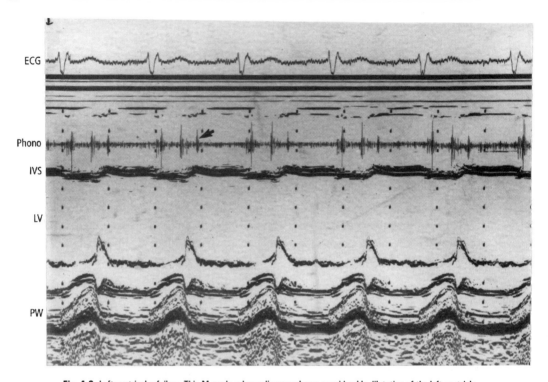

ECG

Phono

IVS

LV

PW

Fig. 4.6 Left ventricular failure. This M-mode echocardiogram shows considerable dilatation of the left ventricle (the vertical dots are a 1-cm scale). Note that the interventricular septum (IVS) is almost akinetic, but the posterior wall (PW) is contracting normally. Regional contractile impairment of this type indicates coronary artery disease and must be distinguished from the global contractile impairment that occurs in cardiomyopathy. The phonocardiogram recorded simultaneously shows normal first and second heart sounds and also a third heart sound (arrowed).

cardiac output is associated with an inappropriately low wedge pressure (see page 140). It may also be useful for haemodynamic monitoring in critically ill patients with cardiogenic shock when initial responses to therapy are unsatisfactory.

Left heart catheterization in heart failure rarely provides diagnostic information that cannot be obtained by non-invasive means. Nevertheless, in patients with surgically correctable disease (e.g. ventricular aneurysm, valvular disease) the surgeon usually requires precise definition of the lesion with haemodynamic measurements and angiography.

Differential diagnosis

Acute left heart failure must be distinguished from other causes of acute-onset dyspnoea, including bronchial asthma, pneumothorax and pulmonary embolism. In none of these conditions, however, does the chest X-ray demonstrate pulmonary oedema.

The differential diagnosis of chronic heart failure includes other causes of dyspnoea and peripheral oedema.

Obstructive pulmonary disease

In bronchitis, a history of winter cough and sputum can usually be obtained. Although typical orthopnoea is unusual, nocturnal symptoms may interrupt sleep if diaphragmatic excursion is restricted by the weight of the abdominal viscera or nocturnal wheezing occurs Respiratory function tests are usually diagnostic in these patients and non-invasive imaging will rule out important heart disease.

Dependent oedema of the elderly

This is common in sedentary patients and is caused by venostasis in the legs, which results from inactivity of the muscle pump, varicose veins and gravitational pooling of blood. Treatment with support stockings and elevation of the legs is usually effective.

TREATMENT

Treatment of acute left ventricular failure (LVF)

General measures

The patient should be nursed in the head-up position. Urgent correction of arrhythmias and hypertension is essential. Treatment of hypoxaemia is directed at maintaining an arterial oxygen tension of at least 7 kPa; if this cannot be achieved despite high concentrations of inhaled oxygen, positive pressure ventilation may be necessary.

Medical therapy (Table 4.3)

Intravenous *opiates* and *diuretics* are the first-line agents. Morphine 10 mg or diamorphine 5 mg relieves dyspnoea by a combination of vasodilatation, respiratory depression and relief of anxiety. Loop diuretics (e.g. frusemide 40 mg) initiate a prompt diuresis which reduces left atrial pressure but, because diuretic activity depends largely on adequate renal perfusion, these drugs are of less value in severe low-output states.

Vasodilators and inotropes

If opiates and diuretics are not rapidly effective, treatment should be directed at improving left ventricular function with vasodilators and inotropes. Agents with a short plasma half-life for intravenous infusion should be chosen. In this way infusion rates can be rapidly adjusted, with the aim of improving peripheral perfusion, as reflected by urine flow and skin temperature, and reducing left ventricular filling pressure such that pulmonary oedema begins to clear. In

Table 4.3 Medical treatment of acute left ventricular failure.

Drug	Action	Indication	Dose	Note
Diuretics				
Frusemide	Diuresis	Pulmonary oedema	40–80 mg	Often unhelpful in severe low-output states
Opiates				
Morphine	Venodilatation Respiratory suppression Relief of anxiety	Pulmonary oedema	5–10 mg	Use cautiously in patients with associated respiratory disease
Vasodilators				
Glyceryl trinitrate	Venodilatation	Pulmonary oedema	0.2–2.0 μg/kg/min	Contraindicated if systolic blood pressure is < 90 mmHg
Inotropes				
Dobutamine	Positive inotropism	Severe low output with hypotension	2.0–10.0 μg/kg/min	Usually only indicated in severe low-output states or cardiogenic shock
Dopamine	Positive inotropism and renal arteriolar dilatation (low dose) Generalized arteriolar constriction (high dose)	Severe low output with oliguria	1.0–10.0 μg/kg/min	Avoid high doses of dopamine

refractory cases, direct measurement of pulmonary artery wedge pressure (indirect left ventricular filling pressure) with a Swan–Ganz catheter is sometimes helpful, with treatment aimed at reducing the wedge pressure to between 15 and 20 mmHg. Further reductions in wedge pressure should be avoided because the reduction in preload lowers cardiac output.

Glyceryl trinitrate is the most widely used vasodilator. It is predominantly a venodilator and causes blood to pool in the abdominal capacitance vessels, reducing venous return to the heart and lowering left atrial pressure. Nitrates also have a minor effect on the peripheral arterioles and may cause a small reduction in blood pressure. Although this tends to increase cardiac output, systolic blood pressure must not be allowed to fall below 90 mmHg because of the risk to vital organ perfusion. Vasodilators are contraindicated in patients who are already hypotensive. There is no role for angiotensin-converting enzyme (ACE) inhibitors in acute LVF.

Dobutamine and *dopamine* are widely used inotropic agents with sympathomimetic activity. Stimulation of cardiac beta-1 adrenoceptors enhances contractility and cardiac output. Dopamine (unlike dobutamine) also has important peripheral vascular effects: low doses (up to 5 μg/kg/min) selectively dilate the renal arterioles and improve renal perfusion but high doses produce widespread alpha-adrenoceptor-mediated arteriolar constriction. This improves blood pressure but further depresses left ventricular function by increasing afterload. Thus dopamine is best used at a low dose for its renal action, whilst dobutamine produces dose-related increments in cardiac output without adverse peripheral vascular effects. Combination therapy with dobutamine and low-dose dopamine is particularly useful for improving both cardiac output and renal perfusion. Simultaneous treatment with diuretics and nitrates is necessary for correction of pulmonary oedema. The risk of cardiac arrhythmias during inotropic therapy demands careful ECG monitoring.

Intra-aortic balloon pump (Fig. 4.7)

This device may be used to provide temporary support in acute LVF. A catheter with a terminal sausage-shaped balloon is introduced into the femoral artery and the tip is positioned in the thoracic aorta just below the left subclavian branch. Pumping is synchronized with the ECG. The balloon inflates in early diastole, thereby augmenting pressure in the aortic root and improving coronary flow; it deflates immediately prior to ventricular systole, producing an abrupt fall in pressure which reduces afterload and improves cardiac output.

Despite the short-term value of the intra-aortic balloon, it is often impossible to wean patients off the device. This limits its clinical application to patients with a surgically correctable cardiac lesion (e.g. ventricular septal defect, acute valvular incompetence) or to patients with a temporarily 'stunned' ventricle following heart surgery. In both groups the device provides valuable haemodynamic support pending corrective surgery or spontaneous recovery of contractile function.

Complications include balloon rupture, peripheral embolism and trauma to the aorta and iliofemoral vessels, with varying degrees of arterial insufficiency.

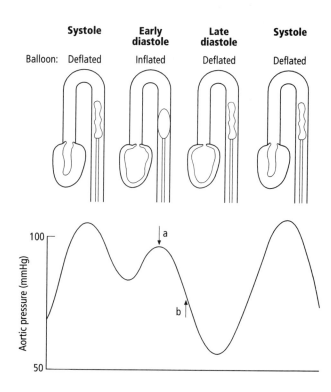

Fig. 4.7 Intra-aortic balloon pump and simultaneous aortic pressure signal. a, balloon inflation in early diastole augments pressure in the ascending thoracic aorta. b, deflation in late diastole leads to an abrupt fall in pressure.

Surgical therapy

Emergency surgery is potentially life-saving when an acute mechanical cardiac lesion produces LVF without substantial myocardial damage. Any delay may cause irrecoverable loss of ventricular contractile function, following which results are less favourable. Thus, endocarditis complicated by LVF is usually an indication for urgent valve replacement. Similarly, papillary muscle or septal rupture following myocardial infarction usually requires immediate surgical correction.

Treatment of chronic congestive heart failure

Although the cause of chronic congestive heart failure can usually be identified, its correction is not always feasible—particularly when ventricular contractile impairment is established. Thus treatment is usually directed towards controlling symptoms and slowing the progression of disease. Although general measures, including arrhythmia and blood-pressure control, are important, most patients require treatment with a diuretic and an ACE inhibitor. Not only does this help to correct symptoms, but the ACE inhibitor may also improve prognosis. In intractable heart failure, the addition of digoxin may be helpful in some cases but, at this stage, prognosis is poor and heart transplantation becomes the only treatment likely to work.

General measures

Simple measures, including control of cardiac arrhythmias, hypertension and anaemia are important. Atrial fibrillation is particularly common and, if resistant to electrical cardioversion, can usually be controlled by digitalis which slows the ventricular response and improves stroke volume. Treatment of hypertension improves left ventricular function by reducing afterload, and correction of anaemia improves oxygen delivery to metabolizing tissues.

Salt and water retention provides a rationale for limiting salt intake but, with the availability of potent diuretics, this is rarely necessary in practice.

Medical therapy (Table 4.4)

All patients with symptomatic left ventricular dysfunction should be given a diuretic and an ACE inhibitor (Box 4.1). Patients who are asymptomatic without signs of fluid retention do not need a diuretic but may still obtain prognostic benefit from an ACE inhibitor, if echocardiography (or any other imaging technique) shows that left ventricular function is severely depressed with an ejection fraction $\leq 35\%$ (Box 4.2).

Diuretics

These promote salt and water excretion which lowers atrial pressures and

Table 4.4 Medical treatment of congestive heart failure.

Drug	Daily oral dose (mg)
Thiazide diuretics	
Bendrofluazide	2.5–10.0
Cyclopenthiazide	0.25–1.0
Loop diuretics	
Frusemide	40–500
Bumetanide	0.5–5.0
Ethacrynic acid	25–150
Potassium-sparing diuretics	
Spinonolactone	100–200
Amiloride	5–20
Triamterene	100–200
Angiotensin-converting enzyme inhibitors	
Captopril	25–150
Enalapril	5–40
Lisinopril	10–40
Quinapril	10–40

corrects pulmonary and systemic congestion. The associated reduction in body weight provides a useful clinical yardstick of the diuretic response. Diuretics do not improve ventricular function; rather, by reducing preload, they tend to have the reverse effect and over-diuresis must therefore be avoided.

Box 4.1 Studies of Left Ventricular Dysfunction (SOLVD): Treatment Trial

Study design Randomized, double-blind, placebo-controlled, multicentre.

Randomization Enalapril, 2.5 or 5 mg b.d., titrated up to 10 mg b.d.; or placebo. Additional non-ACE-inhibitor therapy was allowed.

Inclusion Symptomatic heart failure.

End points Mortality, hospitalization, incidence of myocardial infarction, morbidity, quality of life, ejection fraction.

Patients 2569 (1285 enalapril; 1284 placebo) with symptomatic heart failure (ejection fraction ≤ 35%).

Results After 41.4 months, there were fewer deaths in the enalapril group than in the placebo group (35.2% vs 39.7%), with a risk reduction of 16% ($P = 0.004$). There were also fewer cardiovascular deaths in the enalapril group than in the placebo group (31.1% vs 35.9%) representing a risk reduction of 18% ($P > 0.002$). There were fewer deaths or hospitalizations for congestive heart failure in the enalapril group than in the placebo group (47.7% vs 57.3%), representing a risk reduction of 26% ($P < 0.0001$), but no significant difference in non-cardiovascular deaths (3.8% vs 4.1%).

Conclusions Findings show that addition of enalapril to conventional treatment produces survival benefits in individuals with symptomatic heart failure.

Anonymous (1991) Effects of enalapril on survival in patients with reduced left ventricular ejection fractions and congestive heart failure. *N Engl J Med*; **325**: 293–302.

Box 4.2 Studies of Left Ventricular Dysfunction (SOLVD): Prevention Trial

Study design Randomized, double-blind, placebo-controlled, multicentre.	**Randomization** Enalapril, 2.5 or 5 mg b.d., titrated up to 10 mg b.d.; or placebo. Additional non-ACE-inhibitor therapy was allowed.
Inclusion Asymptomatic heart failure.	**End points** Mortality, hospitalization, incidence of myocardial infarction, morbidity, quality of life.
Patients 4228 (2 111 enalapril; 2 117 placebo) with symptomatic heart failure (ejection fraction ⩽ 35%).	**Results** After an average of 37.4 months follow-up, there was a non-significant trend towards fewer deaths (14.8% vs 15.8%) in the enalapril than the placebo group (14.8% vs 15.8%). There was however, a highly significant reduction in the combined end-point of death or development of symptomatic heart failure in the enalapril group (29.8% vs 38.6%) representing a risk reduction of 29%, $P < 0.001$.

Conclusions Findings show that in patients with asymptomatic left ventricular dysfunction, enalapril reduces the combined risk of death and hospitalization for heart failure.

Anonymous (1992) Effect of enalapril on mortality and the development of heart failure in asymptomatic patients with reduced left ventricular ejection fractions. *N Engl J Med*; **327**: 685–91.

Thiazides increase sodium excretion in the distal renal tubule. They are mild diuretics and, in severe heart failure, the more potent loop diuretics are more effective. These inhibit sodium reabsorption in the ascending loop of Henle, thereby removing the osmotic gradient in the renal medulla and preventing concentration of the urine. In the very oedematous patient, drug absorption from the bowel is unreliable and parenteral administration may be required.

Diuretics increase the sodium concentration in the distal nephron for aldosterone-mediated exchange with potassium. This predisposes to hypokalaemia with the attendant risk of cardiac arrhythmias. Hypokalaemia can be avoided by potassium supplementation or, preferably, by simultaneous prescription of a potassium-sparing diuretic. Spironolactone, an aldosterone inhibitor, is the most effective but, because it causes gastrointestinal side-effects and gynaecomastia, amiloride is usually preferred.

Angiotensin-converting enzyme (ACE) inhibitors

These block the renin-induced conversion of angiotensin I to angiotensin II. Removal of angiotensin II has two important effects: vasodilatation which increases cardiac output by reducing blood pressure (afterload); and removal of the major stimulus for aldosterone secretion, thereby enhancing the renal excretion of salt and water. Thus, by increasing cardiac output and promoting salt and water excretion, ACE inhibitors improve both peripheral perfusion and the congestive manifestations of heart failure. Of particular importance, however, is the finding that these drugs may also improve long-term prognosis in heart failure (see Box 4.1) although the mechanism of this beneficial effect is not known.

Because ACE inhibitors are potent vasodilators they can produce profound hypotension in susceptible patients. Thus, careful monitoring of blood pressure and serum biochemistry is essential early in the course of treatment to guard against prerenal failure. Reductions in diuretic therapy are often required as the ACE inhibitor is introduced, to maintain adequate plasma volume. ACE inhibitors, by reducing aldosterone secretion, conserve potassium so that potassium supplements or potassium-sparing diuretics are not usually necessary.

Vasodilators

Drugs with venodilator (e.g. nitrates), arteriolar dilator (e.g. hydralazine) or both properties (e.g. prazosin) have been widely used in the treatment of chronic congestive heart failure. Venodilatation causes pooling of blood in the abdominal capacitance vessels which reduces venous return to the heart and lowers atrial pressure (preload). Arteriolar dilatation improves cardiac output by reducing blood pressure (afterload). This can improve both pulmonary congestion and peripheral perfusion. Vasodilator therapy is beneficial in acute heart failure (see page 87) but in the longer term efficacy diminishes and these drugs are now rarely used in the management of chronic congestive heart failure.

Inotropic agents

Digoxin is the only orally active inotropic agent licensed for clinical use. Like all other inotropes, it increases the availability of intracellular calcium to the myocardial contractile proteins and increases the force of contraction. However, its inotropic properties are mild and the therapeutic range narrow, increasing the risk of side-effects. The major indication for digoxin is to control the ventricular response in atrial fibrillation, a common arrhythmia in chronic congestive heart failure. For the patient in sinus rhythm, digoxin is now only recommended if heart failure is severe and unresponsive to diuretics and ACE inhibitors when it will sometimes produce limited clinical improvement.

Anticoagulants

Prophylactic anticoagulation with warfarin is necessary for patients in atrial fibrillation, because the risk of thromboembolism is greatest in this group. Anticoagulation is also necessary in patients who have already had a thromboembolic event, regardless of the cardiac rhythm, so long as there are no specific contraindications.

Beta-blockers

Some preliminary work has shown a paradoxically beneficial response to beta-blocker therapy in certain patients with advanced chronic congestive heart failure, not only in terms of symptomatic improvement but also in terms of prognostic benefit. A single randomized controlled trial using carvedilol (a combined alpha- and beta-blocker) has appeared to confirm this and further trials are currently in progress. It must be emphasized, however, that beta-blockers are negatively inotropic and potentially dangerous in heart failure and their clinical role (if any) remains uncertain pending the results of these important trials.

Antiarrhythmic drugs

Digoxin is the treatment of choice for rate control in atrial fibrillation. Amiodarone may also be used and is the treatment of choice for ventricular arrhythmias, because it is less negatively inotropic than type I agents. Randomized controlled trials have not shown unequivocal benefit for *routine* prophylactic amiodarone therapy in patients with heart failure who are rhythmically stable.

Other medical measures

Pleural effusions usually respond well to diuretics but, when large, should be aspirated, particularly if the patient is severely dyspnoeic. Severe oedema, unresponsive to full medical therapy, can be corrected by ultrafiltration, when body water is selectively removed by passing the blood across a highly permeable membrane.

Surgical therapy

Heart failure caused by valvular disease, left ventricular aneurysm or certain congenital defects is potentially correctable by surgery. In some patients with coronary heart disease, coronary bypass surgery improves left ventricular function by restoring contractility in areas of 'hibernating myocardium' (myocardium that is non-contractile but viable late after coronary occlusion). In the majority of patients, however, heart transplantation is the only option, although it is only appropriate in advanced left ventricular disease resistant to all medical therapy. The orthotopic procedure is favoured in most transplant centres. The diseased heart is subtotally excised with preservation of the posterior atrial wall, and suturing of recipient–donor atria to atria and great vessels to great vessels is then undertaken. The operative risk is small compared to the hazards of organ rejection and immunosuppressive therapy. These hazards are greatest during the first year following surgery but, thereafter, the threat of accelerated coronary atherosclerosis (the cause of which is unknown) becomes increasingly important. Due largely to advances in the early recognition and treatment of rejection, the results of heart transplantation have improved rapidly and there is now an 80% 2-year survival rate. The results of heart–lung transplantation (in patients with intractable right-sided failure caused by advanced pulmonary vascular disease) are also improving.

Undoubtedly the major limitation of heart transplantation is the lack of donor organs which ensures that many patients referred for this procedure die on the waiting list before a suitable heart can be found. The future therefore appears to depend on the development of either a genetically engineered animal donor eliciting an attenuated immune response or a totally artificial heart.

Cardiomyoplasty is another new surgical technique in which an electrically stimulated skeletal muscle autograft (usually latissimus dorsi) is applied to the ventricular wall to assist contractile function in advanced heart failure. Early results have looked promising but the long-term tolerance of skeletal muscle to continuous work remains uncertain.

Prognosis

Acute heart failure resulting from a surgically correctable lesion such as valvular incompetence or ventricular septal defect may have an excellent prognosis following definitive treatment. In most cases of chronic congestive heart failure, however, left ventricular contractile impairment is irreversible and the outlook is poor (Fig. 4.8). Survival is closely related to the severity of disease whether assessed symptomatically, haemodynamically, functionally or by its association with arrhythmias. In the most advanced cases (NYHA functional classification III and IV) annual mortality approaches 50%. Death may be the result of progressive deterioration in cardiac function culminating in multiple organ failure, but may also occur suddenly from cardiac arrhythmias at almost any time during the

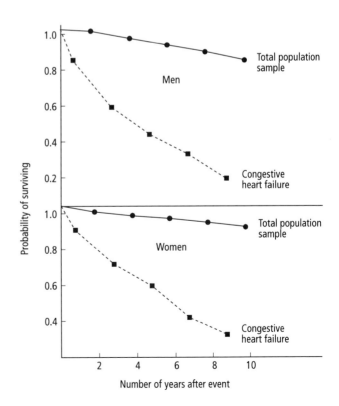

Fig. 4.8 Survival of men and women after the onset of heart failure in the Framingham study. (Reproduced with permission from McKee *et al. N Engl J Med* 1971; 285: 1441.)

natural history of the illness, patients with advanced left ventricular dysfunction being at greatest risk. Specific neurohormonal antagonists may improve survival in these high-risk patients. Evidence is best for ACE inhibitors, and randomized controlled trials have shown a small but significant reduction in mortality in all grades of heart failure from NYHA 1 to 4, although the mechanism is not clear (see Box 4.1). ACE inhibitors should be introduced early in the course of heart failure at the time of initial presentation for maximum benefit. In end-stage disease, heart transplantation is the only treatment likely to provide substantial prognostic improvement.

SHOCK

Shock is a syndrome of critically impaired vital organ perfusion which, if not rapidly corrected, leads to irreversible cell damage with multiple organ failure and death. It is usually caused by severe heart failure (cardiogenic shock), hypovolaemia or septicaemia. The pathogenesis is complex and poorly understood, involving a combination of haemodynamic and toxic factors. Widespread capillary damage intensifies the tissue perfusion deficit, threatening vital organs, including the heart. As myocardial perfusion deteriorates, a 'vicious cycle' of falling cardiac output and worsening end-organ damage becomes established.

Clinically the patient is cold, clammy and cerebrally obtunded with tachycardia, hypotension and oliguria. If urine flow cannot be maintained with volume replacement, inotropic drive, low-dose dopamine and frusemide, tubular damage leads to oliguric renal failure requiring dialysis. Pulmonary oedema is common, even when shock is non-cardiac in origin, and results from capillary damage which allows protein-rich fluid to leak into the lung (adult respiratory distress syndrome—ARDS). Hypoxaemia requires mechanical ventilation, although the increase in intrathoracic pressure reduces venous return to the heart and exacerbates the critical haemodynamic state. Heart failure may respond to inotropic support (intra-aortic balloon pumping is inappropriate in the absence of a surgically correctable lesion), but the improvement is usually only temporary and the prognosis remains very poor with a mortality greater than 80%.

Cardiogenic shock

Any cause of heart failure with severe reduction in cardiac output may lead to cardiogenic shock. The majority of cases, however, are the result of acute myocardial infarction involving damage to at least 40% of the left ventricle. Physiological responses directed at maintaining left ventricular pump function include elevation of left atrial pressure and catecholamine drive. Nevertheless, although these responses help maintain cardiac output by the Starling mechanism and inotropic stimulation, respectively, they also lead to pulmonary oedema and peripheral vasoconstriction which exacerbate hypoxaemia, left ventricular dysfunction and the vital organ perfusion deficit. In acute myocardial infarction, primary angioplasty to reopen the occluded coronary may improve survival. In most cases, however, treatment is aimed at improving left ventricular function with intravenous inotropic agents, which may be given in combination with vasodilators if blood pressure is adequately maintained. Pulmonary artery pressure monitoring with a Swan–Ganz catheter is recommended in these critically ill patients. Arterial oxygen tension should also be monitored and, if this cannot be maintained above 7 kPa with inhaled oxygen, mechanical ventilation is necessary. When cardiogenic shock is the result of a surgically correctable lesion (e.g. mitral regurgitation, ventricular septal defect), intra-aortic balloon pumping provides useful haemodynamic support, but surgery should not be delayed in these cases.

Hypovolaemic shock

This is usually the result of haemorrhage but may also occur in extensive burn injury and severe vomiting or diarrhoea (particularly in children). Important iatrogenic causes include inappropriate diuretic therapy and inadequate fluid replacement following surgery. Modest reductions in blood volume (< 500 ml) elicit an acute sympathoadrenal response which increases heart rate and peripheral resistance so that blood pressure is maintained. Thereafter, increased secretion of antidiuretic hormone and aldosterone encourages salt and water retention which restores the volume deficit. When reductions in blood volume exceed 20% of normal (> 1 l), cardiac output falls abruptly and sympathoadrenal responses are inadequate to maintain blood pressure, despite intense vasoconstriction. The patient becomes agitated and pale with tachycardia, tachypnoea, diaphoresis and oliguria. At this stage there is no compensatory reserve and any further volume loss leads inexorably to severe shock with life-threatening reductions to cardiac output, blood pressure and tissue perfusion. Physiologically, therefore, the condition resembles cardiogenic shock except that atrial pressures are low. Thus, the JVP is not elevated and pulmonary oedema does not develop acutely. These patients are nevertheless prone to ARDS if not treated promptly with plasma volume replacement. This should be titrated against the JVP but, in patients with left ventricular disease, pulmonary artery pressure monitoring provides a better guide to volume requirements.

Septicaemic shock

This is usually caused by Gram-negative organisms, particularly *Escherichia coli*, *Klebsiella* and *Pseudomonas*. Less commonly, Gram-positive infection with *Pneumococcus* or *Streptococcus* is responsible. In Gram-negative septicaemia, the shock syndrome is the result of endotoxins which cause cell damage directly, and also indirectly, by stimulating release of lysosomal enzymes from leucocytes and activating the complement cascade. Severe capillary injury and tissue anoxia is invariable. Haemodynamic changes are complex and difficult to predict. Cutaneous vasodilatation may cause a warm skin, although sequestration of venous blood and capillary damage with loss of plasma protein ensures that cardiac output and vital organ perfusion are critically impaired. Myocardial contractile function is often depressed, not only by coronary hypoperfusion but also by the direct effects of toxaemia. The JVP may be low or elevated and does not usually provide a useful guide to volume requirements, which should be titrated against pulmonary artery wedge pressure measured with a Swan–Ganz catheter. Metabolic changes are also complex, ranging from hyperventilation and respiratory alkalosis in early shock to profound lactic acidaemia and metabolic acidosis as the condition deteriorates. ARDS and disseminated intravascular coagulation, with consumption of clotting factors, commonly accompany the progression of the illness. Treatment is with circulatory and respiratory support and usually requires plasma volume adjustment, inotropic drive and mechanical ventilation. Intravenous antibiotics via a central line are essential and should be started as soon as blood samples for bacteriological culture have been obtained. Ampicillin (6–12 g/day) and gentamicin (titrated against blood levels) provide broad spectrum cover against most Gram-negative organisms and provide initial therapy pending the blood culture result. A penicillinase-resistant penicillin (e.g. flucloxacillin 6–12 g/day) should also be prescribed to cover staphylococcal infection. Glucocorticoids are of no proven clinical value.

FURTHER READING

Barnett DB. Beta-blockers in heart failure: a therapeutic paradox. *Lancet* 1994; 343: 557.

Braunwald E. ACE inhibitors: a cornerstone of the treatment of heart failure. *N Engl J Med* 1991; 325: 351.

Burnett JC. Atrial natriuretic factor: is it physiologically important? *Circulation* 1990; 82: 1523.

Califf RM, Bengtson JR. Cardiogenic shock. *N Engl J Med* 1993; 330: 1724.

Cleland JFG, Swedburg K. Carvedilol for heart failure. *Lancet* 1996; 347: 1199.

Cohn JN. The prevention of heart failure—a new agenda. *N Engl J Med* 1992; 327: 725.

Curfman GD. Inotropic therapy for heart failure—an unfulfilled promise. *N Engl J Med* 1991; 325: 1509.

De Bono D. Digoxin in eurhythmic heart failure: PROVED or 'not proven'? *Lancet* 1994; 343: 128.

Fowler MB. Exercise intolerance in heart failure. *J Am Coll Cardiol* 1991; 17: 1073.

Francis GS. The relationship of the sympathetic nervous system and the renin–angiotensin system in congestive heart failure. *Am Heart J* 1989; 118: 642.

Gottlieb SS. The use of antiarrhythmic agents in heart failure: implications of CAST. *Am Heart J* 1989; 118: 1074.

Grossman W. Diastolic dysfunction in congestive heart failure. *N Engl J Med* 1991; 325: 1557.

Henderson AH. Amiodarone for chronic heart failure. *Lancet* 1994; 344: 489.

Millner RWJ, Pepper JR. Cardiomyoplasty. *Br Med J* 1991; 302: 1353.

Packer M. The search for the ideal positive inotropic agent. *N Engl J Med* 1993; 329: 200.

Parillo JE. Pathogenic mechanisms of septic shock. *N Engl J Med* 1993; 328: 1471.

Pfeffer MA, Stevenson LW. Beta-adrenergic blockers and survival in heart failure. *N Engl J Med* 1996; 334: 1396.

Schofield PM. Indications for heart transplantation. *Br Heart J* 1991; 65: 55.

Smith TW. Digoxin in heart failure. *N Engl J Med* 1993; 329: 51.

Sutton GC. Epidemiologic aspects of heart failure. *Am Heart J* 1989; suppl 6: 1538.

CHAPTER 5

Coronary Artery Disease

CONTENTS

SUMMARY

Coronary artery disease is the most common cause of premature death in this country. Its cause is unknown but a number of risk factors have been identified including cigarette smoking, hypertension and hypercholesterolaemia, correction of which may protect against the development or progression of disease. It is characterized pathologically by the atheromatous plaque which may stenose the coronary arterial lumen sufficiently to cause exertional myocardial ischaemia, experienced by the patient as angina. Plaque rupture provides a focus for platelet deposition and thrombosis, and may result in unstable angina or myocardial infarction, depending on whether the thrombus is subocclusive or occludes the coronary lumen completely.

Angina is best diagnosed from a careful clinical history concentrating on the character, location, radiation and duration of the pain and its relation to provocative stimuli, particularly exertion. It often responds to treatment with nitrates and beta-blockers although some patients require the addition of calcium antagonists and potassium channel openers. In cases of diagnostic uncertainty, stress testing (exercise ECG, thallium perfusion scintigram) is helpful and may also provide useful prognostic information. If symptoms are inadequately controlled by medical treatment, coronary revascularization by angioplasty or bypass surgery should be considered.

Unstable angina presents with recurrent and usually prolonged episodes of angina occurring on minimal exertion or at rest, often associated with reversible ST segment depression on the ECG. Myocardial infarction or death occurs in about 10% of cases within 3 months. The antithrombotic effects of heparin infusion and aspirin have been shown to improve prognosis while glyceryl trinitrate infusion and beta-blockers help relieve chest pain by improving the myocardial oxygen supply–demand imbalance. Early coronary arteriography with a view to angioplasty or bypass surgery is usually recommended, particularly when symptoms fail to settle promptly.

Myocardial infarction is fatal in about 40% of cases, often as a result of ventricular fibrillation before hospital admission. In hospital, where ventricular fibrillation can be corrected by electrical cardioversion, left ventricular failure due to extensive infarction is the most important cause of death. Thus significant reductions in mortality can be achieved by rapid transfer to hospital (ensuring early access to a defibrillator) and by specific treatment with thrombolytic drugs and aspirin, which restore coronary patency and reduce the extent of infarction. Before discharge from hospital, secondary prevention measures should be taken to protect against recurrent myocardial infarction and death. These include lifestyle advice (with particular emphasis on quitting smoking, dietary modification and aerobic exercise) and specific drugs including aspirin, beta-blockers, HMG CoA reductase inhibitors and ACE inhibitors. Coronary rehabilitation courses are recommended for a combination of health education and supervised aerobic exercise. Patients with continuing chest pain or an ischaemic predischarge stress test after myocardial infarction require coronary arteriography with a view to revascularization.

EPIDEMIOLOGY

In 1993, coronary artery disease caused nearly 170 000 deaths in this country (> 25% of all deaths) and was responsible for the loss of an estimated 66 million working days (13% of all days lost due to sickness). Importantly, more than 50 000 of the deaths were premature, occurring in people aged under 70. Death rates are higher in Northern Ireland, Scotland and the north of England than in the south of England. Recent data have shown a downward trend in mortality during the last 10 years probably caused by a decline in both incidence and case fatality rate. A similar, though considerably more substantial, downward trend became established in the US more than 20 years ago, since when mortality has fallen by over 30%. Although the declining mortality here and elsewhere in the developed world is well established, there is no doubt that coronary artery disease will remain a major social and medical challenge in the foreseeable future.

Coronary artery disease in women

The risk of coronary artery disease is low in young women, possibly because of a protective effect of oestrogens, but in elderly women comes close to that of men. Hormone replacement therapy, however, may provide women with continuing protection against coronary artery disease beyond the menopause. There has been recent concern that women with coronary heart disease are investigated less vigorously than men, as reflected by the rates of angiography and coronary revascularization in symptomatic individuals. The reasons for this are not clear but the lower prevalence of coronary disease in women is probably an important factor because it ensures that diagnostic suspicion among doctors is correspondingly low and that non-invasive testing is less helpful (see page 110). Women have been further disadvantaged by the fact that randomized trials of new therapeutic agents have often enrolled only men and caution may be necessary in generalizing treatment benefits across the sexes. However, the finding that women with acute myocardial infarction have a worse prognosis than men is related less to treatment effects than to differences in age and risk factor profiles: women with myocardial infarction tend to be older and are more commonly hypertensive and diabetic.

Coronary artery disease in different racial groups

Compared with the white population of this country, people of Afro-Caribbean origin have had a lower prevalence of coronary artery disease (a difference that is now diminishing) but a higher prevalence of cerebrovascular disease, ensuring a comparable overall cardiovascular mortality. In contrast, both the prevalence of, and mortality from, coronary disease is higher for people of South Asian origin (Indians, Pakistanis, Bangladeshis) living in this country than for whites. Moreover, coronary mortality in South Asians is continuing to rise, unlike other racial groups in whom it is in decline (see above). The susceptibility of South Asians to coronary artery disease has been difficult to explain in terms of conventional risk factors and there is a growing consensus that it is the result of the genetically determined *insulin resistance syndrome*: central obesity, hyperinsulinaemia, hypertrigliceridaemia, reduced plasma high-density lipoprotein cholesterol, and hypertension, with or without non-insulin-dependent diabetes.

RISK FACTORS

Although the cause of atherosclerosis is unknown, a number of 'risk factors' have been identified which, though associated with coronary artery disease, are not essential for its development. Conversely, the absence of risk factors in an individual does not confer immunity against the disease.

Reversible (or potentially reversible) risk factors

These are particularly important because their avoidance or correction may protect against the development or progression of coronary artery disease. Most important are cigarette smoking, hypertension and hypercholesterolaemia.

Cigarette smoking

The risk of coronary artery disease rises in proportion to the number of cigarettes smoked. Stopping smoking reduces the risk, although it remains higher than in individuals who have never smoked. The component(s) of tobacco smoke causing vascular disease and the mechanism of the damage are both unknown.

Hypertension

The risk of coronary artery disease rises in proportion to the level of both systolic and diastolic blood pressure. Thus systolic and diastolic pressures ≥ 160 and ≥ 95 mmHg, respectively, increase risk by 2–3 times. Treatment of hypertension provides some protection against coronary heart disease but significantly greater protection against stroke and heart failure.

Hypercholesterolaemia

Risk rises in proportion to the total blood cholesterol level. For example, at levels of 6.5 and 7.8 mmol/l, the risk rises to two and four times that seen at 5.2 mmol/l. Low-density lipoprotein is the major component of total cholesterol and is particularly atherogenic; high-density lipoprotein, on the other hand, protects against the disease. Reducing total cholesterol levels, and the ratio of LDL to HDL, in the general population (primary prevention) and in patients with coronary artery disease (secondary prevention) reduces risk. Treatment may also slow the progression of established coronary artery disease and in some cases lead to regression of atheromatous plaques.

Hypertriglyceridaemia is not usually regarded as a risk factor for coronary artery disease; however, it is often accompanied by low levels of high-density lipoproteins and may increase risk, particularly in women.

Lipoprotein (a)

This lipoprotein is produced in the liver; blood concentrations above 0.3 g/l are associated with an increased risk of coronary artery disease. To date, there is no effective treatment for reducing raised blood concentrations.

Homocysteine

There is now clear evidence of an independent relation between serum homocysteine concentrations and the risk of coronary artery disease, perhaps due to a direct toxic effect of homocysteine on the vascular endothelium. Inadequate folate intake is an important predisposer to elevated homocysteine concentrations.

Obesity

The increased risk of coronary artery disease in obese individuals is largely due to associated hypertension, hypercholesterolaemia and diabetes.

Physical inactivity

A considerable body of evidence links physical inactivity to an increased risk of coronary artery disease. Until recently, however, this was regarded as a rather minor risk factor operating indirectly through plasma lipid profiles and systemic blood pressure, both of which are adversely affected by physical inactivity. It is now recognized that physical inactivity is an important independent determinant of risk which operates in a graded fashion, the risk of coronary artery disease declining progressively with increased physical fitness.

Irreversible risk factors

Age

The risk of coronary artery disease rises progressively with increasing age.

Male sex

The risk is greater in young men than in women of comparable age, although with advancing years the difference diminishes. Overall, there appears to be a 10-year delay in coronary deaths in women compared with men, with one in three of all men and one in four of all women dying from the disease.

Family history

Although the familial incidence of coronary artery disease is partly explained by a genetic predisposition to hypertension, hypercholesterolaemia and diabetes, it is now well established that family history is itself an independent predictor of increased risk.

Diabetes mellitus and insulin resistance

Diabetes increases the risk of coronary artery disease in both men and women. The syndrome of insulin resistance may account for the high prevalence of coronary artery disease in South Asians (see above).

Personality type

Although the type-A personality (chronic sense of time urgency) has been associated with an increased risk compared with the more placid type-B personality, the evidence remains inconclusive.

PREVENTION OF CORONARY ARTERY DISEASE

Primary prevention

Primary prevention of coronary heart disease aims to prevent its development in asymptomatic individuals. This may be achieved through a *population strategy* by attempting to modify, in the entire population, lifestyle or environmental factors known to increase the risk of disease. Examples include advertising campaigns to discourage smoking or to popularize aerobic exercise. Generally speaking, population strategies are driven by government agencies and fall outside the remit of the doctor. An alternative approach is the selective *high-risk strategy* in which individuals at high risk are targeted and action taken to reduce the risk. Here there is a role for the doctor who might, for example, target asymptomatic family members of patients with myocardial infarction to advise about smoking and screen for hypertension and hypercholesterolaemia, because there is clear evidence that measures of this type are effective in reducing coronary risk (Box 5.1).

Secondary prevention

Secondary prevention aims to prevent disease progression in patients who already have coronary heart disease. It is a more efficient approach than primary

---

Box 5.1 West of Scotland Coronary Prevention (WOSCOP) Study

Study design Randomized, double-blind, placebo-controlled, multicentre.

Randomization Pravastatin 40 mg daily or placebo. All patients received advice about lipid-lowering diet.

Inclusion Hypercholesterolaemia (LDL cholesterol 4.5–6.0 mmol/l on a lipid-lowering diet) in men without known coronary heart disease.

End points Non-fatal myocardial infarction or death from coronary heart disease.

Patients 6595 men aged 45–60 with an LDL cholesterol 4.5–6.0 mmol/l (on a lipid-lowering diet), a normal ECG and no history of myocardial infarction.

Results Over 4.9 years median follow-up, pravastatin lowered plasma cholesterol levels by 20% and LDL cholesterol by 26%; cholesterol was unaffected by placebo. Pravastatin reduced the risk of non-fatal myocardial infarction or death from coronary heart disease by 31% ($P < 0.001$). All-cause mortality was reduced by 22% ($P = 0.051$).

Conclusions Findings suggest that treatment with pravastatin reduces the risk of death and non-fatal myocardial infarction in men with moderate hypercholesterolaemia and no history of myocardial infarction.

Shepherd J (1995) Prevention of coronary heart disease with pravastatin in men with hypercholesterolemia: The West of Scotland Coronary Prevention (WOSCOP) Study. *N Engl J Med*; **333**: 1301–7.

Box 5.2 Scandinavian Simvastatin Survival Study (4S)

Study design Randomized, double-blind, placebo-controlled, multicentre.	**Randomization** Simvastatin 20 mg daily; or placebo. The dose of simvastatin was titrated-up to reduce serum cholesterol to 3.0–5.2 mmol/l. All patients received lipid-lowering diet.
Inclusion Hypercholesterolaemia (serum cholesterol 5.5–8.0 mmol/l on a lipid-lowering diet) in patients with coronary heart disease.	**End points** *Primary:* total mortality. *Secondary:* coronary deaths and non-fatal myocardial infarction.
Patients 4444 patients with angina or previous myocardial infarction and serum cholesterol 5.5–8.0 mmol/l on a lipid-lowering diet.	**Results** Over 5.4 years, simvastatin produced mean changes in total cholesterol, LDL cholesterol and HDL cholesterol of −25%, −35%, and + 8%, respectively. Total mortality in the simvastatin group was 8% compared with 12% in the placebo group (relative risk of death 0.70, $P = 0.0003$). Relative risk of coronary death in the simvastatin group was 0.58, and of myocardial infarction was 0.66 (both $P < 0.0001$). Other benefits of treatment included a 37% reduction in the risk of undergoing myocardial revascularization procedures.

Conclusions Findings suggest that treatment of hypercholesterolaemia with simvastatin in patients with coronary artery disease improves prognosis by reducing the risk of death and non-fatal myocardial infarction.

Anonymous (1994) Randomized trial of cholesterol lowering in 4444 patients with coronary heart disease: The Scandinavian Simvastatain Survival Study (4S). *Lancet*; **344**: 1383–9.

prevention because fewer patients need to be treated to save one life or clinical event. Risk-factor modification is the cornerstone of secondary prevention. Quitting smoking after myocardial infarction reduces the risk of recurrent attacks by up to 50%; it also reduces the risk of myocardial infarction in patients with angina. Similarly, lowering blood cholesterol by a combination of dietary restriction and treatment with an HMG-CoA reductase inhibitor reduces cardiac mortality in post-myocardial infarction and angina patients (Box 5.2). Other drugs, apart from HMG-CoA reductase inhibitors, that are of proven benefit for secondary prevention in acute myocardial infarction include aspirin, beta-blockers and ACE inhibitors.

AETIOLOGY AND PATHOGENESIS

Coronary artery disease is nearly always caused by atherosclerosis; indeed, the two terms are often used synonymously. Other causes of coronary artery disease, listed in Table 5.1, are rare. Thus, a middle-aged or elderly patient with polyarteritis nodosa or syphilis is just as likely to have atherosclerosis causing angina as arteritic or syphilitic involvement of the coronary circulation.

The cause of atherosclerosis is unknown. Epidemiological evidence points to a complex interaction of genetic and environmental influences, the relative importance of which remains speculative. Current understanding of the pathogenesis of atherosclerosis is best described by the *'response-to-injury'* hypothesis which

Table 5.1 Causes of coronary artery disease.

Atherosclerosis
Arteritis
systemic lupus erythematosus
polyarteritis nodosa
rheumatoid arthritis
ankylosing spondylitis
Takayasu disease
Embolism
infective endocarditis
left atrial/ventricular thrombus
left atrial/ventricular tumour
prosthetic valve thrombus
complication of cardiac catheterization
Coronary mural thickening
amyloidosis
radiation therapy
Hurler's disease
pseudoxanthoma elasticum
Other causes of coronary luminal narrowing
aortic dissection
coronary spasm
Congenital coronary artery disease
anomalous origin from pulmonary artery
arteriovenous fistula

sees endothelial injury by any of a variety of potential agents (oxidized low-density lipoproteins, toxic products of tobacco smoke, hypertension, viruses) as the event that triggers the disease process. The oxidized low-density lipoproteins which penetrate the damaged endothelium are scavenged by macrophages which become foam cells. At the same time vascular smooth muscle cells migrate from the media into the intima where they hypertrophy, proliferate and synthesize an extracellular matrix of connective tissue. Extracellular cholesterol accumulates within the matrix which is covered by a fibromuscular cap consisting of smooth muscle cells, collagen and a single layer of endothelial cells.

The final lesion is the atherosclerotic plaque which is the pathological hallmark of coronary artery disease and is responsible directly or indirectly for all its manifestations. These manifestations, however, are variable reflecting the variable size and composition of atherosclerotic plaques. Small fibrous plaques, for example, are often silent but as they increase in size they project into the arterial lumen and, by impeding blood flow, may result in myocardial ischaemia, particularly when oxygen demand increases during exertion or stress. Lipid-rich plaques, on the other hand, with relatively little fibrous tissue (cholesterol 30–40%) are prone to rupture in response to sheer stresses imposed by blood pressure. Exposure of the plaque contents provides a potent thrombogenic stimulus and may precipitate an acute ischaemic event if the coronary artery is totally or subtotally occluded.

PATHOLOGY

The heart is essentially an obligate aerobic organ: without oxygen, energy production fails within seconds and contraction ceases. The capacity of the heart to extract arterial oxygen, though high, is relatively fixed. Thus, under circumstances of increased myocardial oxygen demand (e.g. exercise), oxygen delivery must be increased. This can only be achieved through an increase in coronary flow (Fig. 5.1). Appropriately, therefore, myocardial oxygen demand is the principal regulator of coronary flow: increments in demand stimulate coronary arteriolar dilatation and flow increases accordingly. Coronary artery disease, however, restricts flow and deprives the heart of its primary metabolic substrate, undermining its capacity to function. The left ventricle is particularly vulnerable because its oxygen requirement is greater than that of any of the other cardiac chambers, reflecting its muscle mass and wall tension both of which are major determinants of oxygen demand. Thus, while coronary artery disease may affect oxygen delivery to any part of the heart, the left ventricle (particularly the subendocardium) is worst affected.

The proximal 6 cm of the coronary arteries are usually involved, with relative sparing of the smaller distal vessels. The disease is characterized pathologically by the *atherosclerotic plaque*, a focal proliferation of smooth muscle cells, collagen and cholesterol esters lying within the intimal and medial layers of the arterial wall. The plaque is usually endothelialized but, as it increases in size, it may ulcerate and rupture, providing a focus for platelet deposition and thrombosis.

Myocardial Oxygen supply

Myocardial Oxygen demand

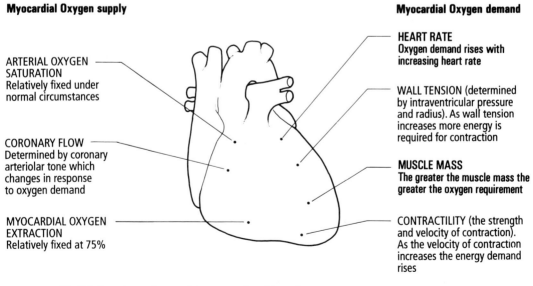

ARTERIAL OXYGEN
SATURATION
Relatively fixed under
normal circumstances

CORONARY FLOW
Determined by coronary
arteriolar tone which
changes in response
to oxygen demand

MYOCARDIAL OXYGEN
EXTRACTION
Relatively fixed at 75%

HEART RATE
Oxygen demand rises with
increasing heart rate

WALL TENSION (determined
by intraventricular pressure
and radius). As wall tension
increases more energy is
required for contraction

MUSCLE MASS
The greater the muscle mass the
greater the oxygen requirement

CONTRACTILITY (the strength
and velocity of contraction).
As the velocity of contraction
increases the energy demand
rises

Fig. 5.1 Determinants of myocardial oxygen supply and demand.

Clinicopathological correlates

Coronary atherosclerosis is often asymptomatic. The development of symptoms is closely related to the size and composition of the atherosclerotic plaque (see above). Four symptom complexes (*syndromes*) are recognized, each associated with characteristic coronary pathology.

1 *Stable angina.* This is associated with a smooth, endothelialized coronary plaque causing luminal stenosis. Stenosis in excess of 70% of the coronary luminal diameter may restrict flow to the extent that myocardial oxygen delivery fails to meet demand. This produces myocardial ischaemia, experienced by the patient as angina.

2 *Variant angina.* This unusual syndrome is associated with a smooth, endothelialized coronary plaque which may be small, causing only trivial luminal stenosis. In up to 30% of cases the artery is normal. However, unprovoked increments in coronary tone (*spasm*) restrict coronary flow sufficiently to cause myocardial ischaemia, experienced by the patient as angina.

3 *Unstable angina.* This is provoked by the abrupt rupture of an atheromatous plaque, exposing its contents and providing a focus for platelet deposition and thrombosis. In unstable angina the thrombus is subocclusive but causes intense myocardial ischaemia. Progression to thrombotic coronary occlusion and myocardial infarction occurs in up to 10% of cases within three months.

4 *Myocardial infarction.* The pathological process is identical to unstable angina, except that the thrombus completely occludes the coronary artery. This usually produces myocardial infarction in the territory subtended by the occluded artery. Nevertheless, a well-developed collateral supply or early spontaneous recanalization may modify the evolution of the infarct, restricting damage to the vulnerable subendocardial layer (see page 128).

CLINICAL MANIFESTATIONS

The major clinical manifestations of coronary artery disease are angina, myocardial infarction and sudden death, which are discussed in this chapter. Others include heart failure and cardiac arrhythmias and are discussed elsewhere.

ANGINA

Angina, the pain that occurs during periods of myocardial ischaemia, consists of a retrosternal constricting discomfort which may radiate to either arm, the throat or the jaw, and may be associated with shortness of breath. It is usually a manifestation of coronary artery disease but any other cause of imbalance between myocardial oxygen supply and demand may also cause angina (Table 5.2). Three anginal syndromes are recognized: stable angina; variant angina; and unstable angina.

Table 5.2 Causes of angina.

> *Reduced myocardial oxygen supply*
> Coronary artery disease (see Table 5.1)
> Severe anaemia
>
> *Increased myocardial oxygen demand*
> Left ventricular hypertrophy
>   hypertension
>   aortic stenosis
>   aortic regurgitation
>   hypertrophic cardiomyopathy
> Rapid tachyarrhythmias

Stable angina

Clinical manifestations

Stable angina may be provoked by any stimulus which increases myocardial oxygen demand through increments in heart rate or blood pressure. Typically, it is provoked by exertion and relieved within 2–10 minutes by rest; other provocative factors are emotion and sexual intercourse. Symptoms are usually worse in the morning, shortly after getting up, probably because blood pressure is at its height at this time of day; for the same reason, symptoms tend to be worse in cold weather and also after a heavy meal which increases heart rate. Surprisingly, the severity of symptoms is not closely related to the extent of coronary artery disease; indeed, extensive disease is sometimes entirely asymptomatic although episodes of 'silent' myocardial ischaemia can often be detected by special techniques.

The examination is usually normal. Nevertheless, elevated blood pressure and evidence of other major risk factors should be noted. Hypercholesterolaemia is associated with tendon xanthoma but ocular manifestations, including corneal arcus and xanthelasma are relatively non-specific, particularly in the elderly. In diabetes, retinopathy and neuropathy are often present. Patients with signs of peripheral vascular disease (e.g. absent pulses, arterial bruits) have associated coronary artery involvement in at least 75% of cases.

Complications

Angina is a symptom and does not itself produce complications. Nevertheless, patients with angina are at risk of all the other manifestations of coronary artery disease, including myocardial infarction and sudden death.

Diagnosis

Figure 5.2 summarizes diagnostic strategy for the evaluation of the patient with chest pain. A careful history—emphasizing the location of the pain, its character and its relation to provocative stimuli—provides the most useful information. If

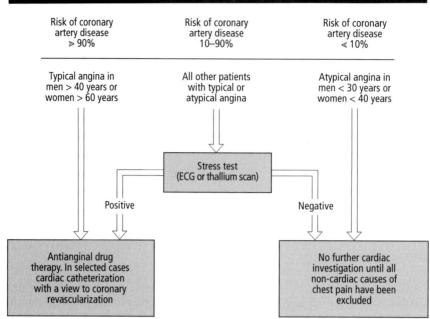

Fig. 5.2 Diagnostic strategy in chronic stable angina.

the history is *typical*, the probability of coronary artery disease is high, rising to above 90% in men over 40 and women over 60. If the history is *atypical*, the diagnostic probability is lower, falling below 10% in men under 30 and women under 40. In patients where the history, age and sex indicate an intermediate probability (10–90%) of coronary artery disease, stress testing helps to confirm or refute the diagnosis. However, it is not an infallible technique, and Bayes' theory of diagnostic probability states that the predicted accuracy of a positive test will vary according to the probability of coronary heart disease in the population under study (Fig. 5.3). Thus, stress testing is generally unhelpful in patients with a very low risk (less than 10%), because misleading false-positive results are common in this group; also, in patients with a very high risk (more than 90%), a positive result—whilst strongly predicting coronary heart disease—can hardly increase the diagnostic probability further. For these reasons, the use of stress testing for *diagnostic* purposes is best reserved for patients in whom the history, age and sex indicate an intermediate probability of coronary heart disease. In patients with established coronary disease, however, stress testing has an additional role for making a *prognostic* assessment, based on criteria summarized below.

Stress testing

Exercise ECG (Fig. 5.4)

This is one of the most widely used tests for evaluating the patient with chest

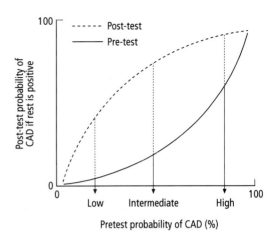

Fig. 5.3 If the pretest probability of coronary artery disease (CAD) is very low (e.g. young patients with atypical chest pain) or very high (e.g. more elderly patients with typical angina), stress testing is generally unhelpful for diagnostic purposes because a positive test does not increase the probability of coronary artery disease very much. In patients with an intermediate probability of disease (e.g. young patients with very typical angina, or older patients with atypical chest pain), however, a positive test produces a much larger increase in the probability of disease.

pain. The patient is usually exercised on a treadmill, the speed and slope of which can be adjusted to increase the workload gradually. The exercise ECG provides important diagnostic and prognostic information.

Diagnosis. The resting ECG is often normal in the patient with coronary artery disease, but as heart rate and blood pressure increase during exercise, myocardial oxygen demand may rise sufficiently to cause ischaemia. Exercise-induced

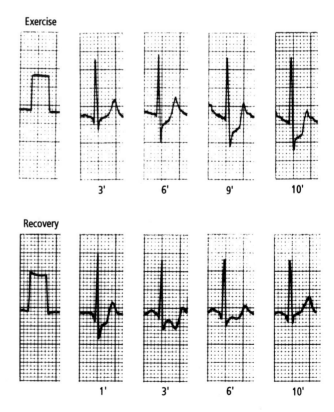

Fig. 5.4 Stress testing—exercise ECG (lead V4). Note the progressive planar depression of the ST segment during exercise. During recovery the ECG slowly reverts to normal after a period of 10 minutes.

horizontal ('planar') or down-sloping ST segment depression is strongly suggestive of myocardial ischaemia—particularly when associated with typical chest pain. Other causes of ST depression unassociated with coronary disease are shown in Fig. 2.13. Note that ST segment changes are usually impossible to interpret in the presence of left bundle branch block, digitalis therapy or paced rhythms, any of which effectively contraindicates the exercise ECG for diagnostic purposes.

Prognosis. Diagnostic ST segment depression at a low workload usually indicates very severe coronary artery disease and a poor prognosis. Exercise-induced ventricular arrhythmias or a paradoxical fall in blood pressure are also bad prognostic signs, sometimes reflecting extensive coronary artery disease but more commonly reflecting advanced left ventricular dysfunction.

Exercise myocardial perfusion scintigraphy (see page 57)

The resting myocardial perfusion scintigram may be normal in coronary artery disease, but exercise-induced ischaemia produces a regional perfusion defect. Reversible perfusion defects of this type are strongly suggestive of myocardial ischaemia caused by coronary artery disease, and must be distinguished from fixed perfusion defects (present at rest and during exercise) which are caused by an area of myocardial infarction. In general, the larger the area of hypoperfusion (fixed or reversible) the worse the prognosis.

Stress radionuclide angiography (see page 57)

In practice, peripheral cold stress with the hand held in iced water (cold pressor test) is used more commonly than exercise during radionuclide angiography. In patients with coronary artery disease, stress-induced myocardial ischaemia produces regional abnormalities of left ventricular wall motion which reverse following withdrawal of the stress.

Stress echocardiography

This recently developed application of echocardiography remains investigational at present. Pharmacological stress with dobutamine is usually used, patients with coronary artery disease showing regional wall-motion abnormality in response to the inotropic stimulus. A potentially interesting development of the technique is its potential for identifying 'hibernating' (and therefore potentially salvageable) myocardium in patients with previous coronary occlusions (see page 94).

Coronary arteriography (see page 65)

This is the definitive diagnostic test (Fig. 5.5). The technique is invasive and not

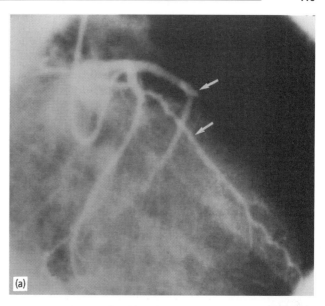

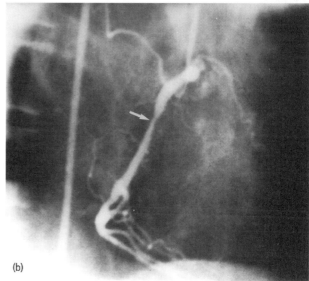

Fig. 5.5 Coronary arteriography. Left (a) and right (b) coronary arteriograms are shown. The left anterior descending coronary artery is occluded after the first septal branch (arrowed) and there is diffuse disease in the obtuse marginal branch of the circumflex artery (arrowed). The right coronary artery has a tight narrowing in its mid portion (arrowed).

without risk (mortality $\leq 0.1\%$), and is not appropriate in every patient. It is usually reserved for patients being considered for coronary artery bypass grafting or coronary angioplasty (Table 5.3).

Differential diagnosis

Careful consideration of the differential diagnosis is essential in the patient with chest pain. Angina is a term which jeopardizes insurance and career prospects and may condemn someone to a life of needlessly restricted activity.

Table 5.3 Indications for coronary arteriography.

Angina unresponsive to medical treatment
Unstable angina
Acute myocardial infarction for treatment by primary angioplasty
Continuing or recurrent cardiac chest pain after myocardial infarction
Cardiac arrhythmias when there is clinical suspicion of underlying coronary artery disease
Preoperatively in patients requiring valve surgery when advanced age (> 40) or angina suggest a high
    probability of coronary artery disease

Neuromuscular disorders

Chest-wall pain from the costochondral junctions or the muscular insertions on the ribs and sternum is common. The pain is usually sharp and localized and may be provoked by coughing or isometric stress such as pushing or pulling.

Upper gastrointestinal disorders

Oesophageal pain caused by acid reflux is retrosternal but, unlike angina, has a burning quality and is provoked by stooping or lying flat, particularly after a meal. Peptic ulceration occasionally causes pain in the lower chest but the history will usually demonstrate a specific relation to eating. Importantly, upper gastrointestinal pain is not provoked by exertion and usually responds to antacids. Oesophageal spasm may be more difficult to distinguish from angina because the pain is retrosternal and may be relieved by glyceryl trinitrate. Nevertheless, symptoms are usually protracted and unrelated to exertion.

Psychological disorders

Neurotic anxiety that focuses on the heart is common and disabling. Symptoms, however, are rarely typical of angina: stabbing pains in the left side of the chest are a common complaint and may be associated with hyperventilation. Time spent discussing the problem with the patient is more productive than extensive investigation, which only serves to reinforce fixed notions of underlying heart disease.

Syndrome X

A number of patients have typical angina but normal coronary arteries and none of the conditions listed in Table 5.2. Definitive diagnosis requires the demonstration of normal angiographic anatomy by cardiac catheterization. The name, syndrome X, adequately describes the lack of understanding which surrounds this condition, although undoubtedly there is some heterogeneity with psychological chest pain. In some cases inadequate coronary vasodilator reserve may be the cause of ischaemia, but anti-anginal drugs are rarely effective. Nevertheless, as a group, patients with syndrome X have an excellent prognosis comparable to that of the general population.

Treatment

General measures

The management of angina should include correction of established risk factors. Conditions which exacerbate angina (e.g. obesity, hypertension, arrhythmias, thyrotoxicosis, anaemia) require prompt attention. Exercise should be encouraged—within limits set by the severity of angina—because it enhances the sense of well-being and also has a training effect that leads to long-term improvement in functional capacity.

Medical therapy (Table 5.4)

Drugs used to treat angina help correct the imbalance between myocardial oxygen supply and demand, most importantly by coronary vasodilatation. However, reductions in oxygen demand may be achieved by reducing heart rate, contractility or left ventricular wall tension as determined by blood pressure. Nitrates and beta-blockers are the first-line agents with calcium antagonists and potassium-channel openers as second choice. In addition, low-dose aspirin (75–150 mg daily) is now recommended in patients with angina to protect against myocardial infarction.

Nitrates. These dilate the coronary arteries and peripheral circulation, improving the myocardial oxygen supply–demand ratio by increasing coronary flow and reducing left ventricular wall tension (blood pressure). Sublingual glyceryl trini-

Table 5.4 Medical treatment of angina.

Drugs	Dose
Nitrates	
Glyceryl trinitrate	
sublingual tablet	0.3 mg as required
aerosol spray	0.4–0.8 mg as required
Isosorbide mononitrate (long acting)	50 or 60 mg once daily
Beta-blockers	
Metoprolol	50–100 mg 3 times daily
Atenolol	50–100 mg once daily
Bisoprolol	5–10 mg once daily
Calcium antagonists	
Nifedipine (long acting)	30 mg daily
Amlodipine	5–10 mg once daily
Diltiazem (long acting)	240 or 360 mg once daily
Potassium-channel openers	
Nicorandil	10–20 mg twice daily

trate, by tablet or spray, should be given to all patients with angina. It is rapidly absorbed through the buccal mucosa, providing relief within 3 minutes, and can also be used prophylactically to prevent angina during vigorous exertion.

Long-term nitrates for regular oral administration are widely used. Isosorbide mononitrate is the preferred agent and extended-release preparations are now available for once-daily administration.

Nitrates are non-toxic and generally well tolerated. Side-effects caused by vasodilatation include headache and postural dizziness.

Beta-blockers. All patients with angina should be given a beta-blocker in the absence of contraindications. These drugs reduce myocardial oxygen demand by slowing the heart rate and reducing contractility and wall tension (blood pressure). A wide variety of agents is available, all with similar anti-anginal efficacy; choice is largely determined by patient acceptability. In general, drugs like atenolol or bisoprolol are preferred because they are long acting (for once-daily administration), cardioselective, and lipid insoluble, preventing entry into the central nervous system. Thus, non-cardiac effects of beta-blockade, including cold extremities and drowsiness, are less troublesome than with non-selective agents such as propranolol. Beta-blockers, regardless of cardiose-lectivity, should never be used in patients with a history of bronchial asthma since they can precipitate severe bronchospasm. They should be used with caution in heart failure, because of their negative inotropic action.

Calcium antagonists. Like nitrates, these are vasodilators and improve myocardial oxygen balance by their effect on coronary flow and blood pressure. The dihydropyridines (e.g. nifedipine) may cause reflex tachycardia and are not recommended as monotherapy in stable angina. In combination with a beta-blocker, however, they are effective although there is an ongoing debate about their long-term safety, particularly in high dosage. The non-dihydropyridine calcium antagonists (diltiazem, verapamil) do not increase heart rate and may be used as monotherapy in patients unable to take beta-blockers; combination therapy with a beta-blocker is not recommended because undue slowing of the heart rate may occur. Calcium antagonists cause variable reductions in contrac-tility and should usually be avoided in heart failure. Side-effects are related to vasodilatation and include facial flushing, headache, postural dizziness and mild ankle oedema.

Potassium-channel openers. Nicorandil is the only drug among this new class of agents available for clinical use. It relaxes vascular smooth muscle and may complement the anti-ischaemic effects of nitrates and calcium antagonists by increasing coronary flow and reducing left ventricular wall tension (blood pressure). The principal side-effect is headache.

Revascularization procedures

These include coronary artery bypass surgery and balloon angioplasty. An essential prerequisite of both is coronary arteriography in order to define the coronary anatomy and select the appropriate revascularization procedure.

Coronary artery bypass surgery. Surgery is usually performed on the arrested heart using full cardiopulmonary bypass. Saphenous vein grafts applied to the ascending aorta may be inserted into the coronary arteries distal to the diseased segments. In left anterior descending disease, however, the left internal mammary artery is preferred because it produces a better long-term result although it is not usually long enough for grafting other coronary arteries.

Coronary bypass surgery provides significant relief from angina in over 80% of cases, and mortality is < 2%, rising to between 5 and 10% for a second procedure. In addition to the symptomatic benefit, prospective studies of bypass surgery vs. medical therapy have shown a clear prognostic benefit for surgery in certain subgroups with 'high-risk' coronary anatomy, including patients with left main disease (Fig. 5.6) and patients with multivessel disease, particularly when the proximal left anterior descending coronary artery is involved.

Saphenous vein grafts have a perioperative occlusion rate of up to 10%, depending largely on the adequacy of 'run-off' which determines flow within the graft. Treatment with aspirin or warfarin helps preserve graft patency in the perioperative period, but late occlusion can be expected in many patients after 10–12 years due to accelerated atherosclerotic disease. Internal mammary grafts, however, usually remain patent for much longer than this.

Surgical strategies currently under investigation include *minimally invasive techniques* for applying the internal mammary artery to the left anterior descending coronary artery through a keyhole incision without cardiopulmonary bypass (not applicable for circumflex or right coronary disease); and *transmyocardial revascularization* in which the surgeon uses a laser source to drill multiple conduits from the left ventricular cavity into the ischaemic myocardium in patients with diffuse, inoperable coronary disease.

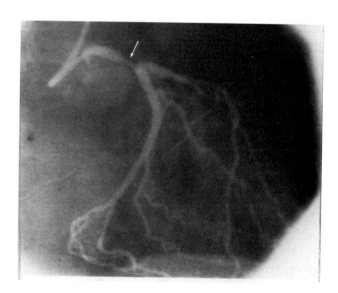

Fig. 5.6 Left main coronary artery disease. This left coronary arteriogram shows a very tight narrowing in the left main stem (arrowed).

Coronary angioplasty and stenting. This now accounts for about 33% of all myocardial revascularization procedures in the UK (about 50% in the US), coronary bypass surgery accounting for the remainder. A catheter with a terminal balloon is introduced percutaneously and directed into the diseased coronary artery over a fine guide-wire. Inflation of the balloon dilates the artery and restores normal flow (Fig. 5.7). The technique is less invasive and less costly than bypass surgery and offers particular advantages to the patient, because hospitalization is brief and immediate return to normal activities is possible. However, only 33–50% of patients with symptomatic coronary artery disease are suitable candidates for angioplasty and results are best in patients with a proximal stenosis involving only one or two major vessels. Excellent results can sometimes be obtained in patients with more extensive disease. Coronary angioplasty provides effective relief from angina in over 80% of cases and carries a low mortality (< 1.5%) comparable to that of bypass surgery.

The major problems with angioplasty are abrupt coronary closure during the procedure (2–5% of cases) and restenosis in the first 6 months afterwards (20–30% of cases), requiring repeat dilatation. Aspirin reduces the risk of abrupt thrombotic closure but to date no pharmacological interventions have been shown to affect the risk of restenosis. The recently introduced coronary stent (an expansile tubular wire-mesh device), however, promises to improve the results of angioplasty considerably. The stent is delivered on a balloon catheter and following inflation across the diseased arterial segment holds the vessel widely patent. Stents provide an effective 'bail-out' technique for dealing with abrupt coronary closure and promise to reduce the risk of restenosis considerably. Their use is increasing rapidly and in coronary vein graft angioplasty, which carries a particularly high restenosis rate, elective stenting is now the recommended approach (Fig. 5.8). Many operators are also stenting electively in high-risk proximal disease of the left anterior descending coronary artery and in all cases where full arterial patency cannot be achieved with conventional balloon angioplasty.

In complete coronary occlusion, conventional balloon angioplasty is successful in only about 50% of cases. Drills and laser devices have been evaluated for these difficult cases but it now looks unlikely that they will have a useful clinical role.

Prognosis

The natural history of coronary artery disease is summarized in Fig. 5.9. In individual patients with angina, the pattern of symptoms may show little change over several years and may even improve as collateral vessels open up. More common is a gradual deterioration in symptoms with an annual mortality of about 4%. Arteriographic findings permit a more precise prediction of prognosis with the annual mortality rising from less than 2% in single-vessel to 12% in multivessel disease.

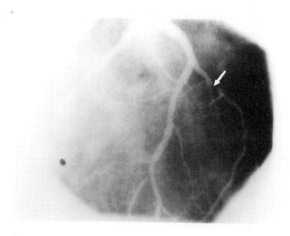

(a)

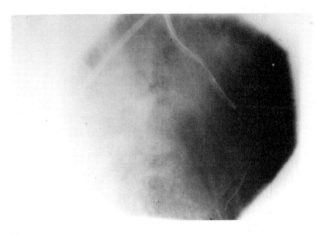

(b)

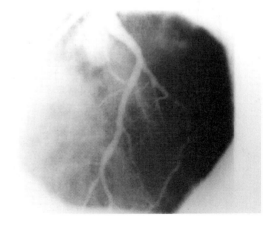

Fig. 5.7 Coronary angioplasty. (a) A tight stenosis in
the left anterior descending coronary artery is shown
(arrowed). (b) During angioplasty. A balloon catheter
has been positioned across the stenosis and inflated.
(c) After angioplasty the stenosis has been
successfully dilated and the left anterior descending
coronary artery is now widely patent.

(c)

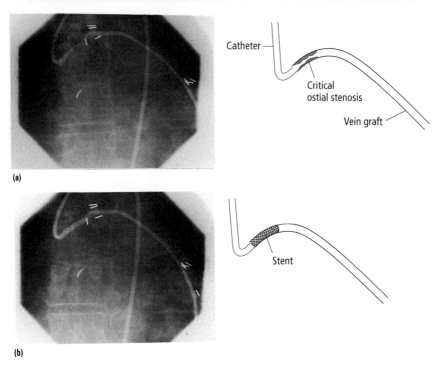

(a)

(b)

Fig. 5.8 Coronary vein graft stenting. (a) Before the procedure a long stenosis is clearly visible involving the ostium of the vein graft to the left anterior descending coronary artery. (b) Successful stent deployment results in a widely patent graft.

Variant angina

This unusual anginal syndrome was first described by Prinzmetal and is characterized by unprovoked episodes of chest pain which may be associated with ST segment elevation on the ECG. Coronary artery disease is present in 70% of cases but in the remainder the coronary arteries appear normal. An exaggerated increase in coronary arterial tone ('spasm') has been demonstrated in these patients during attacks of angina.

The spasm is usually focal in distribution and even in the absence of coronary artery disease can restrict flow sufficiently to produce profound myocardial ischaemia. These patients are at risk of cardiac arrhythmias and prolonged attacks of spasm may result in myocardial infarction. Calcium antagonists prevent spasm and are the treatment of choice. Nitrates are also beneficial but beta-blockers are less so, and may be detrimental if unopposed alpha-adrenergic stimulation further increases coronary tone.

Unstable angina

This is caused by subocclusive coronary thrombosis initiated by rupture of an atheromatous plaque. It presents with recurrent and usually prolonged episodes of angina occurring on minimal exertion or at rest and may be the first

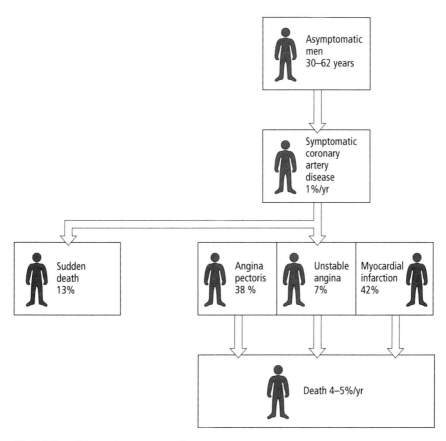

Fig. 5.9 Natural history of coronary artery disease.

manifestation of coronary artery disease or may occur as an abrupt change in an established pattern of chronic stable angina. Attacks of pain are often associated with reversible ST segment depression on the ECG (Fig. 5.10).

Unstable angina is a medical emergency requiring management in the coronary care unit. Myocardial infarction or death occur in up to 30% of cases within 3 months. The antithrombotic effects of heparin infusion and aspirin (independently and in combination) have been shown to improve prognosis by preventing progression of the coronary thrombosis to complete occlusion. Patients should also receive glyceryl trinitrate infusion and beta-blockers to improve the myocardial oxygen supply–demand imbalance. Calcium antagonists are less helpful, particularly dihydropyridines (e.g. nifedipine) which should be avoided because they may increase the risk of myocardial infarction. Early coronary arteriography with a view to angioplasty or bypass surgery is usually recommended, particularly when symptoms fail to settle promptly (Fig. 5.11).

MYOCARDIAL INFARCTION

Myocardial infarction (MI) is caused by occlusive coronary thrombosis initiated

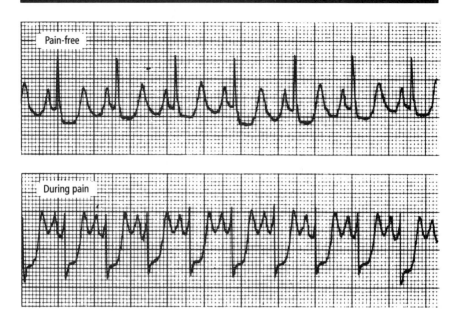

Fig. 5.10 Unstable angina. During chest pain the heart rate increases and marked depression of the ST segment occurs; there is some loss of R-wave amplitude. These changes reverse as chest pain is relieved.

by rupture of an atheromatous plaque. It may be the first manifestation of coronary artery disease or may occur against a background of chronic stable angina, often with the recent development of unstable symptoms.

Clinical manifestations

Clinical manifestations of acute MI are largely attributable to the direct effects of

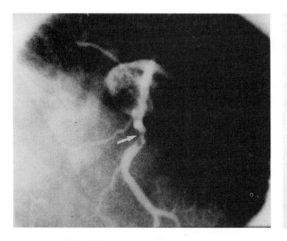
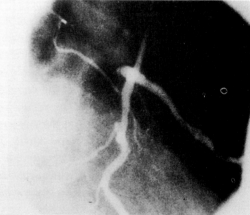

Fig. 5.11 Unstable angina treated by coronary angioplasty. The patient had continuing severe chest pain despite medical treatment. Coronary arteriography showed a subocclusive thrombus clearly visible as a filling defect in the circumflex coronary artery (arrowed). Angioplasty (right panel) restored arterial patency and relieved symptoms.

ischaemic myocardial damage and to autonomic disturbance. The effects of complications are discussed on pages 135–145.

Myocardial damage

Chest pain is the most prominent manifestation of ischaemic myocardial damage. It is characteristically unprovoked, unaffected by glyceryl trinitrate and prolonged, often lasting several hours. Like angina, the pain has a band-like constricting quality which is retrosternal and may radiate into the arms, neck and jaw. In an estimated 10% of cases, symptoms are so trivial that medical attention is not sought. Asymptomatic infarction of this type is more common in the elderly and in diabetic patients with sensory neuropathy. Other manifestations of ischaemic myocardial damage include a palpable dyskinetic impulse over the left precordium (more common in anterior infarction) and a fourth heart sound. Pyrogens released from the damaged myocardium cause low-grade pyrexia for the first 3 days and during this period the white cell count and erythrocyte sedimentation rate (ESR) are commonly elevated.

Autonomic disturbance

Manifestations of autonomic disturbance may include sweating, vomiting or syncope. Sympathoadrenal activation causes tachycardia and elevation of blood pressure, but these usually settle with pain relief. Sympathoadrenal activation also stimulates glycogenolysis and lipolysis leading to hyperglycaemia and hyper-triglyceridaemia with lowering of blood cholesterol. The blood cholesterol may remain lowered for up to 12 weeks. Hypokalaemia is also common and is caused by stimulation of sodium–potassium exchange at the cell membrane.

Diagnosis

Early diagnosis of MI is essential to allow prompt intervention with specific treatment to limit infarct size. In most cases the clinical history and the presenting ECG provide sufficient information. However, confirmation of the diagnosis requires documentation of the typical evolution of ECG and serum enzyme changes over a period of 2–3 days. Non-invasive imaging techniques are only rarely helpful in diagnosis.

ECG

This provides the most convenient and reliable method of early diagnosis. The typical evolution of changes is shown in Fig. 5.12. Peaking of the T wave and ST segment elevation occur within seconds of coronary occlusion and are often associated with 'reciprocal' ST segment depression in the opposite ECG leads. These 'hyperacute' changes resolve over a period of 18–24 hours, or much more rapidly if spontaneous or drug-induced coronary recanalization occurs. During

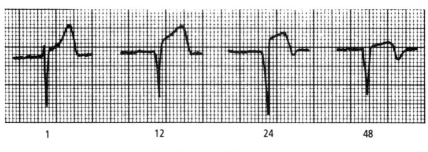

1   12   24   48

Hours after onset of chest pain

Fig. 5.12 Evolution of ECG changes in acute myocardial infarction.

this period a pathological Q wave (see page 34) develops which usually persists indefinitely, and is pathognomonic of infarction. T-wave inversion may also occur at the time of Q-wave formation. Occasionally, changes are restricted to the ST segment and T wave without the development of a Q wave. Non-Q-wave infarction of this type often denotes more limited myocardial damage.

Because coronary occlusion affects different regions of the left ventricle, depending on the artery involved, the ECG provides a useful guide to infarct location. Left anterior descending coronary occlusion causes anterior infarction with the characteristic evolution of changes in the anteroseptal (V1–V3) or anterolateral (V1–V6) leads, depending on the extent of damage (Fig. 5.13). The right coronary artery usually supplies the inferior wall of the ventricle by its posterior descending branch and occlusion causes the characteristic evolution of

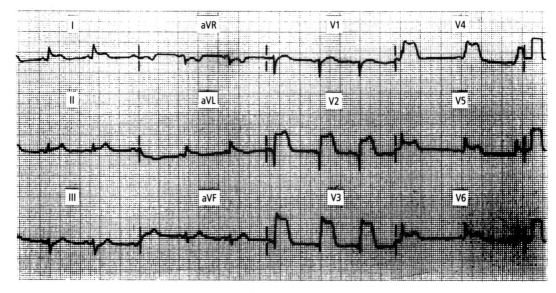

Fig. 5.13 Acute anteroseptal myocardial infarction. The ECG shows marked ST segment elevation in leads V1–V3 with the development of pathological Q waves. There is also ST elevation in leads I, AVL and V4 indicating some lateral extension of the infarct. The ST depression in leads II, III and aVF is 'reciprocal'.

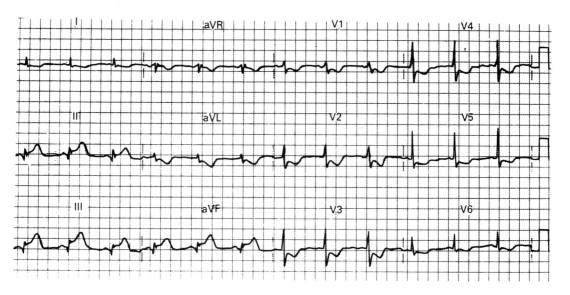

Fig. 5.14 Acute inferoposterior myocardial infarction. ST segment elevation in leads II, III and AVF is associated with 'reciprocal' ST depression in leads I, AVL and V1–V4. Posterior extension of the infarct is indicated by the dominant R waves in leads V1 and V2.

ECG changes in leads II, III and aVF (Fig. 5.14). Circumflex occlusion causes lateral infarction with ECG changes in leads I, aVL and V6. It may also cause inferior damage in the 15% of people in whom the posterior descending artery arises from the circumflex rather than the right coronary artery. If the high posterior wall of the ventricle is involved in the infarct ECG changes may be difficult to detect but dominant R waves in leads V1 and V2 often develop (see Fig. 5.14).

The ECG is of little diagnostic value in patients with left bundle branch block or paced ventricular rhythms. Previous infarction with extensive Q waves and persistent ST segment changes may also make ECG interpretation difficult. Very occasionally patients with acute infarction present with a normal ECG although serial recordings almost invariably reveal the development of diagnostic changes. A persistently normal ECG is rarely consistent with the diagnosis of MI.

Serum enzymes

Electron microscopy has identified disruption of the sarcolemmal membrane as one of the earliest histological manifestations of MI. Disruption allows intracellular enzymes and other proteins to escape into the circulation for use as biochemical markers of infarction. Serial measurements are required to show diagnostic changes in blood concentrations (Fig. 5.15).

Creatine kinase (CK)

Blood activities do not rise above normal until 6–10 hours after the onset of

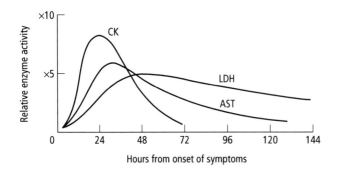

Fig. 5.15 Serum enzyme activity (relative to normal values) in acute myocardial infarction.

symptoms, peaking at 17–24 hours. This is earlier than other enzymatic tests but, nevertheless, limits its value for very early diagnosis. Skeletal-muscle CK may cause false-positive results in patients who have received intramuscular injections or external cardiac massage and, in difficult cases, the isoenzyme MB (specific for myocardial CK) can be measured.

Aspartate transaminase (AST)

Serum levels peak on the second day. The enzyme, however, is non-specific, and liver, lung or brain disorders may give false-positive results.

Lactic dehydrogenase (LDH)

Because serum levels remain elevated for 2 weeks, this is useful for patients who present late. Red cells are rich in LDH and traumatic venesection or other causes of haemolysis may give false-positive results.

New serum markers of myocardial injury

New serum markers of myocardial injury currently being evaluated include troponin T, troponin I, and myosin light chains. Potential advantages include the early release of these proteins from injured cardiac myocytes which may permit rapid diagnosis of infarction when the ECG is non-diagnostic.

Non-invasive imaging

Non-invasive imaging techniques are of limited diagnostic value. Echocardiography reliably identifies abnormal left ventricular wall motion in the zone of infarction, but the finding is not diagnostic because the same abnormality may reflect old infarction or acute ischaemia without irreversible damage. Radionuclide imaging with infarct-avid agents (usually technetium-99m pyrophosphate, see Fig. 3.13) has not been useful clinically, largely because uptake of isotope is rarely adequate for diagnostic purposes until 24 hours after the onset of symptoms. Moreover, false-positive results may occur in unstable angina. The role of immunoscintigraphy with radio-labelled antimyosin antibody fragments has also been investigated but again it is unlikely to have a useful clinical role because cardiac imaging cannot be done until 24 hours after the administration of antibody to permit its clearance from the blood.

Differential diagnosis

Acute MI must be differentiated from other conditions presenting with chest pain and ECG changes, particularly pericarditis and pulmonary embolism. In these, however, the character of the chest pain is usually different and the typical ECG and enzyme changes do not occur. Aortic dissection may also cause ECG changes if the dissection occludes a coronary artery producing coincidental MI.

Treatment

The main aims of treatment are to correct symptoms, especially chest pain, and prevent death. MI has an estimated 35–40% mortality. About half of these deaths occur within 2 hours of the onset of symptoms, before hospital admission, and in most cases are the result of ventricular fibrillation, although myocardial rupture also contributes. In hospital, however, lethal arrhythmias can be corrected by defibrillation and the most important cause of death is left ventricular failure (LVF) due to extensive infarction. Patients with large infarcts are also at increased risk of death in the year following hospital discharge. Thus significant reductions in the mortality from acute MI can be achieved by ensuring early access to a defibrillator and by intervention with specific drugs to prevent myocardial rupture and reduce infarct size.

General measures

Early access to a defibrillator prevents death from ventricular fibrillation. This requires prompt hospital admission and patients with unrelieved cardiac chest pain should be encouraged to call an ambulance immediately. Most front-line ambulances are equipped with a defibrillator and carry specially trained paramedical personnel. Following admission, the patient should be managed in the coronary care unit where facilities are available for continuous ECG monitoring and cardiopulmonary resuscitation. Pain relief and sedation with intravenous (IV) diamorphine (2.5–5.0 mg) are essential, and drug-induced nausea and vomiting is prevented by IV prochlorperazine (25–50 mg). Anticoagulation with heparin is recommended, not only as an adjunct to thrombolytic therapy (see below), but also to guard against thromboembolism by preventing deep venous thrombosis and mural thrombosis within the left ventricle. If the early course is uncomplicated, the patient should be transferred to the general ward after 24 hours and mobilized, with a view to discharge within 5 days.

Treatment to prevent myocardial rupture

Hypertensive patients appear to be at special risk of myocardial rupture in the first 24 hours. Early treatment with an IV beta-blocker reduces hospital mortality by about 15%, possibly because reductions in left ventricular wall tension and the force of contraction reduce the risk of rupture. Current recommendations are for IV metoprolol or atenolol (5 mg) in patients with a systolic blood pressure > 160 mmHg. The dose should be repeated every 15 minutes, titrated against the blood pressure and heart-rate responses. Treatment is contraindicated in patients with asthma, severe bradycardia (< 60 beats/minute), or LVF.

Treatment to reduce infarct size

MI is a dynamic process and, although the subendocardium infarcts within 30 minutes of coronary occlusion, outward extension to involve the full thickness of the left ventricular wall may take several hours. Restoration of antegrade flow in the infarct-related artery during this 'window of opportunity', before the trans-mural spread of infarction is complete, is now seen as the primary goal of hospital treatment because it allows reperfusion and salvage of the threatened myocardium with reduction of eventual infarct size. This may be achieved by thrombolytic therapy or by coronary angioplasty.

Thrombolytic therapy

Spontaneous thrombolysis and coronary recanalization occur in about 15% of cases, accounting for many of the small non-Q-wave infarcts encountered in clinical practice. Thrombolytic therapy, however, increases the recanalization rate to 60–70% and randomized trials have shown that treatment can reduce mortality by up to 50% if given within an hour of the onset of chest pain; diminishing (but still substantial) benefit can be demonstrated for patients treated within 12 hours of the onset of chest pain (Fig. 5.16). Aspirin also reduces mortality, probably because its effects on platelet function favour coronary patency (Fig. 5.17 and Box 5.3). Current recommendations are for IV infusion of streptokinase (1.5 million units over 1 hour) and oral aspirin (75–150 mg) to be given as soon as possible after admission. There is evidence that tissue-type plasminogen activator (tPA or alteplase) may be more effective than streptokinase in producing coronary recanalization and reducing mortality. Thus, despite its greater cost, it is often preferred, particularly for high-risk patients with anterior infarction (15 mg by IV injection, followed by a total of 85 mg by IV infusion over the next 90 minutes). Heparin infusion (1000 units/hour) helps maintain coronary patency after treatment with tPA and most physicians continue to recommend its use after streptokinase until the patient starts to mobilize, with maintenance aspirin treatment thereafter.

Contraindications to thrombolytic therapy include active peptic ulceration, prolonged resuscitation, and surgery within the previous 4 weeks. Cerebrovas-

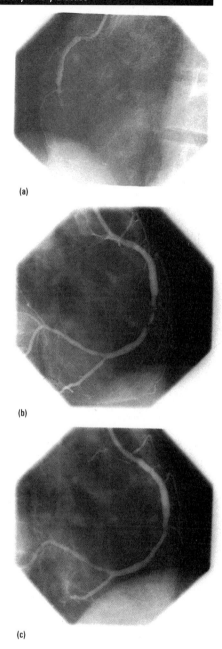

(a)

(b)

(c)

Fig. 5.16 Thrombolytic therapy in acute myocardial infarction. (a) Before thrombolytic therapy. The right coronary artery is occluded (arrowed). (b) After intravenous streptokinase 1.5 million units. The coronary artery has recanalized, but there remains a very tight stenosis in its mid portion which caused continuing ischaemic chest pain in this case. (c) After coronary angioplasty. In order to correct ongoing ischaemia, 'rescue' coronary angioplasty has been performed.

cular accident within the previous three months is also a contraindication. Streptokinase is antigenic and elicits an antibody response which, in the event of re-exposure to the drug, neutralizes its thrombolytic activity and predisposes to anaphylaxis. Thus patients with acute MI who have received streptokinase previously should be treated with the non-antigenic alteplase which is synthesized by recombinant DNA technology to resemble the tissue plasminogen activator normally secreted by human endothelial cells.

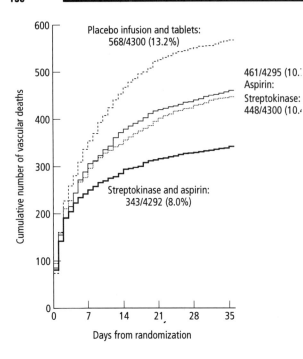

Fig. 5.17 ISIS-II Study (see Box 5.3): the study showed a > 20% mortality reduction at 5 weeks for patients who received either streptokinase or aspirin as monotherapy. The beneficial effects of these drugs were additive, and patients who received both agents showed > 40% mortality reduction. (Reproduced with permission from *Lancet* 1988; ii: 349–61.)

Box 5.3 International Study of Infarct Survival (ISIS II)

Study design Randomized, double-blind, placebo-controlled, multicentre.

Randomization Streptokinase (1.5 mega-units IV over 1 hour); or aspirin (162.5 mg/day); or both; or placebo. Any additional therapy was allowed.

Inclusion Suspected acute myocardial infarction in previous 24 hours.

End points 5-week vascular mortality, stroke, reinfarction, need for transfusion.

Patients 17 187 (4300 streptokinase; 4295 aspirin; 4292 both; 4300 placebo) who had a suspected myocardial infarction in previous 24 hours.

Results At 5 weeks, 9.2%, 9.4% and 8.0% of the patients in the streptokinase, aspirin, and streptokinase plus aspirin groups had died as a result of vascular causes, respectively, compared with placebo deaths of 12%, 11.8% and 13.2%. These represented odds ratio reductions of 25%, 23% and 42% (all $P < 0.00001$). Streptokinase was associated with a greater need for transfusion compared with the placebo group (0.5% vs 0.2%), but fewer strokes (0.6% vs 0.8%). Aspirin was associated with fewer non-fatal reinfarctions compared with placebo (1.0% vs 2.0%) and fewer non-fatal strokes (0.3% vs 0.6%).

Conclusions Findings suggest that streptokinase and aspirin both improve survival, when administered within 24 hours of myocardial infarction, but their use in combination is even more effective.

Anonymous (1988) Randomized trial of intravenous streptokinase, oral aspirin, both, or neither among 17,187 cases of suspected acute myocardial infarction. *Lancet*; ii: 349–60.

Primary coronary angioplasty

Coronary angioplasty may also be used to restore coronary patency in patients with MI presenting early after the onset of symptoms. This is called 'primary' coronary angioplasty to distinguish it from strategies of 'early' coronary angioplasty for patients pretreated with thrombolysis (rarely helpful), and 'rescue' coronary angioplasty for patients treated with thrombolysis who have ongoing chest pain (often helpful, see Fig. 5.16). Primary angioplasty is only feasible in centres with the appropriate facilities and expertise, but the results of comparative trials indicate that the outcome in terms of early mortality and recurrent infarction may be as good if not better than for thrombolytic therapy. Coronary angioplasty appears particularly useful for the treatment of cardiogenic shock where non-controlled data suggest that mortality can be reduced from > 80% to < 50%.

Secondary prevention

In the year after MI, recurrent infarction or sudden death occurs in 10–15% of cases. There is now clear evidence that lifestyle modification and drug therapy can reduce the incidence.

Lifestyle modification

Patients who quit smoking reduce their risk of recurrent events by up to 50%. Modification of dietary fat intake is also beneficial, and while obesity itself may not be an independent risk factor for further coronary events, there is general agreement about the indirect benefits of weight reduction on blood pressure, cholesterol and glucose tolerance. Finally, the benefits of exercise rehabilitation following MI have been demonstrated to the satisfaction of most, particularly in terms of psychological recovery but perhaps also in terms of reduced mortality. For this reason formal coronary rehabilitation courses are now provided by most centres, providing a combination of health education and supervised aerobic exercise. Most patients can return to work after 2–3 months. Patients should not drive for 1 month; vocational drivers must inform the DVLA. Sexual intercourse can usually be resumed once patients are able to undertake moderate exercise without symptoms.

Drugs for secondary prevention

Randomized trials have shown that daily aspirin significantly reduces the risk of reinfarction and death. A daily dose of 75–150 mg is recommended. Beta-blockers also reduce the risk of reinfarction and death and are recommended for all patients without contraindications (Box 5.4). The recent Scandinavian '4S' trial (see Box 5.2) showed that the use of dietary restriction plus an HMG-CoA reductase inhibitor (simvastatin) to lower blood cholesterol produced substantial reductions in coronary mortality following MI; similar benefits have been con-

Box 5.4 BHAT: The Beta-Blocker Heart Attack Trial	
Study design Randomized, double-blind, placebo-controlled, multicentre.	**Randomization** Propranolol, 60 or 80 mg t.d.s.; or placebo, 5–21 days after myocardial infarction.
Inclusion Acute myocardial infarction.	**End points** All-cause mortality, cardiovascular mortality, atherosclerotic heart disease including sudden cardiac death, haemodynamics, non-fatal reinfarction, symptomatic heart failure.
Patients 3837 (1916 propranolol; 1921 placebo) mean age 54.8 years who had experienced myocardial infarction 5–21 days before enrolment.	**Results** All-cause mortality at 25 months was 7.2% in the propranolol group and 9.9% in the placebo group ($P < 0.005$). Cardiovascular mortality was also lower in the propranolol group (6.6% vs 8.9%; $P < 0.01$) as was death from atherosclerotic heart disease (6.2% vs 8.5%; $P < 0.01$) and sudden cardiac death (3.3% vs 4.6%; $P < 0.05$). Non-fatal reinfarction was 15.6% lower in the propranolol group compared with the placebo group.
Conclusions Findings suggest that administration of propranol 5–21 days after myocardial infarction significantly reduces medium-term mortality and the risk of reinfarction.	

A randomized trial of propranolol in patients with acute myocardial infarction. 1. Mortality results and 2. Morbidity results. *J Am Med Assoc* 1982; **247**: 1707–14 *and* 1983; **250**: 2814–19.

firmed with pravastatin. Finally, randomized trials of ACE inhibition after MI have shown significant mortality benefits, particularly in patients with clinical evidence of heart failure (Box 5.5).

Risk stratification

Nearly 50% of all patients admitted to hospital with MI die or suffer a recurrent ischaemic event (MI or unstable angina) in the ensuing 3 years. Identification of high-risk patients permits targeting of treatment (and finite resources) on the group in whom the potential benefits are greatest. Tests used for risk stratification should meet the following requirements:
• ready availability in hospitals that treat the bulk of patients;
• suitability for use early after infarction to anticipate the period of greatest risk; and
• high sensitivity (low false-negative results) and high positive predictive accuracy.

Stress testing (radionuclide or ECG)

This is readily available in most hospitals and can usually be performed before discharge. Patients with evidence of residual ischaemia are commonly referred for cardiac catherization with a view to revascularization on the grounds that they are at risk of recurrent ischaemic events. However, the sensitivity of stress testing (particularly the stress ECG) and its positive predictive accuracy are both low, and although it is widely used, there is little evidence that it is of clinical value for risk stratification.

Box 5.5 AIRE: The Acute Infarction Ramipril Efficacy Trial	
Study design Randomized, double-blind, placebo-controlled, multicentre.	**Randomization** Ramipril, 2.5 mg b.d. for 2 days, then 5 mg b.d., if tolerated; or placebo, administered between days 3 and 10 after myocardial infarction.
Inclusion Myocardial infarction complicated by heart failure.	**End points** *Primary:* all-cause mortality. *Secondary:* death, progression to severe/resistant heart failure, reinfarction or stroke.
Patients 1986 (1004 ramipril; 982 placebo) with heart failure after acute myocardial infarction.	**Results** After an average follow-up of 15 months, all cause mortality was lower in the ramipril group than in the placebo group (17% vs 23%) representing a 27% ($P = 0.002$) risk reduction. Ramipril was also associated with a 19% reduction in the risk of a secondary outcome ($P = 0.008$): death (9% vs 12%), severe/resistant heart failure (10% vs 14%), reinfarction (7% vs 7%), stroke (2% vs 2%).
Conclusions Findings suggest that the administration of ramipril to patients with clinical evidence of heart failure 3–10 days after myocardial infarction causes a highly significant and substantial reduction in all-cause mortality that is evident as early as 30 days after starting treatment.	

Anonymous (1993) Effect of ramipril on mortality and morbidity on survivors of acute myocardial infarction with clinical evidence of heart failure. *Lancet*; **342**: 921–9.

Measurement of left ventricular ejection fraction

Ejection fraction is a measure of left ventricular function (see page 74) which in turn is the major determinant of prognosis. It can be measured by echocardiography or radionuclide blood-pool imaging, both of which are readily available in most hospitals and can be performed before discharge. Measurement of ejection fraction is now widely recommended because it can be used to guide requirements for ACE inhibition which in turn can improve prognosis (see below).

Other tests for risk stratification

These include the signal-averaged ECG in which late potentials are a poor prognostic sign and reduced vagal tone as evidenced by reductions in heart-rate variability (see page 41). More recently, studies of Holter monitoring (see page 38) early after MI have shown that patients with ventricular arrhythmias or prolonged periods of ischaemic ST depression (with or without chest pain) may be at high risk of recurrent infarction and death. The extent to which treatment of these high-risk individuals affects outcome is unclear although early cardiac catheterization with a view to revascularization is usually recommended.

Management strategies after MI

Asymptomatic patient (Fig. 5.18)

The asymptomatic patient with uncomplicated infarction should be discharged

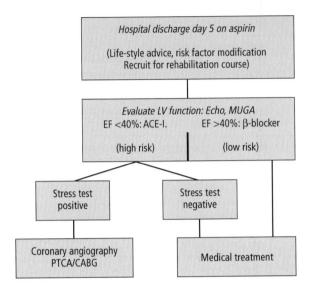

Fig. 5.18 Simple management strategy for asymptomatic patients recovering from acute myocardial infarction. Note that patients with ongoing or recurrent chest pain after myocardial infarction should always be considered for coronary arteriography.

after 5 days, having received lifestyle advice, an appointment for the rehabilitation programme and a prescription for aspirin. Because left ventricular function is the major determinant of prognosis, it should be evaluated by either echocardiography or radionuclide blood-pool imaging. Those with an ejection fraction of > 45% are a relatively low-risk group to whom beta-blockers can be safely given. Those with an ejection fraction of < 45% are a high-risk group for whom ACE inhibitors (in addition to beta-blockers, if possible) are of proven benefit. Stress testing (radionuclide or ECG) in this high-risk group may be used to identify those with residual ischaemia who might benefit from coronary arteriography with a view to revascularization by angioplasty or bypass surgery. All patients should have fasting blood cholesterol measured at 3 months (earlier testing produces spuriously low values), those with a cholesterol > 5.4 mmol/l, despite diet, requiring treatment with an HMG–CoA reductase inhibitor.

Symptomatic patient

The patient with continuing (or recurrent) ischaemic chest pain after thrombolytic therapy requires urgent cardiac catheterization with a view to 'rescue' angioplasty of the infarct-related artery or, if necessary, coronary bypass surgery. Patients with intractable heart failure have a very poor prognosis, but may also benefit from urgent revascularization to revitalise 'stunned' myocardium in the zone of infarction. Prognosis is also poor in patients with ventricular arrhythmias > 48 hours after MI. Extensive myocardial damage is almost invariable in this group who are at high risk of sudden death. Antiarrhythmic therapy with type III agents (amiodarone) is usually recommended although evidence of benefit from randomized trials is wanting. Treatment with an implantable defibrillator (see page 250) is a more expensive, and probably more effective, alternative.

Prognosis

MI is fatal in approximately 40% of cases.

Pre-hospital mortality (20%)

This is due to primary ventricular fibrillation (VF) in an estimated 75% of cases, with fulminant LVF and myocardial rupture accounting for the remainder. Primary VF does not necessarily reflect extensive infarction and the prognosis for those patients who are successfully resuscitated is only slightly worse than that for other early survivors.

Hospital mortality (12–15%)

This is closely related to infarct size and with the introduction of thrombolytic and aspirin therapy has fallen from 15–25% to between 12 and 15%. Nevertheless, when infarction is sufficiently extensive to cause LVF, mortality exceeds 30%, rising to 80% for cardiogenic shock. Other factors, in addition to overt heart failure, are also predictive of a poor prognosis (Table 5.5) but, apart from advanced age and diabetes, these are variably related to extensive myocardial damage, emphasizing the important relation between infarct size and prognosis.

Post-hospital mortality (10% in first year)

Prognosis after discharge is also influenced by infarct size, and patients with poor left ventricular function have a considerably higher 1-year mortality.

Complications

Arrhythmias

Patients with acute MI are at high risk of cardiac arrhythmias. Arrhythmia provocation is enhanced by autonomic responses, metabolic abnormalities and drug actions (Table 5.6). Management must include modification of these

Table 5.5 Adverse prognostic features in myocardial infarction.

Advanced age
Diabetes
Left ventricular failure
Systolic hypotension
Anterior full-thickness infarction
Left bundle branch block
History of previous myocardial infarction
Complex ventricular arrhythmias (particulary those occurring late (> 36 hours) after myocardial infarction

Myocardial ischaemia/infarction
Heightened sympathoadrenal activity
pain
anxiety
heart failure
Metabolic abnormalities
hypoxaemia—pulmonary congestion
acidosis—low cardiac output
hypokalaemia—diuretics
hypomagnesaemia—diuretics
Drugs
sympathomimetic agents
digitalis
beta-adrenergic blockers

Table 5.6 Arrhythmogenic factors in myocardial infarction.

provocative factors but specific treatment is usually only required if the arrhythmia intensifies ischaemia or embarrasses left ventricular function.

Atrial arrhythmias

Abnormalities of sinus rhythm rarely require specific treatment. Severe *sinus bradycardia* may occur in inferior infarction and, if associated with low cardiac output, usually responds to intravenous atropine (0.3–0.6 mg). Treatment of *sinus tachycardia* should be directed at the underlying cause, particularly unrelieved pain, anxiety and heart failure.

Atrial premature beats occur commonly and require no treatment. *Atrial fibrillation* affects up to 15% of patients in the first 24 hours. Untreated, it usually reverts spontaneously to sinus rhythm but, meanwhile, the ventricular rate should be controlled with digoxin. There is no evidence that therapeutic doses of digoxin increase the risk of ventricular arrhythmias but amiodarone is sometimes preferred for patients in whom ventricular arrhythmias have been troublesome.

Ventricular arrhythmias

Ventricular premature beats occur in all patients after MI but require no treatment, unless they are so frequent that they cause significant impairment of left ventricular function.

Ventricular tachycardia (VT) is defined as three or more consecutive ventricular premature beats at a rate in excess of 120 beats/minute. It occurs in up to 40% of patient with acute MI and is associated with increased mortality. If VT complicates an excessively slow heart rate, atropine or pacemaker therapy is indicated; otherwise, paroxysmal attacks require suppression with lignocaine or amiodarone. Sustained VT usually produces severe LVF and requires urgent direct-current cardioversion followed by lignocaine infusion. In most patients, antiarrhythmic therapy can be safely discontinued during mobilization on the ward. However, 'late' VT (> 24 hours after admission) usually reflects extensive

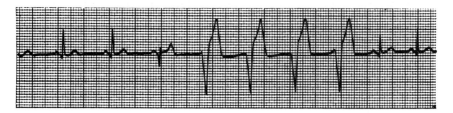

Fig. 5.19 Accelerated idioventricular rhythm. After the second sinus beat there is a fusion beat (part sinus, part ventricular in origin) followed by a short four-beat run of accelerated idioventricular rhythm before the sinus node re-establishes itself.

infarction and is a poor prognostic sign. Prophylactic antiarrhythmic treatment is not always helpful, and the proarrhythmic effects of some drugs may adversely affect prognosis (see page 244). Amiodarone is preferred, but if this fails to control the cardiac rhythm, electrophysiological studies to provoke the arrhythmia and to test the efficacy of treatment should be undertaken before discharge from hospital (see page 40).

Accelerated idioventricular rhythm (rate 60–120 beats/minute) commonly complicates acute MI, but is rarely seen in other contexts (Fig. 5.19). The accelerated ventricular ectopic focus is usually in continuous competition with the sinus node, such that the idioventricular rhythm is typically intermittent, alternating with episodes of sinus rhythm. Treatment is unnecessary because the ventricular rate is, by definition, slow and haemodynamic stability is usually well maintained.

Ventricular fibrillation (Fig. 5.20) may be a primary electrical event (occurring within the first 24–48 hours of infarction) or may be secondary to severe left ventricular dysfunction (often occurring late after infarction). Urgent direct-current cardioversion is mandatory to prevent death. Primary VF affects up to 15% of patients in the coronary care unit and it is now clear that those patients successfully resuscitated have only a slightly increased risk of late mortality. Prophylactic antiarrhythmic therapy is unnecessary after primary VF but is mandatory after secondary VF because of the high incidence of sudden death during early follow-up. The choice of prophylactic treatment is influenced by the same considerations as for 'late' VT (see above).

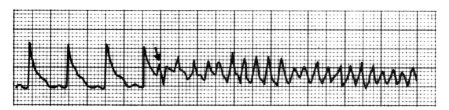

Fig. 5.20 Primary ventricular fibrillation. The first four complexes are sinus beats with marked ST segment elevation indicating acute myocardial infarction. A very early ('R-on-T') ventricular premature beat (arrowed) initiates ventricular fibrillation.

Table 5.7 Indications for pacemaker therapy in myocardial infarction.

Third-degree (complete) AV block complicating inferior myocardial infarction and any of the following if unresponsive to atropine:
   rate < 40 per minute
   low-output state
   unreliable escape rhythm
   bradycardia-dependent ventricular arrhythmias
Third-degree or Mobitz type II second-degree block complicating anterior infarction
Acute bifascicular block

Heart block

MI may damage the specialized conduction tissues, causing an excessively slow heart rate, and a temporary pacemaker may be necessary (Table 5.7).

Atrioventricular nodal block

Bradyarrhythmias and conduction defects are common in inferior MI because of autonomic reflexes which tend to slow the sinus rate and delay conduction through the atrioventricular (AV) node. Treatment, if necessary, is nearly always a temporary measure and recovery of normal conduction can be expected within 10 days. First-degree AV block, characterized by prolongation of the PR interval (> 0.20 seconds), requires no treatment. Second-degree AV block is nearly always Mobitz type 1 (Wenckebach) in which successive sinus impulses find the AV node increasingly refractory until AV conduction fails (Fig. 5.21). No treatment is necessary unless the ventricular rate is very slow, when atropine will increase AV conduction. In third-degree (complete) AV block, complicating inferior infarction, a junctional pacemaker (low AV node, bundle of His) takes over in most instances (Fig. 5.22). The escape rhythm is usually reliable and cardiac output is well maintained, so that treatment is required only if the ventricular rate is very slow. Junctional pacemakers often respond to atropine

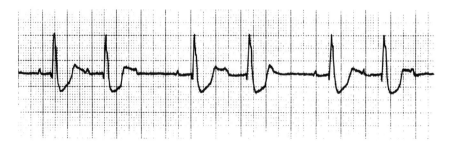

Fig. 5.21 Mobitz type I (Wenckebach) second-degree heart block in acute myocardial infarction. The patient has suffered a recent inferior infarct. Three Wenckebach cycles are shown, in each of which progressive prolongation of the PR interval culminates in a dropped beat.

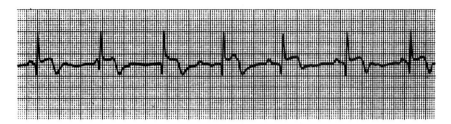

Fig. 5.22 Third-degree (complete) AV block. The lead is aVF and shows changes consistent with acute inferior myocardial infarction. There is complete failure of AV conduction evidenced by the dissociation of the P waves and QRS complexes. The block is at the level of the AV node and a junctional focus has taken over pacemaker activity. Thus the QRS complexes are narrow and the rate is well maintained.

but, if this fails to increase the heart rate, temporary pacing may be necessary until recovery of AV conduction occurs.

When AV block complicates anterior MI, damage is always extensive and mortality high. Block is usually below the bundle of His, involving both bundle branches and, whether it is intermittent (Mobitz type II) or complete, the ventricular rate is slow and there is a significant risk of prolonged asystole. Temporary pacing is mandatory and, because recovery of normal AV conduction does not always occur, a permanent pacemaker may be required in the long term.

Bundle branch block

Left or right bundle branch block complicating MI is an adverse prognostic sign but requires no specific treatment. Similarly, left or right axis deviation (indicating selective damage to the anterior or posterior divisions of the left bundle, respectively) requires no specific treatment. But when axis deviation ('hemiblock') and right bundle branch block occur together ('bifascicular block'), AV conduction is dependent upon the remaining division of the left bundle (Fig. 5.23). The risk of progression to complete heart block is considerable and temporary prophylactic pacing is indicated.

Heart failure

Heart failure is the principal cause of death in the coronary care unit, affecting about 30% of all patients admitted to hospital with MI.

Left ventricular failure

The severity is closely related to infarct size. When about 40% of the left ventricle is damaged, cardiogenic shock develops, characterized by cold, clammy skin, tachycardia, hypotension and oliguria. The principal clinical manifestations of LVF are pulmonary oedema and peripheral hypoperfusion, caused by elevated left atrial pressure and reduced cardiac output, respectively. Pulmonary oedema

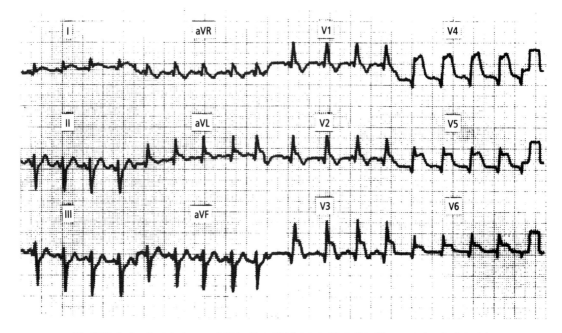

Fig. 5.23 Acute anterolateral myocardial infarction with bifascicular block. Note ST segment elevation in leads I, aVL and V1–V6. The rSR configuration in lead V1 indicates right bundle branch block. In addition there is marked left axis deviation indicating damage to the anterior division of the left bundle branch. AV conduction is dependent upon the posterior division of the left bundle.

occurs when left atrial pressure rises above 18 mmHg and is best assessed by observation of the chest X-ray. Peripheral hypoperfusion occurs when cardiac output falls below 3.5 l/minute and is best assessed by measurement of urine output and skin temperature. Four subsets of patients have been identified based on these clinical observations and defined by a left atrial (pulmonary artery wedge) pressure of 18 mmHg and a cardiac output of 3.5 1/minute (Fig. 5.24).

1 Well-preserved left ventricular function requiring no specific therapy.

2 Dominantly 'backwards' failure with pulmonary oedema but well-maintained cardiac output. Treatment with morphine and diuretics is usually effective.

3 Dominantly 'forwards' failure without pulmonary oedema. Left atrial (pulmonary artery wedge) pressure is inappropriately low and oliguria and hypotension may be corrected by infusion of a plasma volume expander which increases cardiac output by the Starling mechanism. A therapeutic challenge with 500 ml of crystalloid (e.g. N saline) is usually safe because it rapidly disperses throughout the body water without a prolonged effect on plasma volume. Prompt clinical improvement provides indication for colloid infusion (e.g. plasma or gelatin solution), but if the saline challenge is ineffective further volume should not be given for fear of provoking pulmonary oedema. In difficult cases, monitoring of pulmonary artery wedge pressure with a Swan–Ganz catheter is recommended to prevent overloading the circulation. Pulmonary oedema develops if the wedge pressure rises above 18 mmHg.

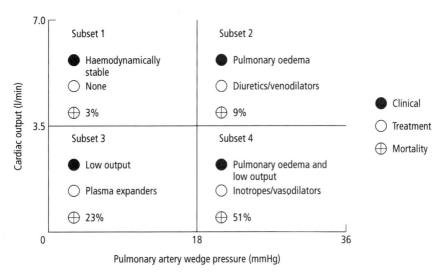

Fig. 5.24 Haemodynamic subsets in acute myocardial infarction. The clinical therapeutic and prognostic correlates of subset classification are demonstrated.

4 Low cardiac output and pulmonary oedema occurring together. Treatment must be directed towards improving left ventricular function with vasodilators and inotropes (see page 87), which should be given by controlled intravenous infusion to correct pulmonary oedema and improve cardiac output. In critically ill patients failing to respond to these measures, pulmonary artery pressure monitoring with a Swan–Ganz catheter is sometimes helpful (see page 67).

It is important to emphasize that *clinical* and *radiographic* assessment of the patient with LVF complicating MI is satisfactory in the large majority of cases. Measurement of urine output and assessment of skin temperature with review of the chest X-ray will nearly always permit an accurate subset allocation without the need for pulmonary artery pressure monitoring. Subset classification provides not only a useful basis for therapeutic decision-making but also a means of predicting prognosis. Mortality rises from < 5% in subset 1 to > 50% in subset 4.

Right ventricular failure

When right coronary occlusion causes inferior infarction it is occasionally associated with variable right ventricular damage which, if severe, may produce significant right ventricular failure (RVF) with low cardiac output and elevation of the right atrial and jugular venous pressures. Useful increments in cardiac output can be achieved by further increasing right atrial pressure with infusion of a plasma volume expander, which increases the output of the right ventricle by the Starling principle. A therapeutic challenge with 500 ml of crystalloid should first be given and if this produces prompt clinical improvement it should be followed by colloid infusion (see above). Again, monitoring of the pulmonary artery wedge pressure with a Swan–Ganz catheter may be helpful in difficult cases to guard against overloading the circulation and precipitating pulmonary oedema.

Myocardial rupture

This is an important cause of death early after MI but may occur any time during the first 10 days. When rupture involves the free wall of the left ventricle, it produces severe tamponade which is nearly always rapidly fatal. Sudden haemodynamic deterioration, associated with the development of a pansystolic murmur, is caused by rupture of either the interventricular septum or a papillary muscle. This results in a ventricular septal defect or torrential mitral regurgitation, respectively. Clinically they are difficult to distinguish (Table 5.8) but accurate differential diagnosis is possible with colour-flow Doppler imaging which identifies the high-velocity jet from left to right across the septum or backwards through the mitral valve, depending on the lesion. In most cases, however, urgent cardiac catheterization is required to define both the lesion and the coronary anatomy to assess the potential for surgical correction. Mortality is high and, although temporary haemodynamic support can be provided with the intra-aortic balloon pump, surgery should not be delayed unduly.

Thromboembolism

Deep venous thrombosis and intracardiac mural thrombosis (overlying the infarcted ventricular myocardium) are potential sources of pulmonary and systemic thromboembolism, respectively. Heparin should be used prophylactically.

Pericarditis

Pericarditis is a common cause of persistent chest pain the first 3 days following full-thickness MI. It is a direct consequence of the underlying muscle damage and usually resolves within a week. During this period, the temperature may remain elevated and a pericardial friction rub is intermittently audible. Pericarditic pain can usually be distinguished from ongoing ischaemic pain by its

Table 5.8 Differential diagnosis of ventricular septal defect and papillary muscle rupture.

	Ventricular septal defect	Papillary muscle rupture
Murmur	Left stenal edge	Apex
Heart failure	Dominantly right-sided—often with minimal pulmonary oedema	Dominantly left-sided—always with severe pulmonary oedema
Infarct location	Anterior or inferior	Inferior
Right heart catheter	'Step-up' in oxygen saturation in right ventricle	Dominant 'V' wave in pulmonary artery wedge pressure trace
Echocardiography	Permits direct visualization of defect in some cases	Demonstrates flail valve leaflet
Doppler study	Demonstrates high-velocity jet across defect	Demonstrates high-velocity regurgitant jet

sharp quality and its relation to deep inspiration, coughing or changes in posture. Anti-inflammatory analgesics such as aspirin or indomethacin provide effective symptomatic relief.

Dressler's syndrome

Less than 4% of patients develop a pyrexial illness, often with pericarditis and pleurisy, 2–12 weeks after MI. A similar illness is sometimes seen following heart surgery (post-cardiotomy syndrome). The cause is uncertain but autoimmune mechanisms seem likely: elevation of the ESR and leucocytosis occur in most cases. Anti-inflammatory analgesics are effective and, in severe cases, corticosteroids may shorten the course of the illness. Relapses may occur up to 2 years after MI.

Left ventricular aneurysm

Following acute infarction, shrinkage and scarring of the damaged myocardium is usually complete within 6 weeks. In about 10% of cases, however, the healing process is inadequate and a thin-walled ventricular aneurysm develops. This may be associated with persistent ST segment elevation on the ECG. The risk of rupture is negligible and in many cases the aneurysm is of little consequence. However, left ventricular aneurysm can be a cause of cardiac arrhythmias, heart failure or clot embolization. If these complications cannot be controlled medically, excision of the aneurysm may be required.

SUDDEN DEATH

The majority of sudden deaths in the community occur in association with coronary artery disease and are presumed to be due to VF. The coronary artery disease usually involves all three major vessels and myocardial scars indicating old infarction may be present. In many cases death occurs as a result of the abrupt rupture of an atheromatous plaque and coronary thrombosis. However, when successful resuscitation is achieved, there may be no evidence of fresh infarction, indicating that severe ischaemia is the mechanism responsible for VF in some cases.

Following successful resuscitation, the patient requires full in-hospital investigation. This will usually involve cardiac catheterization with a view to myocardial revascularization (bypass surgery, angioplasty) or aneurysmectomy, if appropriate. Programmed electrical stimulation studies using intracardiac electrode catheters, in order to provoke the ventricular arrhythmia and to test the efficacy of antiarrhythmic therapy, may also be necessary (see page 40). Only when a treatment regimen has been selected to protect against dangerous ventricular arrhythmias should the patient be discharged from hospital. Increasingly, patients of this type are being treated with implantable cardioverter defibrillators (see page 250).

FURTHER READING

PREVALENCE, RISK FACTORS AND PREVENTION

Curfman GD. Is exercise beneficial—or hazardous—to your heart? *N Engl J Med* 1993; 329: 1730.

Garber AM, Avins AL. Triglyceride concentrations and coronary heart disease. *Br Med J* 1994; 309: 2.

Gupta S, de Belder A, Hughes LO. Avoiding premature coronary deaths in Asians in Britain. *Br Med J* 1995; 311: 1035.

Jackson G. Coronary artery disease and women. *Br Med J* 1994; 309: 555.

Kannel WB. Update on the role of cigarette smoking in coronary artery disease. *Am Heart J* 1981; 101: 319

Levine GN, Keaney JF, Vita JA. Cholesterol reduction in cardiovascular disease—clinical benefits and possible mechanisms. *N Engl J Med* 1995; 332: 512.

Loscalzo J. Regression of coronary atherosclerosis. *N Engl J Med* 1990; 323: 1337–9.

Marmot M. The cholesterol papers. *Br Med J* 1994; 308: 350.

Mason JE, Tosteson H, Ridker PM *et al.* The primary prevention of myocardial infarction. *N Engl J Med* 1992; 326: 1406.

Oliver M, Poole-Wilson P, Shepherd J, Tikkanen MJ. Lower patients' cholesterol now. *Br Med J* 1995; 310: 1280.

Rich-Edwards JW, Manson JE, Hennekens CH, Buring JE. Primary prevention of coronary heart disease in women. *N Engl J Med* 1995; 332: 1758.

Scott J. Lipoprotein (a). *Br Med J* 1991; 303: 663–4.

Simpson RJ, White A. Getting a handle on the prevalence of coronary heart disease. *Br Heart J* 1990; 64: 291.

Stampfer MJ, Malinow MR. Can lowering homocysteine levels reduce cardiovascular risk? *N Engl J Med* 1995; 332: 328.

Steinberg D. Antioxidant vitamins and coronary heart disease. *N Engl J Med* 1993; 328: 1487.

Stott N. Screening for cardiovascular risk in general practice. *Br Med J* 1994; 308: 285.

Tunstall Pedoe DS. Exercise and heart disease: is there still a controversy? *Br Heart J* 1990; 64: 293.

Wenger NK, Speroff L, Packard B. Cardiovascular health and disease in women. *N Engl J Med* 1993; 329: 247.

PATHOGENESIS

Bateman AC. Pathogenesis of sudden ischaemic cardiac death. *Lancet* 1996; 347: 70.

Chesebro JH, Fuster V. Thrombosis in unstable angina. *N Engl J Med* 1992; 327: 192.

Davies MJ. Detecting vulnerable coronary plaques. *Lancet* 1996; 347: 1422.

Fuster V, Badimon L, Badimon JJ, Chesebro JH. Pathogenesis of coronary artery disease and the acute coronary syndromes (2 parts). *N Engl J Med* 1992; 326: 242 (part 1) and 310 (part 2).

Hamsten A. Hemostasis and coronary artery disease. *N Engl J Med* 1995; 332: 677.

Hanlin RI. Platelets and coronary artery disease. *N Engl J Med* 1996; 334: 1126.

Luscher TF. The endothelium and cardiovascular disease—a complex relation. *N Engl J Med* 1994; 330: 1083.

ANGINA

Borow RO. Prognostic applications of exercise testing. *N Engl J Med* 1991; 325: 887.

Brady AJB, Warren JB. Angioplasty and restenosis. *Br Med J* 1991; 303: 729.

Cameron EWJ, Walker WS. Coronary artery bypass surgery. *Br Med J* 1990; 300: 1219.

Campbell S. Silent myocardial ischaemia. *Br Med J* 1988; 297: 751.

Cannon RO. Chest pain and normal coronary angiograms. *N Engl J Med* 1993; 328: 1706.

Douglas PS, Ginsberg GS. Evaluation of chest pain in women. *N Engl J Med* 1996; 334: 1311.

Hillis LD, Rutherford JD. Coronary angioplasty compared with bypass surgery. *N Engl J Med* 1994; 331: 1086.

Killip T. Twenty years of coronary bypass surgery. *N Engl J Med* 1988; 319: 366.

Landau C, Lange RA, Hillis LD. Percutaneous transluminal coronary angioplasty. *N Engl J Med* 1994; 330: 981.

Loop FD. Internal-thoracic-artery grafts: biologically better coronary arteries. *N Engl J Med* 1996; 334: 263.

Masseri A. Syndrome X: still an appropriate name. *J Am Coll Cardiol* 1991; 17: 1471.

Pepine CJ. Prognostic implications of silent myocardial ischemia. *N Engl J Med* 1996; 334: 113.

Petch MC. Coronary bypasses 10 years on. *Br Med J* 1991; 303: 661.

Timmis AD. Probability analysis in the diagnosis of coronary artery disease. *Br Med J* 1985; 291: 1443.

Topol EJ. Caveats about elective coronary stenting. *N Engl J Med* 1994; 331: 539.

Underwood MJ, More RS. The aspirin papers. *Br Med J* 1994; 308: 71.

ACUTE ISCHAEMIC SYNDROMES

Anonymous. Magnesium for acute myocardial infarction. *Lancet* 1991; 338: 667.

Anonymous. Predictors of sudden death after myocardial infarction. *Lancet* 1991; 338: 727.

Cairns JA. Medical management of unstable angina. *Lancet* 1995; 346: 1644.

Chua TP, Lipkin DP. Cardiac rehabilitation. *Br Med J* 1993; 306: 731.

Cobbe SM. Thrombolysis in acute myocardial infarction. *Br Med J* 1994; 308: 216.

Davies MJ, Thomas AC. Plaque fissuring—the cause of acute myocardial infarction, sudden ischaemic cardiac death, and crescendo angina. *Br Heart J* 1985; 53: 363.

Fuster V. Coronary thrombolysis—a perspective for the practicing physician. *N Engl J Med* 1993; 329: 723.

Grines CL, Weaver WD. Treating myocardial infarction: importance of early reperfusion. *Lancet* 1994; 344: 490.

Ham CW. New serum markers for acute myocardial infarction. *N Engl J Med* 1994; 331: 607.

Herbert P. Suspected myocardial infarction and the GP. *Br Med J* 1994; 308: 734.

Keung EC. Antiarrhythmic treatment and myocardial infarction. *J Am Coll Cardiol* 1990; 16: 1719.

Kinch JW, Ryan TJ. Right ventricular infarction. *N Engl J Med* 1994; 330: 1211.

Lamas GA, Pfeffer MA. Left ventricular remodeling after acute myocardial infarction: clinical course and beneficial effects of angiotensin-converting enzyme inhibition. *Am Heart J* 1991; 121: 1194.

Lange RA, Hillis LD. Immediate angioplasty for acute myocardial infarction. *N Engl J Med* 1993; 328: 726.

Lubsen J. Medical management of unstable angina: what have we learnt from the randomized trials? *Circulation* 1990; 82 (suppl II): 82.

Mayou R. Rehabilitation after heart attack. *Br Med J* 1996; 313: 1498.

Muller JE, Verrier RL. Triggering of sudden death—lessons from an earthquake. *N Engl J Med* 1996; 334: 460.

Northridge DB, Hall RJC. Post-myocardial-infarction exercise testing in the thrombolytic era. *Lancet* 1994; 343: 1175.

Pfeffer MA. ACE-inhibition in acute myocardial infarction. *N Engl J Med* 1995; 332: 118.

Pringle SD, Boon NA. Immediate coronary angioplasty for acute myocardial infarction. *Br Med J* 1993; 306: 1489.

Schoenfeld MH. Sustained ventricular arrhythmias after infarction: when should the worrying begin? *J Am Coll Cardiol* 1991; 17: 327.

Timmis AD. Early diagnosis of acute myocardial infarction. *Br Med J* 1990; 301: 941.

Topol EJ, Calitt RM. Thrombolytic therapy for elderly patients. *N Engl J Med* 1992; 327: 45.

Uren NG, Chronos NAF. Intracoronary stents. *Br Med J* 1996; 313: 892.

Vannan MA, Taylor DJE, Webb-Peploe MM, Korstan MA. ACE inhibitors after myocardial infarction. *Br Med J* 1993; 306: 531.

Verheugt FWA. Primary angioplasty for acute myocardial infarction. *Lancet* 1996; 347: 1276.

White H. Thrombolytic therapy for recurrent myocardial infarction. *Br Med J* 1991; 302: 429–30.

White HD. Angioplasty versus bypass surgery. *Lancet* 1995; 346: 1174.

Wilcox RG. Coronary thrombolysis: round two and beyond. *Br Heart J* 1991; 65: 175.

Yusuf S, Sleight P, Held P, McMahon S. Routine medical management of acute myocardial infarction: lessons from overviews of recent randomized controlled trials. *Circulation* 1990; 82 (suppl II): 117.

Cardiomyopathy and Specific Heart-Muscle Disorders

C O N T E N T S

SUMMARY

Cardiomyopathy is defined as chronic heart-muscle disease not caused by ischaemic, hypertensive, congenital or valvular disease. Indeed, in most cases the cause is unknown. *Dilated cardiomyopathy* is characterized by ventricular dilatation and hypertrophy with global impairment of systolic function. It may be the result of viral infection, chronic alcohol abuse or doxorubicin toxicity but in most cases it is idiopathic, although some evidence exists for an infectious–immune aetiology related to myocarditis. It presents with the symptoms and signs of congestive heart failure. The chest X-ray and echocardiogram help confirm the diagnosis, and treatment with ACE inhibitors and diuretics is the same as for other causes of heart failure. *Hypertrophic cardiomyopathy* is usually a familial disorder characterized anatomically by left ventricular hypertrophy, histologically by myocyte disarray, and physiologically by impaired diastolic relaxation. The echocardiogram is usually diagnostic. Hypertrophic cardiomyopathy may cause dyspnoea or angina requiring treatment with beta-blockers but in many cases it presents with sudden death caused by ventricular arrhythmias. Thus all patients should undergo ambulatory ECG monitoring and those with arrhythmias should be protected with amiodarone. *Restrictive cardiomyopathy* is rare in this country. It may be caused by a variety of pathological processes, particularly amyloidosis, but also haemochromatosis and glycogen deposition. Endomyocardial fibrosis is an uncommon cause in this country where it may be associated with cryptogenic hypereosinophilia. Physiologically it resembles constrictive pericarditis but differential diagnosis is usually possible by computed tomography which demonstrates normal pericardial thickness in patients with restriction. Restrictive cardiomyopathy presents with symptoms of heart failure requiring treatment with diuretics. Steroids may improve prognosis in patients with endomyocardial fibrosis associated with hypereosinophilia.

CARDIOMYOPATHY

The cardiomyopathies are a group of chronic heart-muscle disorders, excluding those that are secondary to ischaemic, hypertensive, congenital or valvular disease. In most cases the cause is unknown.

Dilated cardiomyopathy

Dilated cardiomyopathy is characterized by ventricular dilatation and hypertrophy associated with impaired systolic function. It occurs more commonly in the Third World than in developed countries.

Aetiology

A variety of systemic disorders affect the myocardium to produce a cardiac lesion that is often indistinguishable from idiopathic dilated cardiomyopathy (Table 6.1). The most common of these disorders (viral infection, alcohol and doxorubicin toxicity) are discussed below; others are discussed in Chapter 16. In most cases of dilated cardiomyopathy, however, the cause is unknown but some evidence exists for an infectious–immune aetiology related to myocarditis. Heart-reactive antibodies and other serological markers of autoimmunity can occasionally be

Toxic
Alcohol
Doxorubicin
Cobalt

Infective
Viral, e.g. Coxsackie A and B, influenza, varicella, mumps, herpes simplex
Protozoal, e.g. trypanosomiasis (Chagas' disease)

Metabolic
Thiamine deficiency (beriberi)
Kwashiorkor

Endocrine
Thyrotoxicosis
Myxoedema
Diabetes mellitus

Connective tissue disease
Polyarteritis nodosa
Systemic lupus erythematosus

Neuromuscular disease
Muscular dystrophy

Miscellaneous
Peripartum cardiomyopathy
Obesity

Table 6.1 Common causes of dilated cardiomyopathy.

demonstrated in dilated cardiomyopathy. Moreover, myocardial biopsy specimens show histological features typical of myocarditis in over 15% of cases; in some of these, antibody tests for Coxsackie B virus are positive. Thus it is possible that in certain cases abnormal immunological responses to common viral infections result in myocardial damage leading to dilated cardiomyopathy.

Viral myocarditis

Myocarditis occurs in a variety of infective disorders but viral disease is the most important cause in this country. Although viruses have never been unequivocally recovered from human myocardium, serological studies have identified Coxsackie B as the most common. Others include influenza and herpes simplex. Transient ECG changes (usually T-wave inversion) commonly occur during viral infection and probably reflect subclinical myocardial involvement. Occasionally symptoms and signs of congestive heart failure develop, usually while other signs of viral infection are subsiding. Cardiac arrhythmias and pericarditis may also occur. The chest X-ray shows variable cardiac enlargement and the echocardiogram confirms ventricular dilatation and contractile impairment. In most cases there is complete recovery within a week but, rarely, fulminant heart failure and death occurs. The relationship between viral myocarditis and dilated cardiomyopathy remains speculative but it may well be that many of the idiopathic cases are mediated by an immune response to occult viral infection (see above).

Alcoholic cardiomyopathy

The acute and chronic effects of alcohol poisoning on the heart must be distinguished. Acutely, alcohol intoxication causes cardiac arrhythmia, usually AF, which reverts spontaneously to sinus rhythm as blood-alcohol levels decline. Indeed, alcohol intoxication is probably the most common cause of AF in young adults. Much more serious is chronic alcohol abuse which, over a period of 10 years or more, can lead to dilated cardiomyopathy. In some cases, nutritional deficiencies (e.g. thiamine) or toxic beer additives (e.g. cobalt) may contribute to myocardial damage. In the large majority of cases, however, the toxic effects of alcohol or its metabolites are directly responsible. AF occurs more commonly in alcoholic cardiomyopathy than idiopathic cases, but in all other respects cardiac manifestations are identical. A history of heavy alcohol consumption is highly suggestive of an alcoholic aetiology, particularly when other manifestations of alcohol abuse are present. Abstinence may prevent progression of alcoholic cardiomyopathy and, in some cases, results in variable improvement; complete regression occasionally occurs if treatment is started early.

Doxorubicin-induced cardiomyopathy

The myocardial toxicity of the cytotoxic drug doxorubicin (and related compounds epirubicin and daunorubicin) is largely dose-related and rarely occurs if the total cumulative dose is less than 500 mg/m^2, a level normally achieved after 6–8 months of therapy. Children appear particularly susceptible, and even relatively small doses can lead to a lifelong reduction in myocardial mass that may result in decreased cardiac reserve. Other factors such as mediastinal irradiation may have synergistic cardiotoxic effects in patients receiving doxorubicin. Cardiomyopathy usually presents acutely, with symptoms and signs of severe congestive heart failure. The response to antifailure treatment is almost invariably unsatisfactory and death usually occurs within a few weeks of presentation. Once symptomatic heart failure is established, withdrawal of doxorubicin does not halt progression of the cardiomyopathy. Endomyocardial biopsy is the most sensitive means of identifying early doxorubicin toxicity but this is not feasible in most centres. Regular non-invasive monitoring by echocardiography or radionuclide ventriculography is recommended, with a view to doxorubicin withdrawal at the first sign of left ventricular dysfunction.

Pathophysiology

In dilated cardiomyopathy, the relative degree of left and right ventricular impairment is variable, but in advanced cases severe biventricular failure is usually present. Enhanced sympathoadrenal activity is a 'hallmark' of the disease and may be regarded as a compensatory phenomenon directed at maintaining systolic function and increasing ventricular filling by central redistribution of flow. Nevertheless, the inotropic responsiveness of the failing heart diminishes progressively, possibly as a result of adrenoceptor down-regulation (see page 79). As cardiac output and renal perfusion deteriorate, secondary aldosteronism leads to salt and water retention which not only further increases ventricular filling but also causes worsening systemic and pulmonary congestion.

Thus the heart is exposed to a considerably exaggerated volume load. This results in progressive dilatation, hypertrophy and fibrosis of all the cardiac chambers. Atrial fibrillation (AF) commonly supervenes, particularly in alcoholic cardiomyopathy, and stretching of the atrioventricular valve rings can lead to functional incompetence of the mitral and tricuspid valves, which causes additional impairment of ventricular function.

Clinical manifestations

Dilated cardiomyopathy often remains asymptomatic in its early stages but, with progression of the disease, symptoms and signs of congestive heart failure develop, particularly effort-related fatigue and dyspnoea. Orthopnoea and peripheral oedema develop later in the course of the illness. At this stage, tachycardia and signs of cardiac enlargement are invariably present. The jugular venous pulse (JVP) is elevated, often with a giant 'v' wave due to tricuspid regurgitation. Auscultation reveals a third heart sound; pansystolic murmurs of mitral and tricuspid regurgitation may also be present.

Complications

Cardiac arrhythmias are common in dilated cardiomyopathy, particularly AF and ventricular premature beats. More complex ventricular arrhythmias account for the significant incidence of sudden death in this condition. Systemic and pulmonary thromboembolism arising from the dilated left- and right-sided cardiac chambers may also occur (Fig. 6.1).

Diagnosis

The ECG is invariably abnormal in dilated cardiomyopathy but the changes are non-specific and may include arrhythmias (see above), bundle branch block and T-wave flattening or inversion. The chest X-ray shows cardiac enlargement with dilated upper lobe veins, progressing to pulmonary oedema. The echocardiogram is the most useful diagnostic investigation and shows four-chamber dilatation and global left ventricular contractile impairment (Fig. 6.1). Doppler studies often reveal mitral and tricuspid regurgitation.

Differential diagnosis

The differential diagnosis includes ischaemic, hypertensive, congenital or valvular disease. Ischaemic disease is suggested by a history of angina or MI, associated with pathological Q waves on the ECG. Valvular and congenital disease can usually be diagnosed by echocardiography, although mitral regurgitation can present difficulties as it can be both the cause and the result of left ventricular failure. In hypertensive disease, the history is often helpful and the examination may reveal other non-cardiac manifestations of end-organ injury.

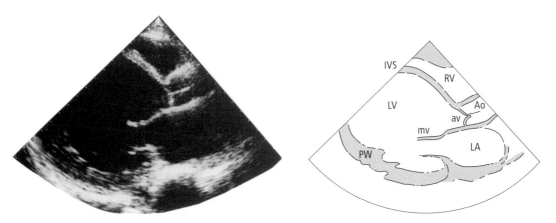

Fig. 6.1 Dilated cardiomyopathy. Echocardiogram. Note the severe left ventricular dilatation with global contractile impairment.

Treatment

Management is the same as for congestive heart failure although additional measures may be necessary in those cases where a specific cause can be identified (see below). ACE inhibitors have a clear prognostic benefit and should be introduced when the diagnosis is made. In patients with evidence of fluid retention diuretics are also required.

Prophylactic anticoagulation with warfarin is necessary for patients in AF, because the risk of thromboembolism is greatest in this group. Anticoagulation is also necessary in patients who have already had a thromboembolic event, regardless of the cardiac rhythm, so long as there are no specific contraindications.

Ventricular arrhythmias—particularly ventricular tachycardia—should be suppressed with an appropriate agent, although it is not known whether this prevents sudden death. Amiodarone is the drug of choice because it is less negatively inotropic than class 1 antiarrhythmic agents (see page 246). Treatment should be monitored with ambulatory ECG monitoring (see page 37).

Prognosis

The prognosis in dilated cardiomyopathy is variable, depending upon the degree of left ventricular dysfunction and the incidence of ventricular arrhythmias. Once symptoms of heart failure develop, the average 5-year survival is less than 50%.

Hypertrophic cardiomyopathy

Hypertrophic cardiomyopathy is known by a variety of other names (e.g. hypertrophic obstructive cardiomyopathy, idiopathic hypertrophic subaortic stenosis, asymmetrical septal hypertrophy), all of which should now be discarded since they make inaccurate assumptions about the nature of the disease. Hypertrophic cardiomyopathy is characterized *anatomically* by ventricular hypertrophy of unknown cause, usually with disproportionate involvement of the interventricular septum. *Physiologically* the disorder is one of impaired diastolic relaxation of the non-compliant ventricles; systolic function is well preserved and usually hyperdynamic. *Pathologically* there is extensive disarray and disorganization of cardiac myocytes.

Aetiology

Hypertrophic cardiomyopathy shows an autosomal dominant pattern of inheritance in some families, although the expression of disease within the family is very variable. The disease has protean manifestations and it is now uncertain whether there is one genetic abnormality, or several, all of which produce abnormal left ventricular hypertrophy. The difficulties of producing a unifying genetic aetiology are heightened by the observation that in some patients the disease is present from a very young age while in others born with apparently normal hearts it does not develop until adulthood. Further complexity is introduced by recent autopsy findings in young previously healthy patients who died suddenly and whose families were known to have hypertrophic cardiomyopathy. There was extensive myocardial disarray typical of the disease without evidence of hypertrophy. Whether these patients would have gone on to develop the morphological features of hypertrophic cardiomyopathy is unknown.

Pathophysiology

Disordered diastolic function is the principal pathophysiological feature. The hypertrophic, non-compliant ventricle exhibits profoundly impaired diastolic relaxation (see Fig. 4.2). Thus, adequate ventricular filling is dependent upon high diastolic pressure. Atrial systole is particularly important for maintaining adequate filling and the development of AF (or atrioventricular dissociation) can produce abrupt deterioration in cardiac output (Fig. 6.2).

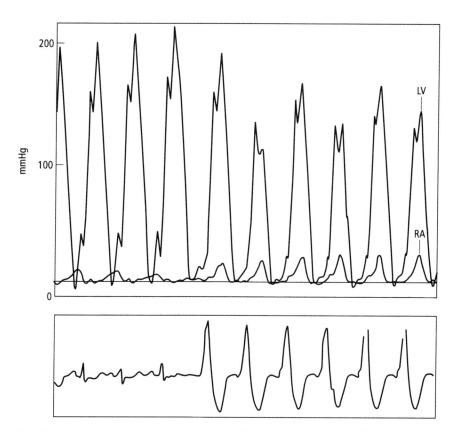

Fig. 6.2 Hypertrophic cardiomyopathy—ventricular pacing. Simultaneous recordings of the ECG and left ventricular (LV) and right atrial (RA) pressure signals are shown. Ventricular pacing produces a broad complex rhythm with AV dissociation. The loss of synchronized atrial contraction at end-diastole impairs LV filling and causes abrupt deterioration in function evidenced by pulsus alternans, a fall in LV pressure and a rise in RA pressure.

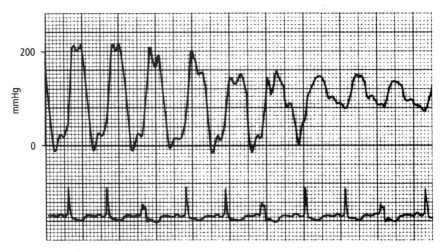

Fig. 6.3 Hypertrophic cardiomyopathy—left ventricular outflow gradient. The catheter has been pulled back from the apex of the left ventricle into the aorta during simultaneous pressure recording. After the fourth beat there is an abrupt drop in left ventricular systolic pressure, representing a subvalvular gradient of about 50 mmHg. Note that there is no systolic pressure gradient across the aortic valve itself.

Systolic function is always vigorous in hypertrophic cardiomyopathy and the left ventricular ejection fraction is usually in excess of 90%. Ventricular emptying is not only more complete than in the normal ventricle, it is also more rapid. Thus, 80% of the stroke volume is ejected in the first half of systole compared with 57% in the normal ventricle.

In many (not all) cases of hypertrophic cardiomyopathy there is a subvalvular aortic pressure gradient caused by the bulky interventricular septum and the systolic anterior motion of the mitral valve leaflets obstructing the left ventricular outflow tract in systole (Fig. 6.3). The obstruction is *dynamic* and can be provoked or exaggerated by physiological stimuli (extrasystoles, Valsalva) or inotropic drugs (Fig. 6.4). This must be distinguished from the *fixed* outflow obstruction caused by aortic stenosis.

The importance of the subvalvular pressure gradient in hypertrophic cardio-myopathy may have been exaggerated. The obstruction caused by the anterior motion of the mitral valve leaflets occurs too late to impede left ventricular ejection, 80% of which is complete by mid-systole. Although symptoms may be improved by surgical debulking of the interventricular septum, this is as likely to reflect improved diastolic relaxation as relief of outflow obstruction. Importantly, neither symptoms nor prognosis are related to the presence or severity of the subvalvular pressure gradient.

Clinical manifestations

Hypertrophic cardiomyopathy is often asymptomatic. The most common com-plaint is exercise-related dyspnoea, due to the elevated left atrial pressure required to fill the stiff, non-compliant ventricle. In advanced cases, frank congestive heart

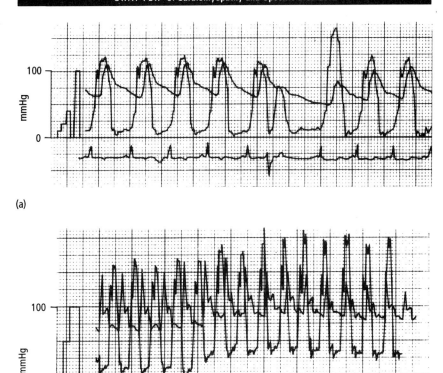

(a)

(b)

Fig. 6.4 Hypertrophic cardiomyopathy—provocation of left ventricular outflow gradient. Simultaneous recordings of the left ventricular and aortic pressure signals are shown. (a) Ventricular premature beat. After the fifth sinus beat there is a ventricular extrasystole. Note that in the post-extrasystolic beat marked exaggeration of the subvalvular pressure gradient occurs. (b) Valsalva manoeuvre. During Valsalva (evidenced by the rise in left ventricular diastolic pressure) there is a progressive increase in the subvalvular pressure gradient.

failure occasionally develops. Angina, due to the excessive oxygen demand of the hypertrophied ventricle, may also be troublesome.

Examination reveals a 'jerky' carotid pulse, due to forceful ejection early in systole. The apical impulse is forceful and often has a double thrust, due to a palpable fourth heart sound. Auscultatory features include the fourth heart sound and a mid-systolic murmur in the aortic area, due to turbulent flow in the left ventricular outflow tract. Mitral regurgitation affects nearly 50% of cases, causing an apical pansystolic murmur.

Complications

Cardiac arrhythmias are the major complication. AF causes abrupt clinical deterioration (see page 153). Paroxysmal ventricular arrhythmias produce dizziness and syncope (Stokes–Adams attacks) and may herald sudden death.

Diagnosis

In the majority of patients, the ECG shows ventricular hypertrophy with prominent voltage deflexions in the chest leads (see Fig. 12.1). A broad-notched P wave reflects left atrial enlargement. Q waves unrelated to infarction are found in up to 30% of cases, usually in the infero-lateral leads. The chest X-ray is normal.

The echocardiogram is usually diagnostic (Fig. 6.5) and shows left ventricular hypertrophy, often with disproportionate involvement of the interventricular septum (*asymmetrical septal hypertrophy*). The two-dimensional recording is required for accurate assessment of the extent and distribution of left ventricular hypertrophy (Fig. 6.5). Other echocardiographic manifestations of hypertrophic cardiomyopathy include systolic obliteration of the left ventricular cavity, systolic anterior motion (SAM) of the mitral valve and mid-systolic closure of the aortic valve.

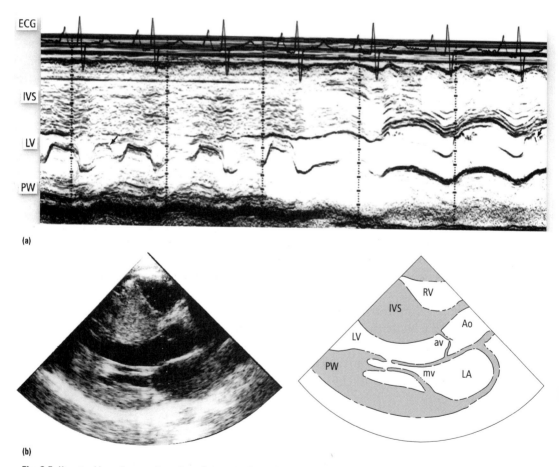

(a)

(b)

Fig. 6.5 Hypertrophic cardiomyopathy—echocardiogram. (a) The M-mode recording shows marked hypertrophy of the interventricular septum with a normal posterior wall. Systolic anterior motion of the mitral valve and early closure of the aortic valve are indicated by the arrows. (b) A better appreciation of the septal hypertrophy is provided by the two-dimensional recording.

Cardiac catheterization is rarely necessary for diagnostic purposes. The left ventricular angiogram shows a hypertrophic ventricle with systolic cavity obliteration. Haemodynamic studies may demonstrate the pressure gradient in the left ventricular outflow tract.

Differential diagnosis

The symptoms, signs and ECG findings in hypertrophic cardiomyopathy resemble those in aortic stenosis, although the character of the carotid pulse is different (jerky versus slow rising). The echocardiogram is particularly helpful, and in aortic stenosis shows a thickened valve associated with left ventricular hypertrophy but not with other features of hypertrophic cardiomyopathy.

Other important differential diagnoses are coronary artery disease and hypertensive heart disease. In patients with angina, exclusion of coronary artery disease may require coronary arteriography. Hypertensive heart disease is suggested by a history of hypertension and by evidence of hypertensive injury elsewhere in the body, particularly the optic fundus and the kidneys.

Treatment

No drugs have been shown to affect disease progression in hypertrophic cardiomyopathy; treatment is aimed at correcting symptoms and preventing sudden death: beta-blockers (e.g. atenolol) are first-line agents. By slowing the heart rate they control angina and improve diastolic filling of the left ventricle. Calcium antagonists (e.g. verapamil) improve diastolic relaxation and are sometimes helpful in patients who fail to respond to beta-blockers.

Surgical procedures involving debulking of the interventricular septum in the outflow tract have been shown to correct symptoms (see above), but do not affect long-term prognosis and should be reserved for patients with intractable symptoms. Recently, a catheter technique has been described for selective infarction of the interventricular septum by injection of sclerosant into the first septal perforator. This effectively relieves outflow obstruction but whether it produces long-term clinical benefit is not known.

All patients with hypertrophic cardiomyopathy should undergo ambulatory ECG monitoring for at least 48 hours. If ventricular arrhythmias are detected, amiodarone is the drug of choice because preliminary evidence suggests that it may prevent sudden death. Because hypertrophic cardiomyopathy is inherited, the patient should receive genetic counselling and members of the family should be screened.

Prognosis

Hypertrophic cardiomyopathy has an annual mortality of about 2.5% in adults, but the prognosis is worse in children, about 6% of whom die each year. The majority of deaths occur suddenly, presumably caused by VF.

Restrictive cardiomyopathy

Aetiology

Amyloidosis

Amyloidosis associated with myeloma affects the heart quite commonly, as does the organ-limited 'senile' amyloidosis seen usually in the elderly. Familial amyloidosis may also affect the heart, but the reactive amyloidosis caused by chronic infectious or inflammatory conditions rarely does so.

Other metabolic disorders

Haemochromatosis and glycogen deposition are rare causes of restriction.

Endomyocardial fibrosis

This causes progressive obliteration of the ventricular cavities. It is rare in this country (where it has been called Loffler's endocarditis) and is nearly always associated with cryptogenic hypereosinophilia. It occurs more commonly in the tropics, but usually without hypereosinophilia. Endomyocardial damage induced by local release of eosinophilic granules has been postulated as a pathogenic mechanism, but this is unlikely to provide the full explanation since an identical cardiac lesion occurs in the tropical form of the disease.

Pathophysiology

The pathophysiology is almost identical to that of constrictive pericarditis (see page 179). The ventricle relaxes normally in early diastole, but by mid-diastole becomes virtually indistensible. Thus ventricular filling is at first rapid but is abruptly checked in mid-diastole, producing a characteristic dip-and-plateau configuration on the ventricular diastolic pressure recording obtained at cardiac catheterization (Fig. 6.6). With progression of disease, ventricular filling deteriorates, despite elevation and equalization of the filling pressures on both sides of the heart. Occasionally, the normal differential between right- and left-sided filling pressures is preserved, such that right atrial pressure, though elevated, remains lower than left atrial pressure throughout the cardiac cycle. This is in contrast to constrictive pericarditis, in which equalization of the ventricular filling pressures on both sides of the heart always occurs (see Fig. 7.6).

Clinical manifestations

Restrictive cardiomyopathy presents with congestive heart failure. The patient complains of peripheral oedema and effort-related fatigue and dyspnoea. The JVP is elevated, with an unusually dynamic waveform due to a prominent 'y'

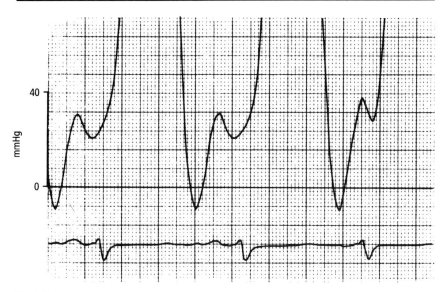

Fig. 6.6 Restrictive cardiomyopathy—left ventricular pressure signal. The rapid rise in diastolic pressure is checked abruptly in mid-diastole by the restrictive effect of the left ventricle. This gives the diastolic pressure signal its characteristic 'dip-and-plateau' contour.

descent (rapid ventricular filling in early diastole), and Kussmaul's sign is present (see page 14). Auscultation reveals third or fourth heart sounds.

Complications

Cardiac arrhythmias are less common than in other types of cardiomyopathy. Systemic and pulmonary thromboembolism from the affected ventricles may occur.

Diagnosis

In most cases, confirmation of the diagnosis is dependent upon demonstration of typical restrictive physiology at cardiac catheterization (Fig. 6.6). Endomyocardial biopsy during the catheter procedure provides the histological diagnosis.

Differential diagnosis

Constrictive pericarditis mimics restrictive cardiomyopathy clinically and haemo-dynamically. Differential diagnosis depends upon computed tomography which shows pericardial thickening in constriction but not in restriction.

Treatment

In restriction caused by amyloid and other metabolic disorders, diuretics for heart failure and anticoagulants to guard against thromboembolism are the only therapeutic measures of value although they do not affect disease progression. In endomyocardial fibrosis associated with hypereosinophilia, steroids or cytotoxic agents lower the eosinophil count and may halt disease progression and produce significant symptomatic improvement. Surgical excision of the fibrotic endocardium may be helpful in advanced cases, presumably because the reduction in myocardial mass improves diastolic relaxation.

Prognosis

The prognosis in cardiac amyloid is very poor, most patients dying within a year of diagnosis. Prognosis is also poor in the rarer metabolic disorders causing restrictive cardiomyopathy but, in endomyocardial fibrosis, patients who respond well to definitive medical and surgical treatment (see above) may have a good prognosis. Progressive fibrosis, however, with worsening congestive heart failure, has a less favourable outlook.

FURTHER READING

Alcoholic myopathy and cardiomyopathy. *N Engl J Med* 1989; 320: 458.

Anonymous. Cardiac biopsy in myocarditis. *Lancet* 1990; 336: 283.

Anonymous. Dilated cardiomyopathy and enteroviruses. *Lancet* 1990; 336: 971.

Caforio ALP, Stewart JT, McKenna WJ. Idiopathic dilated cardiomyopathy. *Br Med J* 1990; 300: 890.

Chahine RA. Surgical versus medical therapy of hypertrophic cardiomyopathy: is the perspective changing? *J Am Coll Cardiol* 1991; 17: 643.

Clark AL, Coats AJS. Screening for hypertrophic cardiomyopathy. *Br Med J* 1993; 306: 409.

Curfman GD. Molecular insights into hypertrophic cardiomyopathy. *N Engl J Med* 1992; 326: 1149.

Davies MJ. Hypertrophic cardiomyopathy: one disease or several? *Br Heart J* 1990; 63: 263.

Dec GW, Fuster V. Idiopathic dilated cardiomyopathy. *N Engl J Med* 1994; 331: 1564.

Doroshow JH. Doxorubicin-induced cardiotoxicity. *N Engl J Med* 1991; 324: 843.

Kelly DP, Strauss AW. Inherited cardiomyopathies. *N Engl J Med* 1994; 330: 1724.

Parrillo JE. Heart disease and the eosinophil. *N Engl J Med* 1990; 323: 1560.

Wilmshurst PT, Katritsis D. Restrictive cardiomyopathy. *Br Heart J* 1990; 63: 323.

CHAPTER 7

Pericardial Disease

SUMMARY

Pericarditis, the most common pericardial disorder, is usually idiopathic or viral in origin, occasionally reflecting more serious systemic disease. Typically, it presents with sharp central chest pain aggravated by deep inspiration, coughing and changes in posture. The ECG shows widespread 'concave' ST elevation. Treatment is with anti-inflammatory analgesics and recovery can normally be expected within a few days. Almost any cause of pericarditis can lead to effusion, and *tamponade* may develop if the fluid collects rapidly, leading to critical elevation of pressure in the pericardial sac and restriction of ventricular filling. This is particularly common when malignant disease of the breast or lung invades the pericardium. In tamponade the diastolic filling pressures of both right and left ventricles rise and equilibrate with loss of the normal differential. The patient presents with dyspnoea and hypotension; a paradoxical pulse is invariable, the JVP is elevated and Kussmaul's sign is commonly present. Treatment is by pericardiocentesis. When pericarditis leads to fibrosis and shrinkage of the pericardial sac, *constriction* may occur. This impedes diastolic relaxation and restricts ventricular filling, with physiology similar to that of tamponade. It is a chronic, debilitating illness, characterized by elevation of the JVP, a positive Kussmaul's sign and fluid retention with oedema and ascites. Cardiac catheterization demonstrates elevation and equalization of the ventricular filling pressures and computed tomography or magnetic resonance imaging confirm thickening of the pericardium. Diuretics are helpful for controlling fluid retention, but definitive treatment requires pericardiectomy.

INTRODUCTION

The pericardium envelops the heart and the proximal portions of the great arteries and veins. The visceral pericardium is intimately attached to the epicardial surface of the heart and is separated from the parietal pericardium by the pericardial space, which is filled by the heart in diastole. Further dilatation of the heart is resisted by the relatively indistensible pericardial sac. The pericardium plays an important role in preventing rapid cardiac dilatation when ventricular diastolic pressures rise acutely but, in contrast to its effect on diastolic function, does not influence the systolic function of the heart.

ACUTE PERICARDITIS

Aetiology

Causes of pericarditis are listed in Table 7.1. Viral infection probably accounts for the majority of cases, including many of those idiopathic cases in which a specific cause cannot be positively identified. Purulent bacterial pericarditis (e.g. *Staphylococcus, Streptococcus*) has become considerably less common, as has tuberculous pericarditis. Pericarditis is a frequent complication of advanced renal failure and is not always prevented by regular dialysis; the cause is unknown. In acute myocardial infarction (MI), pericarditis usually denotes extensive full-thickness damage but it may also occur late following infarction, when Dressler's syndrome is the likely diagnosis (see page 143). Polyserositis involving the pericardium characterizes many connective tissue disorders, particularly rheumatoid disease and systemic lupus erythematosus. Patients with neoplastic disease may develop pericarditis due either to cardiac metastases or to therapeutic irradiation of the chest. Pericarditis is an inevitable consequence of opening the pericardial sac during heart surgery, and may also occur following accidental chest trauma.

Table 7.1 Causes of acute pericarditis.

Idiopathic
Infective
viral (Coxsackie B, influenza, mumps, varicella) bacterial (*Staphylococcus, Streptococcus, Mycobacterium tuberculosis*)
Connective tissue disease—systemic lupus erythematosus, rheumatoid arthritis
Myocardial infarction
Following myocardial infarction or cardiac surgery—Dressler's syndrome
Uraemia
Neoplastic disease—breast, lung, lymphoma, leukaemia
Radiation therapy

Clinical manifestations

In acute pericarditis, chest pain is the predominant symptom and commonly follows an upper respiratory tract infection in viral pericarditis. It is retrosternal in most cases but differs from the pain of MI by its sharp quality which is aggravated by deep inspiration, coughing and changes in posture (particularly lying flat). Occasionally, the pain has an aching quality and radiates into the shoulders or arms making it more difficult to distinguish from ischaemic cardiac pain. Auscultation of the heart typically, though not invariably, reveals a pericardial friction rub which confirms the diagnosis. The rub has a high-pitched scratching quality and may be audible during any phase of the cardiac cycle. Its intensity is influenced by respiration and changes in posture.

Complications

The major complication is pericardial effusion which may cause tamponade. Pericarditis can also progress to pericardial constriction although this may not manifest itself for several years. Atrial arrhythmias are reported to occur commonly in pericarditis but this has been difficult to confirm in prospective studies.

Diagnosis

The chest X-ray is usually normal in pericarditis, except when pericardial effusion produces cardiac enlargement. The ECG may also be normal but in most cases there is ST segment elevation, reflecting epicardial injury (Fig. 7.1). The ST segment elevation affects any or all of the standard or precordial leads (except aVR) depending on the site of inflammation, and is characteristically concave upwards (unlike myocardial infarction) returning towards baseline as pericardial inflammation subsides. T-wave inversion is common, but the evolution of ST segment and T-wave changes seen in myocardial infarction does not occur. Importantly, Q waves never develop in pericarditis.

The aetiological diagnosis in viral pericarditis depends upon the demonstration of elevated viral antibody titres in acute serum samples, which decline during convalescence. Virus may sometimes be cultured from throat swabs and stools. In connective tissue disorders there is usually evidence of multisystem disease; specific serology, including rheumatoid or antinuclear factors, may be positive. Purulent pericarditis is often associated with infective foci elsewhere in the body, particularly the lungs, and cultures of sputum and blood samples should be obtained. Recognition of tuberculous pericarditis is difficult if the chest X-ray is normal. When the aetiology is doubtful, pericardial fluid (if present) may be aspirated for bacteriological, cytological and serological examination.

Differential diagnosis

Important differential diagnoses in acute pericarditis are MI and pleurisy. The

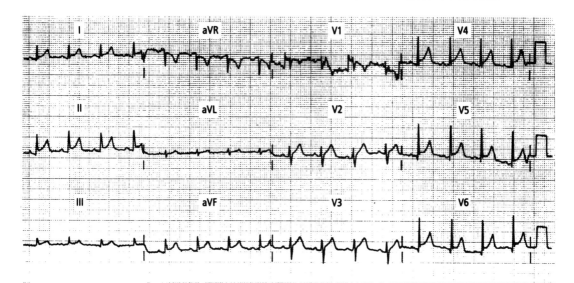

Fig. 7.1 ECG in acute pericarditis. Note the concave ST segment elevation present in multiple leads.

quality of pericarditic pain, the widespread (nonregional) ST change, the failure of Q waves to develop, and the absence of serum enzyme changes, are usually sufficient to rule out MI. Pleuritic pain is similar in quality to pericarditis but its location is different: a pleural rub is often audible over the painful area and signs of pleural effusion may also be present. In making the differential diagnosis, remember that pericarditis may occur in association with both MI and pleurisy.

Treatment

Treatment is directed at relieving chest pain and, if possible, correcting the underlying cause. Non-steroidal anti-inflammatory analgesics (e.g. aspirin, indomethacin) are drugs of choice for controlling symptoms. In viral pericarditis, no other treatment is necessary. Bacterial pericarditis requires vigorous antibiotic treatment, which in tuberculosis should be continued for at least a year.

Pericarditis may be recurrent, particularly in Dressler's syndrome, connective tissue disorders and idiopathic disease. When it is frequent and troublesome, low-dose steroid therapy offers effective prophylaxis.

Prognosis

Pericarditis is usually a benign disorder and the prognosis relates to the underlying cause. Nevertheless, any cause of pericarditis can lead to pericardial effusion and tamponade which may be lethal if not corrected. Pericarditis can also progress to pericardial constriction and heart failure.

PERICARDIAL EFFUSION AND TAMPONADE

Aetiology

The major causes of cardiac tamponade are haemopericardium following heart surgery, and pericardial effusion complicating neoplastic disease (Table 7.2). Nevertheless, almost any other cause of pericardial haemorrhage or effusion may lead to tamponade, depending principally on the rate of fluid accumulation within the pericardial sac.

Pathophysiology

Gradual accumulation of fluid permits progressive stretching of the pericardial sac, such that a substantial effusion may develop without significant elevation of intrapericardial pressure. However, rapid accumulation of fluid leads to critical elevation of pressure which impedes diastolic relaxation of both ventricles equally. Thus, adequate ventricular filling depends on the end-diastolic pressures in both ventricles rising to equilibrate with the intrapericardial pressure. The normal differential between ventricular filling pressures is therefore lost and the filling pressure on the right side of the heart comes to equal that on the left (Fig.7.2). As tamponade worsens, progressive increments in ventricular filling pressures become inadequate to maintain cardiac output.

Clinical manifestations

Tamponade occurs abruptly following haemorrhage into the pericardial sac, but the onset may be more gradual in patients with pericardial effusion. Shortness of breath and fatigue are the principal complaints. The examination reveals tachycardia, elevated jugular venous pulse (JVP), hypotension and signs of reduced

Table 7.2 Causes of tamponade.

Pericarditis
Neoplastic disease
Connective tissue disease (particularly rheumatoid)
Any other cause of pericarditis when pericardial effusion in a complication (see Table 7.1)
Haemopericardium
Heart surgery—postoperative haemorrhage
Myocardial infarction—rupture of free wall of ventricle
Aortic aneurysm—rupture into pericardial sac
Aortic dissection—rupture into pericardial sac
Chest trauma—penetrating or non-penetrating injury
Anticoagulant therapy
Chylopericardium
Idiopathic
Heart surgery—postoperative accumulation of lymph
Malignant disease—obstruction of lymphatics draining the heart

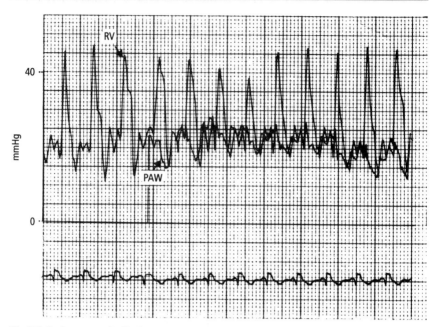

Fig. 7.2 Cardiac tamponade. Simultaneous recordings of the right ventricular (RV) and pulmonary artery wedge (PAW) pressure signals. Note that during diastole pressures are elevated and the recordings are effectively superimposed with loss of the normal differential. Equalization and elevation of the right- and left-sided ventricular filling pressures are characteristic of tamponade but also occur in constrictive pericarditis and restrictive cardiomyopathy.

cardiac output; frank cardiogenic shock may occur. A paradoxical pulse is invariable in cardiac tamponade and in many patients Kussmaul's sign also occurs (see Fig. 1.7). The waveform of the JVP is unusually dynamic due to an exaggerated 'x' descent (see page 16). Auscultation reveals faint heart sounds.

Diagnosis

Pericardial effusion produces globular enlargement of the cardiac silhouette (Fig. 7.3). The diagnosis should always be considered if an abrupt increase in heart size is demonstrated on serial chest X-rays (see Fig. 16.2). The ECG shows diminished voltage deflections and an alternating electrical axis may be present caused by movement of the heart within the fluid-filled pericardial sac (Fig. 7.4). Echocardiography confirms pericardial effusion (Fig. 7.5). In difficult cases, right heart catheterization is helpful, demonstrating equilibration of the right- and left-sided filling pressures as reflected by the right ventricular diastolic and pulmonary capillary wedge pressures, respectively (Fig. 7.2).

Differential diagnosis

Tamponade must be differentiated from other causes of low cardiac output and shock, including MI, pulmonary embolism and septicaemia. This is not difficult if a paradoxical pulse and pericardial effusion can be demonstrated.

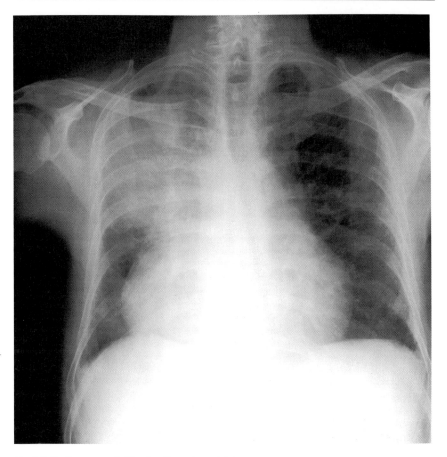

Fig. 7.3 Cardiac tamponade. The chest X-ray shows globular cardiac enlargement with segmental consolidation in the right upper lung field. Bronchoscopy confirmed a right hilar carcinoma which had infiltrated the pericardium causing tamponade.

Treatment

Pericardiocentesis should be undertaken at the earliest opportunity in order to decompress the heart. This is best performed by the subxiphisternal route while the patient reclines at 45°. Following infiltration of local anaesthetic, a needle is introduced into the angle between the xiphisternum and the left costal margin, and is advanced beneath the costal margin towards the left shoulder. Continuous suction applied to the syringe ensures that pericardial fluid is aspirated as the needle enters the effusion. The effusion is then aspirated to dryness.

When pericardial effusion is the result of neoplastic infiltration of the pericardium, fluid commonly reaccumulates following pericardiocentesis. In order to prevent reaccumulation, a drainage catheter can be left in the pericardial sac pending definitive treatment. The catheter is usually introduced over a guide-wire which can be inserted through the lumen of the aspiration needle. If cytotoxic therapy fails to prevent recurrent effusion, surgical excision of a pericardial segment may be necessary. This provides a 'window' through which

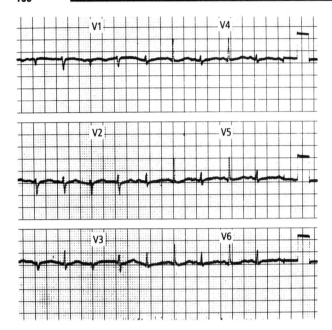

Fig. 7.4 Acute tamponade. The ECG shows diminished voltage deflexions and also an alternating electrical axis—beat-to-beat variation in R-wave amplitude most prominent in leads V4–V6.

the effusion drains, to be absorbed into the pleural and mediastinal lymphatics. An alternative means of improving pericardial drainage is to create a tear in the pericardium by inflating a balloon catheter across the pericardium.

CONSTRICTIVE PERICARDITIS

Constrictive pericarditis is no longer a common disease in developed countries, largely due to the declining incidence of tuberculosis which was responsible for most cases in the past.

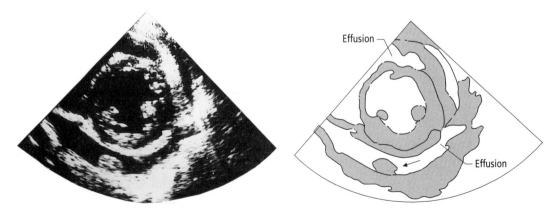

Fig. 7.5 Pericardial effusion. Two-dimensional echocardiogram, short axis view. The effusion produces an echo-free space around the heart. The patient had chicken-pox (a rare cause of pericardial effusion) and a pox lesion (arrowed) is visible on the parietal layer of the pericardium.

Aetiology

Pericarditis of any type may lead to constriction. Nevertheless, in developed countries, most cases are idiopathic in origin.

Pathophysiology

Constrictive physiology is very similar to that seen in restrictive cardiomyopathy and tamponade (see Fig. 4.2). Fibrosis and shrinkage of the pericardial sac impedes diastolic relaxation of the ventricles and prevents adequate filling. Compensatory increments in filling pressures occur and, because constriction usually affects both ventricles equally, the filling pressures also equilibrate. Thus atrial pressures and ventricular diastolic pressures on both sides of the heart are elevated and equal in constrictive pericarditis (Fig. 7.6). Systolic function is usually normal, but may be impaired in some cases due to myocardial involvement in the disease process.

Clinical manifestations

Constrictive pericarditis is a chronic debilitating illness. Though symptoms and signs of low cardiac output are usually present, the consequences of elevated systemic venous pressure, together with salt and water retention, dominate the clinical picture. The appearance is that of severe right heart failure with distension of the neck veins, hepatomegaly, ascites and peripheral oedema. Kussmaul's sign is invariably present but a paradoxical pulse is seen less commonly. The waveform

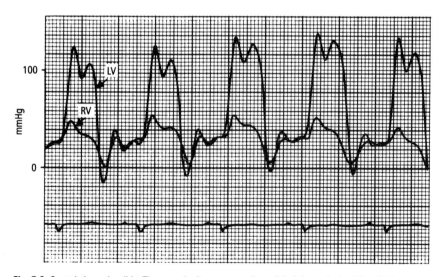

Fig. 7.6 Constrictive pericarditis. These are simultaneous recordings of the left ventricular (LV) and right ventricular (RV) pressure signals. Note the 'dip-and-plateau' configuration during diastole (*cf.* restrictive cardiomyopathy) with equalization of the diastolic pressures in both chambers. Equalization of left- and right-sided filling pressures also occurs in restrictive cardiomyopathy and cardiac tamponade.

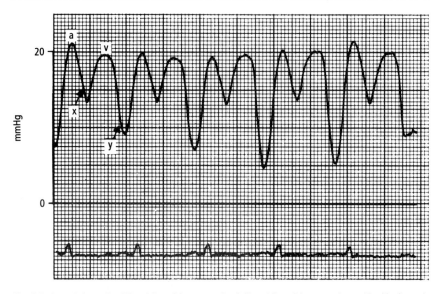

Fig. 7.7 Constrictive pericarditis—right atrial pressure signal. Note right atrial pressure is considerably elevated, with prominence of the 'y' descent.

of the JVP is unusually dynamic due to prominence of both the 'x' and the 'y' descent; the former, however, may be less marked in cases with impaired systolic function (Fig. 7.7). Auscultation reveals an early third heart sound (pericardial 'knock') due to rapid ventricular filling early in diastole.

Diagnosis

The ECG usually shows diminished voltage deflexions with non-specific ST segment and T wave changes. The chest X-ray may be normal; indeed, the combination of a normal heart size and signs of severe right-sided failure is suggestive of constriction. So is the presence of pericardial calcification (best seen on the lateral chest X-ray) although this is relatively uncommon in non-tuberculous constriction. The echocardiogram is rarely helpful. A better indication of pericardial thickening and calcification is provided by computed tomography (Fig. 7.8). Cardiac catheterization shows that the diastolic filling pressures in both ventricles are equal and elevated and have a characteristic dip-and-plateau configuration (see Fig. 7.6).

Differential diagnosis

This includes other causes of right heart failure, and cirrhosis of the liver. In most cases of right heart failure, the heart is enlarged and right ventricular dilatation can be demonstrated by echocardiography. Associated pulmonary vascular or left ventricular disease is often present. Cirrhosis produces ascites and debilitation, but does not show the cardiovascular manifestations of constrictive pericarditis. The

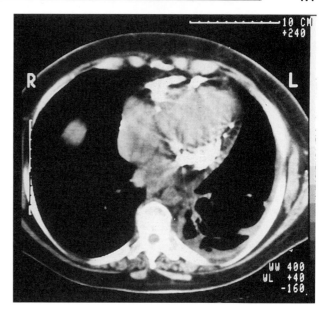

Fig. 7.8 Constrictive pericarditis—computed tomography. This transverse thoracic tomogram at the level of the heart shows dense pericardial calcification (arrowed) particularly in the interventricular groove anteriorly and posteriorly. The calcified pericardium has a white appearance similar to that of bone.

differentiation of constrictive pericarditis from restrictive cardiomyopathy is difficult, because both produce almost identical physiological changes. Nevertheless, computed tomography or magnetic resonance imaging usually permit reliable differential diagnosis by demonstrating a thickened, sometimes calcified, pericardium in constriction, but a normal pericardium in restriction.

Treatment

Diuretics can be used to control salt and water overload, and in some cases no other treatment is necessary. However, it should be recognized that diuretics do nothing to correct the constriction and by reducing ventricular filling may exacerbate the fundamental haemodynamic derangement. Thus, if symptoms are severe, pericardiectomy is the treatment of choice. The procedure is technically difficult but if excision of the diseased pericardium is successful the results are excellent.

FURTHER READING

Cameron J, Westerle SN, Baldwin JC, Hancock EW. The etiologic spectrum of constrictive pericarditis. *Am Heart J* 1987; 113: 354.

Hawkins JW, Vacek JL. What constitutes definitive therapy of malignant pericardial effusion? Medical versus surgical treatment. *Am Heart J* 1989; 118: 428.

Kralstein J, Frishman W. Malignant pericardial diseases: diagnosis and treatment. *Am Heart J* 1987; 113: 785.

Permanyer-Miralda G, Sagrista-Sauleda J, Soler-Soler J. Primary acute pericardial disease: a prospective series of 231 consecutive patients. *Am J Cardiol* 1985; 56: 623.

C H A P T E R 8

Rheumatic Fever and Infective Endocarditis

CONTENTS

SUMMARY

Rheumatic fever is an inflammatory condition usually occurring between the ages of 5 and 15 that affects the heart, joints, skin and brain. It probably represents an autoimmune response to pharyngeal infection with group A haemolytic *Streptococcus*. Once the commonest cause of valvular heart disease in this country, its incidence has now declined due to complex environmental factors and changes in the *Streptococcus* itself. It presents with fever and arthralgia; evidence of carditis (particularly murmurs of mitral or aortic regurgitation) is found in 50% of cases although heart failure is rare. Polyarthritis, erythema marginatum and chorea may also occur. Diagnosis is by application of Jones' criteria in patients with serological evidence of recent streptococcal infection. Treatment is with aspirin and recovery can be expected in about 6 weeks. However, in patients with carditis, progressive scarring and shrinkage of the valve cusps may lead to chronic rheumatic heart disease 15–20 years later.

Infective endocarditis usually involves the left-sided heart valves although any other endocardial location may also be affected. High-risk groups include the elderly; patients with pre-existing heart defects, valve lesions or prostheses; intravenous drug abusers; and immunosuppressed patients. *Streptococcus viridans* from the upper respiratory tract is the commonest infective agent but a wide range of other bacterial and fungal organisms have also been implicated. Infective endocarditis is characterized pathologically by accumulations of blood products ('vegetations') at the site of infection and by progressive destruction of the affected valve. It may present acutely with toxaemia and heart failure, particularly when caused by *Staphylococcus aureus*, but in the commoner *Streptococcccus viridans* cases it is an insidious influenza-like illness associated with the heart murmur of mitral or aortic regurgitation. Major complications include heart failure, embolization of vegetations, mycotic aneurysm and immune complex disease with vasculitis, arthritis, glomerular nephritis and renal failure. The diagnosis is clinical and should be considered in every patient with fever and a heart murmur. Early treatment with bacteriocidal antibiotics for 4–6 weeks is potentially life-saving and in suspected cases should not be delayed beyond the time necessary to collect three blood cultures. Treatment should start with intravenous benzyl penicillin and gentamicin on the assumption that *Streptococcus viridans* is the infective agent but may need adjusting when the results of blood cultures are available. Severe valvular regurgitation causing heart failure requires surgical treatment. Antibiotic prophylaxis against endocarditis is essential in all patients with valvular heart disease or other endocardial defects in order to prevent bacteraemia during dental surgery and other non-sterile invasive procedures.

RHEUMATIC FEVER

Rheumatic fever is an inflammatory disease that follows pharyngeal infection by group A haemolytic streptococci. The major organs and tissues affected are the heart, joints, skin and central nervous system.

Aetiology

One per cent of patients with group A haemolytic streptococcal pharyngitis develop rheumatic fever 2–3 weeks later. Evidence implicating the streptococcus in the aetiology of rheumatic fever is based upon:
• epidemiological studies;
• serological testing in acute rheumatic fever which usually provides evidence of recent streptococcal infection; and
• the efficacy of penicillin prophylaxis in patients with streptococcal pharyngitis.

However, the precise pathogenic role of the streptococcus is unknown. A direct infective process is unlikely because organisms are never present in the lesions of rheumatic fever; similarly there is no evidence of toxic tissue damage. A number of features suggest an autoimmune process, including: (i) the characteristic latency period between throat infection and the development of rheumatic fever; (ii) the demonstration of gamma globulins in the myocardial sarcolemma of patients who have died during the illness; (iii) the immunological cross-reaction between streptococcal antigens and myocardial sarcolemma; and (iv) the demonstration of circulating heart-reactive antibodies in a relatively high proportion of patients with rheumatic carditis. It must be emphasized, however, that many of these features are as likely to be the consequence of cardiac damage as they are to be its primary cause. Thus the role of autoimmunity in the pathogenesis of rheumatic fever remains unproven.

Epidemiology

Rheumatic fever occurs most commonly between the ages of 5 and 15 years. Its incidence in developed countries has declined dramatically during the last 50 years, but elsewhere in the world it continues to be a major health problem.

Environmental, bacteriological and host factors affect susceptibility to rheumatic fever. Crowding and social deprivation encourage the spread of streptococci and are the principal environmental factors predisposing to the disease. The nature of the organism itself is important because, when rheumatic fever does occur in developed countries, it is usually much less severe than in underdeveloped countries. This may also relate to host susceptibility. Thus the tendency for rheumatic fever to be familial and the high incidence of recurrence following an initial attack indicate heightened susceptibility in certain individuals, possibly due to genetic predisposition.

The declining incidence in developed countries cannot be attributed to any single factor. Improvements in housing and welfare are important but do not provide the full explanation because the incidence has fallen in all social strata, including the socially deprived inner-city areas. Penicillin, highly effective against streptococci, became widely available only after the declining incidence of rheumatic fever was well established. The virulence of the organism itself may have changed, since rheumatic fever is now not only less common but also less severe.

Pathology

Rheumatic fever may affect any of the cardiac tissues, including the myocardium, pericardium and endocardium. Myocardial involvement is characterized by the Aschoff body, a granulomatous lesion which persists long after the acute illness has subsided. Rheumatic pericarditis is usually transient, and may produce a fibrinous effusion, but tamponade and constriction are very rare.

Rheumatic endocarditis is the most important cardiac lesion. Inflammation and oedema of the valve cusps is associated with verrucous nodules which develop along the lines of valve closure. Acutely, this may cause severe valve damage but, more commonly, valve function remains little affected in this phase of the illness. During healing, however, progressive scarring of the valve apparatus may occur.

Non-cardiac disease

Arthritis is characterized by an exudative synovitis which does not produce long-term damage to the joints. Subcutaneous nodules are granulomatous and disappear following the acute illness. The cerebral pathology responsible for Chorea has not been identified.

Clinical manifestations

Fever and arthralgia are often the only symptoms. These may be attributed to a trivial, influenza-like illness which is soon forgotten by the patient.

Carditis

Although carditis affects about half of all patients with a first attack of rheumatic fever, it rarely causes symptoms. Thus, many patients who present with valvular disease later are unaware that they had rheumatic carditis during childhood. Chest pain due to pericarditis is the most common symptom but, in fulminant cases, symptoms of heart failure also occur. The examination reveals tachycardia and a gallop rhythm, both of which are non-specific responses to fever in children. Heart murmurs are heard in the majority of cases, particularly the pansystolic apical murmur of mitral regurgitation. An apical mid-diastolic murmur (Carey–Coombs) also indicates mitral involvement but does not always predict mitral stenosis in later life. The early diastolic murmur of aortic regurgitation is somewhat less common but, like the mitral murmurs, is strongly suggestive of rheumatic carditis. On the other hand, soft mid-systolic (ejection) murmurs usually reflect hyperkinetic flow, caused by fever, and do not necessarily indicate rheumatic carditis.

Other major manifestations

Polyarthritis usually affects the large joints of the extremities. Joints are often affected in turn and, as one recovers, others become involved. Subcutaneous nodules are small and painless and often go unnoticed by the patient. They occur over the extensor tendons of the hands, feet, knees and elbows and also over the spinal column.

Erythema marginatum is an evanescent rash characteristic of rheumatic fever. The lesions vary in size and have a pink serpiginous margin, often with a clear centre, usually occurring on the trunk but never on the face.

Chorea (Sydenham's chorea, St. Vitus' dance) is a late manifestation of rheumatic fever which may occur several months after pharyngitis. Its severity is variable but, in mild cases, the involuntary movements and grimaces are often mistaken for insolence by parents or teachers. At its worst, however, violent jerky movements of the entire body demand specially padded beds to prevent serious injury.

Diagnosis

Rheumatic fever tends to be over-diagnosed in children with fever, arthralgia and

Major criteria	Minor criteria
Carditis	Fever
Polyarthritis	Arthralgia
Erythema marginatum	Previous rheumatic fever
Chorea	Elevated erythrocyte sedimentation rate
Subcutaneous nodules	Prolonged PR interval

Table 8.1 Jones' criteria for the diagnosis of rheumatic fever.

soft ejection murmurs, all of which are non-specific manifestations of viral illness. Nevertheless, if recent streptococcal infection can be confirmed, by demonstration of elevated serum antistreptolysin O-titre, then Jones' criteria may be used (Table 8.1). The presence of two major criteria, or one major and two minor, indicates a high diagnostic probability.

Differential diagnosis

This includes other causes of childhood arthritis, bacterial endocarditis and viral pericarditis. Still's disease—the major cause of childhood arthritis—runs a chronic course and other criteria for rheumatic fever are not present. Bacterial endocarditis, although associated with fever and heart murmurs, causes relentless clinical deterioration and positive blood cultures and other stigmata of the condition should be sought. Simple viral pericarditis is never associated with valvular disease, unlike rheumatic pericarditis, in which valvular involvement and heart murmurs are always present.

An unusual but difficult diagnostic problem is the child with penicillin sensitivity following treatment of streptococcal pharyngitis. This often produces fever and arthritis similar to rheumatic fever. An urticarial or maculopapular rash, however, is strongly suggestive of drug sensitivity.

Treatment

Rheumatic fever may be prevented by prompt treatment of streptococcal throat infections with penicillin. A single intramuscular injection of 0.6–1.2 mega-units of benzylpenicillin is painful but effective if given within 9 days after the onset of sore throat.

In established rheumatic fever, no specific treatment cures or changes the course of the illness. Bed-rest is necessary in the acute phase, particularly if there are signs of carditis: a course of penicillin should be given to eradicate residual streptococcal infection. Salicylates are highly effective for treatment of fever and arthritis: aspirin, starting at 100 mg/kg/day in children, is given in sufficient dosage to relieve symptoms without causing frank toxicity (tinnitus, headache, hyperventilation). In patients unable to tolerate salicylates, steroids are equally effective and are preferred by some physicians when active carditis is present. There is no evidence to suggest that steroids are more beneficial than salicylates, however, or that either treatment prevents chronic valvular damage. Steroid dosage is variable, but an initial dose of prednisone 60–120 mg daily may be necessary to suppress symptoms; thereafter the dose can be gradually reduced.

Rheumatic chorea is unaffected by salicylates and steroids. Mental and physical rest in bed reduces the severity of choreiform attacks. Mild sedatives such as diazepam are often helpful.

Following rheumatic fever, long-term prophylactic penicillin therapy should be continued up to the age of 25 or for at least 5 years in patients over 20. Recommended regimens are a monthly intramuscular injection of benzyl penicillin (1.2 mega-units) or oral penicillin V (125 mg twice daily). Oral sulphadiazine (1 g daily) may be used in penicillin-sensitive individuals.

Course and prognosis

Acute rheumatic fever usually subsides within 6 weeks. Occasionally, however, the illness lasts 6 months or longer, particularly in patients with intractable carditis or chorea. Carditis probably affects the majority of young children with rheumatic fever but is less common in older patients; recurrent attacks occur frequently and, in patients with carditis, these exacerbate cardiac damage and increase susceptibility to heart failure and death. In most cases, however, heart failure is delayed until the development of chronic rheumatic heart disease several years later. Chorea and arthritis rarely produce chronic sequelae.

Chronic rheumatic heart disease

Following an attack (or recurrent attacks) of rheumatic fever, cardiac function usually returns to normal. During healing of the inflamed valves, however, progressive scarring may lead to chronic rheumatic heart disease, although this does not usually present until 15–20 years later. Adhesion of the valve commissures and shrinkage of the cusps and the subvalvular apparatus produce variable stenosis and regurgitation, exacerbated by valvular calcification. By the age of 30, many patients have had their first attack of congestive heart failure, which is often precipitated by the onset of AF or the stress of pregnancy. The mitral valve is most commonly affected, and is often associated with disease of the aortic valve. Functional impairment of the tricuspid valve is unusual and rheumatic pulmonary valve disease is almost never seen.

INFECTIVE ENDOCARDITIS

Infective endocarditis usually involves the heart valves (native or prosthetic) but may also occur in association with congenital or acquired defects; occasionally, infection develops in relation to pacemaker electrodes (Fig. 8.1). Infection of the endothelial lining of arterial aneurysms or arteriovenous fistulae is rare but produces a similar illness.

Aetiology

Endocarditis is now seen increasingly in the elderly, unlike 50 years ago when it was more common in young adults. Organisms implicated in the aetiology of

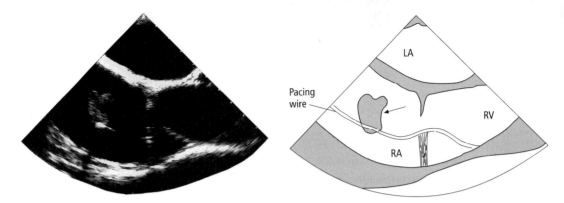

Fig. 8.1 Infective endocarditis in relation to pacing wire. This transoesophageal echocardiogram shows a large vegetation (arrowed) lying within the cavity of the right atrium (RA) adherent to the pacing wire. LA, left atrium; RV, right ventricle.

endocarditis are shown in Table 8.2. The most common of these is *Streptococcus viridans*, a normal commensal of the upper respiratory tract. This is a relatively indolent organism which produces a chronic, subacute, illness. Other more virulent organisms, notably *Staphylococcus aureus*, produce an acute, rapidly progressive, illness. Regardless of the organism, however, the outcome is invariably fatal if endocarditis is not treated.

Endocarditis may affect healthy patients with entirely normal hearts. Nevertheless patients at greater risk are those with pre-existing valvular disease or congenital or acquired cardiac defects. Other high-risk groups are shown in Table 8.3. High-velocity flow favours the endothelial deposition of organisms in bacteraemic patients. Thus, aortic and mitral valve disease, ventricular septal defect and patent ductus arteriosus are the conditions most commonly associated

Table 8.2 Organisms causing endocarditis. The pathogens most commonly implicated are shown in **bold**.

	Typical source of infection	First-choice antibiotics (pending sensitivity studies)
SUBACUTE DISEASE		
Streptococcus viridans	Upper respiratory tract	Penicillin, gentamicin
Streptococcus faecalis	Bowel and urogenital tract	Ampicillin, gentamicin
Anaerobic streptococci	Bowel	Ampicillin, gentamicin
Staphylococcus epidermidis	Skin	Flucloxacillin, gentamicin
Fungi—*Candida*, histoplasmosis	Skin and mucous membranes	Amphotericin B*, 5-fluorocytosine*
Coxiella burnetti	Complication of Q fever	Chloramphenicol*, tetracycline
Chlamydia psittacosi	Contact with infected birds	Tetracycline*, erythromycin
ACUTE DISEASE		
Staphylococcus aureus	Skin	Flucloxacillin, gentamicin
Streptococcus pneumoniae	Complication of pneumonia	Penicillin, gentamicin
Neisseria gonorrhoeae	Venereal	Penicillin, gentamicin

* These drugs are not cidal and valve replacement is nearly always necessary to eradicate infection.

Table 8.3 Groups at increased risk of endocarditis.

The elderly (> 60 years)
Patients with intrinsic cardiovascular disease. High-risk lesions are:
ventricular septal defect
aortic regurgitation
mitral regurgitation
aortic stenosis
patent ductus arteriosus
coarctation of the aorta
Patients with valve prostheses, tissue grafts and other intracardiac foreign material
Main-lining drug addicts—right-sided valvular endocarditis occurs relatively commonly in this group
Immunosuppressed patients: acquired immunodeficiency syndrome; immunosuppressive drugs

with infective endocarditis. Right-sided endocarditis is rare, usually affecting mainlining drug addicts.

The source of infection cannot usually be identified. *Streptococcus viridans* bacteraemia is almost invariable during dental surgery (drilling, scaling, extractions) but less than 15% of patients with endocarditis give a history of this. Instrumentation of the genitourinary (GU) or gastrointestinal (GI) tracts also causes bacteraemia but is not often implicated. Drug addicts commonly use dirty needles and expose themselves to a variety of organisms which may infect the left- or right-sided heart valves, and infected intravenous cannulae are a potential cause of staphylococcal endocarditis in hospitalized patients.

Pathology

Endocarditis leads to accumulation of fibrin, platelets and other blood products at the site of infection. This produces a vegetation which is relatively avascular and tends to isolate the infective organism from host defences and antimicrobial agents. Valve destruction produces worsening regurgitation and commonly leads to heart failure. In staphylococcal endocarditis, valve destruction is rapid but in less aggressive infections (e.g. *Streptococcus viridans*) the progression of disease is slower and large craggy vegetations develop. Embolization to any of the major organs or the extremities is common and may cause metastatic abscesses, particularly in the spleen or brain. Pulmonary embolism, from right-sided cardiac lesions, also occurs. Extension of infection into the adjacent myocardial or arterial walls produces conduction defects, valve-ring abscesses or mycotic aneurysms. The chronic infection that characterizes endocarditis may lead to immune-complex disease with vasculitic involvement of the kidneys, joints or skin.

Clinical manifestations

In acute bacterial endocarditis caused by *Staphylococcus aureus*, the onset is often dramatic, with severe prostration leading rapidly to heart failure and septicaemic shock. In subacute disease, the onset is insidious, with influenza-like symptoms including fever, night sweats, arthralgia and fatigue. Petechial haemorrhages in the skin and under the nails ('splinter haemorrhages') are a common but non-specific finding. Valvular endocarditis produces regurgitant murmurs (typically aortic or mitral) due to destruction of the valve leaflets. Other 'classical' manifestations of endocarditis, including Osler's nodes (tender erythematous nodules in the pulps of the fingers), Janeway lesions (painless erythematous lesions on the palms), clubbing of the fingers and splenomegaly, are now rarely seen.

Complications

Heart failure is the major complication of endocarditis and the usual cause of death. Vegetations may embolize peripherally, threatening limbs or major organs, and metastatic abscesses may occur, particularly in the spleen or brain. Embolization in the vasa vasorum causes mycotic aneurysm which may be infected or sterile. These often develop locally in the sinuses of Valsalva, but may also occur in the peripheral circulation. Rupture can occur during the acute phase of the illness or at any time following. Local abscess formation in the aortic valve ring may produce heart block by damaging the conduction tissue in the interventricular septum. Right-sided endocarditis is commonly associated with pneumonia caused by infected embolization to the lungs.

Immune-complex disease complicating infective endocarditis is a cause of vasculitic rash and arthritis. More important, however, is glomerulonephritis which may progress to renal failure.

Diagnosis

Endocarditis is predominately a clinical diagnosis and should be considered in every patient with fever and a heart murmur. Laboratory findings include leucocytosis, usually with neutrophilia, and normochromic normocytic anaemia is almost invariable. Urinalysis commonly reveals haematuria due to glomerulonephritis. Blood cultures are positive in the majority of cases and should always be obtained before antibiotic treatment is started. Aerobic, anaerobic and fungal cultures should be performed. Occasionally, bone-marrow cultures are helpful for detection of *Candida* and *Brucella* endocarditis. *Coxiella* and *Chlamydia* can never be cultured from the blood and must be diagnosed by serological tests. Failure to detect bacteraemia may be due to:
• pretreatment with antibiotics;
• inadequate sampling—up to six blood samples should be taken over 24 hours; or
• infection with unusual micro-organisms.

The echocardiogram identifies underlying valvular disease, and vegetations may also be seen if these are large enough (Fig. 8.2). The transoesophageal technique is helpful, particularly in prosthetic valve endocarditis and in patients

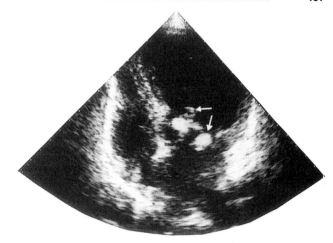

Fig. 8.2 Infective endocarditis. This two-dimensional echocardiogram (apical four-chamber view) shows dense vegetations adherent to both leaflets of the mitral valve (arrowed).

suspected of having abscess formation in the aortic valve ring (Fig. 8.3). Doppler studies identify regurgitant jets through the damaged valves. It should be emphasized, however, that failure to image vegetations by echocardiography does not rule out the diagnosis of endocarditis.

Differential diagnosis

Infective endocarditis must be differentiated from other causes of fever and heart murmurs. Rheumatic fever is no longer common in the developed world but, in children, may be difficult to distinguish from endocarditis. Fever from any cause may be associated with soft ejection systolic murmurs due to hyperkinetic circulation. Nevertheless, if murmurs of valvular regurgitation do not develop, the diagnosis of valvular endocarditis is unlikely.

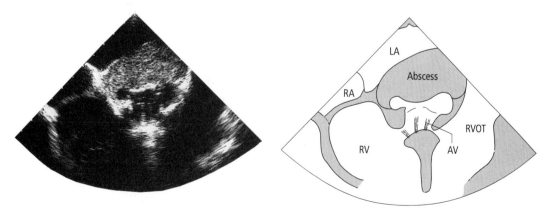

Fig. 8.3 Infective endocarditis with abscess in relation to prosthetic aortic valve. This transoesophageal echocardiogram shows a large abscess in the wall of the aorta closely related to the infected prosthesis.

Treatment

Initial diagnosis is made on clinical grounds and treatment must not be delayed beyond the time necessary to obtain three to four blood samples for culture. Bacteriocidal antibiotic therapy should then be started and the course should continue for at least 4 weeks, or up to 6 weeks in complicated cases of prosthetic valve infection. It is recommended that, for the first 2 weeks, combination therapy is given, with two antibiotics injected intravenously. During this time, serially diluted blood samples should be back-titrated against the cultured organism in the bacteriology laboratory to ensure adequate cidal activity. After 2 weeks of intravenous treatment the course may be completed with oral drugs using a single antibiotic.

Streptococcal infection accounts for over 70% of cases. Thus, while the results of blood culture are awaited, initial treatment should be with benzylpenicillin—12 mega-units daily—and low-dose gentamicin (60–80 mg twice daily), which enhances penicillin activity. The dose of gentamicin must be titrated against blood concentrations in order to achieve peak and trough valves of 3–5 mg/l and <1 mg/l, respectively. When the results of blood culture become available, alternative antibiotics may be necessary. In culture-negative cases treatment with penicillin and gentamicin should continue while a search for unusual organisms such as fungi, *Coxiella* and *Chlamydia* is undertaken.

Fever usually settles within a few days of starting treatment but persistent elevation of the erythrocyte sedimentation rate (ESR) for up to 4 weeks is common. Recurrence of fever is often the result of antibiotic sensitivity but it may also indicate superinfection with a new organism. Fungi are particularly troublesome and difficult to treat. For this reason a weekly injection of amphotericin is often recommended during the course of treatment. Any sign of infection around an intravenous site demands removal of the catheter; the tip should be sent for culture and a new line inserted under full aseptic conditions.

The valve damage caused by endocarditis may require surgical treatment which, if possible, should be delayed until antibiotic therapy has cleared the infection, although the development of heart failure may demand more urgent valve replacement. Conduction defects, recurrent embolism and resistant infection, particularly in prosthetic valve endocarditis, are other relative indications for early surgery. Fungal endocarditis usually requires surgical treatment because all the available antifungal drugs are fungistatic (not fungicidal). Eradication of fungal infection by medical treatment is therefore very difficult.

Prophylaxis

Antibiotic prophylaxis against endocarditis is required for all patients with valvular heart disease, or other endocardial defects caused by acquired or congenital disease. Patients with mitral valve prolapse only need prophylaxis when there is an associated systolic murmur of mitral regurgitation. A permanent pacemaker in patients with conduction tissue disease is not an indication for prophylaxis.

The purpose of prophylaxis is to prevent bacteraemia during dental surgery and other non-sterile invasive procedures. A single oral dose of amoxycillin 3 g should be given 1 hour before dental work (scaling, filling, extraction) to protect against *Streptococcus viridans* infection. In patients allergic to penicillin a single oral dose of clindamycin 600 mg should be substituted. For patients undergoing instrumentation or surgery of the upper respiratory tract (e.g. bronchoscopy) prophylaxis requirements are the same as for dental procedures. Instrumentation or surgery of the GI and GU tracts does not require prophylaxis unless the patient has a prosthetic heart valve or gives a history of previous endocarditis, when amoxycillin combined with intramuscular gentamicin 120 mg is recommended. During childbirth antibiotic prophylaxis is unnecessary for normal vaginal deliveries but is amoxycillin and gentamicin are recommended for instrumented deliveries and for all mothers with prosthetic valves or a history of previous endocarditis.

Prognosis

When penicillin therapy was introduced, mortality in endocarditis fell from 100% to about 30%. Since that time, mortality has shown little tendency to decline further despite the increasing availability of powerful antibiotics. This is probably the result of multiple factors, including the emergence of antibiotic-resistant organisms, the introduction of prosthetic heart valves, the widespread use of immunosuppressive therapy, the worsening problems of intravenous drug abuse and the older, more debilitated age-group that is now at risk. Probably the major impediment to effective treatment in endocarditis is delay in diagnosis. The insidious onset of the illness often causes the correct diagnosis to be overlooked until it is too late. Thus, endocarditis must be considered in all patients with a feverish illness and a heart murmur, particularly those patients known to be at high risk.

FURTHER READING

Bayliss R, Clark C, Oakley CM *et al.* Incidence, mortality and prevention of infective endocarditis. *J R Coll Physicians Lond* 1986; 20: 15.

Bisno AL. Acute rheumatic fever: forgotten but not gone. *N Engl J Med* 1987; 316: 476.

Bisno AL. Group A Streptococcal infections and acute rheumatic fever. *N Engl J Med* 1991; 325: 783.

Durack DT. Prevention of infective endocarditis. *N Engl J Med* 1995; 332: 38.

Gray IR. Infective endocarditis 1937–1987. *Br Heart J* 1987; 57: 211.

Stollerman GH. Rheumatic carditis. *Lancet* 1995; 346: 390.

Tunkel AR, Kaye D. Endocarditis with negative blood cultures. *N Engl J Med* 1992; 326: 1215.

Working Party of the British Society for Antimicrobial Therapy. Antibiotic prophylaxis of infective endocarditis. *Lancet* 1990; 335: 88.

C H A P T E R   9

Valvular Heart Disease

C O N T E N T S

SUMMARY

Valvular heart disease adversely affects ventricular loading and tends to diminish cardiac output. Compensatory mechanisms will often preserve haemodynamic stability but, if the lesion is severe, heart failure eventually supervenes. Diagnosis can usually be made clinically, but echocardiography and Doppler technology permit more precise assessment of lesion severity without the need for cardiac catheterization. Surgery has revolutionized the management of valvular heart disease and, if timed before ventricular dysfunction or pulmonary hypertension have become irreversible, can produce complete haemodynamic correction.

Mitral stenosis is always rheumatic and is associated with progressive increments in left atrial pressure that establish a pressure gradient across the valve to maintain left ventricular (LV) filling. As pressure rises dyspnoea gets worse, deteriorating abruptly with the onset of atrial fibrillation (AF). Auscultation reveals a loud first heart sound, and an opening snap in early diastole followed by a low-pitched mid-diastolic murmur. Treatment is with diuretics but, if dyspnoea remains troublesome, balloon valvuloplasty or surgery is necessary. Patients in AF require digoxin to control the ventricular rate and anticoagulants to protect against systemic embolization.

Mitral regurgitation may be caused by valvular, subvalvular or dilating LV disease. The regurgitant jet causes left atrial pressure to rise and volume-loads the left ventricle which dilates. AF is common and presentation is with dyspnoea and an apical pansystolic murmur, often associated with a third heart sound. Treatment is initially medical, as for mitral stenosis, with surgery in reserve for worsening LV dilatation and symptomatic deterioration.

Aortic stenosis is usually calcific, involving either a congenitally bicuspid valve in the 40–60 age group or, sometimes, a previously normal valve in the very elderly. Rheumatic disease is now less common in the developed world. The left ventricle hypertrophies to generate a pressure gradient across the aortic valve sufficient to preserve forward flow. In end-stage disease the left ventricle dilates and fails, and a paradoxical reduction in the pressure gradient may then occur. Presentation is with dyspnoea, angina and, in severe cases, syncope and left ventricular failure. The carotid pulse has a slow upstroke and auscultation reveals a mid-systolic murmur and a fourth heart sound. The development of symptoms heralds a poor prognosis and is an indication for surgery.

Aortic regurgitation may be caused by valve-leaflet or aortic root disease. The regurgitant jet volume-loads the left ventricle which dilates and, in severe cases, eventually fails. It is commonly an incidental finding but, when severe, causes dyspnoea and angina. The carotid pulse has a sharp upstroke with a wide pulse pressure, and auscultation reveals a high-pitched, early diastolic murmur at the aortic area associated with a mid-systolic flow murmur. Treatment with vasodilators and diuretics is helpful, with surgery in reserve for worsening LV dilatation and symptomatic deterioration.

Tricuspid stenosis is nearly always rheumatic but is rare, unlike *tricuspid regurgitation* which is common and usually a functional consequence of right ventricular failure. The jugular venous pulse is elevated with giant 'v' waves and auscultation reveals a pansystolic murmur at the left sternal edge. Treatment is with diuretics and surgery is rarely required.

Pulmonary stenosis is one of the commoner congenital heart defects and, if severe, may require treatment by balloon valvuloplasty. *Pulmonary regurgitation* is usually a result of severe pulmonary hypertension and requires no specific treatment, being of negligible haemodynamic significance.

INTRODUCTION

The heart valves open and close in response to cyclical changes in intracardiac and arterial pressures, directing the cardiac output forwards into the pulmonary and systemic circulations without impeding flow. Valvular dysfunction is the result of incompetence or stenosis which produce backward flow (regurgitation) or impeded flow, respectively. Regurgitant valve lesions volume-load the heart, whilst stenotic lesions of the ventricular outflow valves (aortic, pulmonary) pressure-load the ventricles. Stenosis of the ventricular inflow valves (mitral, tricuspid) impede filling and reduce preload. The abnormal loading which results from valve dysfunction commonly leads to heart failure, although this may be delayed by the effects of compensatory mechanisms (see page 78). Nevertheless, because full development of these compensatory mechanisms takes time, chronic valve lesions are better tolerated than acute.

The important role of echocardiography in the diagnosis of valvular heart disease has already been emphasized. When it is used in conjunction with Doppler studies, the severity of valvular stenosis and regurgitation can be evaluated. These non-invasive investigations make cardiac catheterization unnecessary for diagnostic purposes, but it is recommended in men over 35 and women over 45 to rule out coronary artery disease. This not only adds precision to the diagnosis of the valve lesion, but also permits coronary arteriography so that, when necessary, bypass grafting can be performed at the same time as valve replacement.

Surgery has revolutionized the management of valvular heart disease and can produce complete haemodynamic correction. The timing of valve surgery is important. If it is delayed until ventricular dysfunction or pulmonary hypertension has become irreversible, the risks are greater and the results less satisfac-

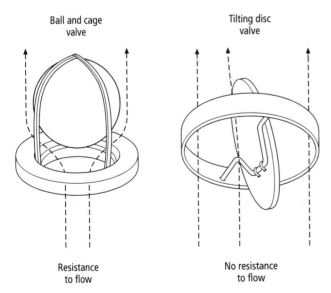

Ball and cage
valve

Tilting disc
valve

Resistance
to flow

No resistance
to flow

Fig. 9.1 Prosthetic heart valves. The ball-and-cage prosthesis causes greater resistance to flow than the tilting disc prosthesis.

tory. In mitral stenosis, dilatation of the valve (valvotomy) is effective if the valve is competent and not calcified. Regurgitation through the atrioventricular valves can sometimes be corrected by repair procedures. In most cases of valvular heart disease, however, surgical correction requires replacement of the valve with a tissue graft or a prosthesis. Porcine xenografts are widely used because, unlike prostheses, they are not thrombogenic and do not expose the patient to the inconvenience and risk of long-term anticoagulation. Nevertheless, tissue grafts usually calcify and fail within 7–10 years. For this reason, prostheses are often preferred—usually ball-and-cage or tilting disc mechanisms. Both types are reliable but tilting disc valves present less obstruction to flow (Fig. 9.1). Long-term anticoagulation is essential following insertion of a prosthetic valve.

It is convenient to consider each of the important valve lesions separately. It must be recognized, however, that an individual valve may be both incompetent and stenosed. Moreover, disease involving more than one valve is not uncommon, particularly in rheumatic disease and endocarditis. Multivalvular disease increases the haemodynamic burden on the heart and produces heart failure earlier.

MITRAL STENOSIS

Aetiology

Mitral stenosis (MS) is nearly always rheumatic in origin, rarely occurring as a congenital defect.

Pathophysiology

In adults the normal mitral valve orifice is 4–6 cm^2. However, flow across the valve remains unimpeded until the valve area is about half this. As stenosis worsens, adequate LV filling demands a progressive increase in left atrial pressure which establishes a diastolic pressure gradient across the mitral valve (Fig. 9.2). Left ventricular contraction is unaffected but, because filling is impeded, adequate cardiac output cannot always be maintained, particularly during exercise.

As pressure rises in the left atrium it dilates and is prone to fibrillate. This compromises LV filling still further, due partly to the loss of atrial systole and partly to the rapid heart rate which reduces diastolic filling time. Thus, the onset of atrial fibrillation (AF) often produces abrupt clinical deterioration.

MS, therefore, is associated with a chronically elevated and labile left atrial pressure, causing pulmonary congestion and pulmonary hypertension that leads to right ventricular failure (RVF). In advanced MS, obliterative disease in the pulmonary arterioles increases pulmonary vascular resistance and exacerbates pulmonary hypertension and RVF. Following the development of obliterative pulmonary vascular disease, pulmonary hypertension is irreversible and remains unaffected by mitral valve surgery.

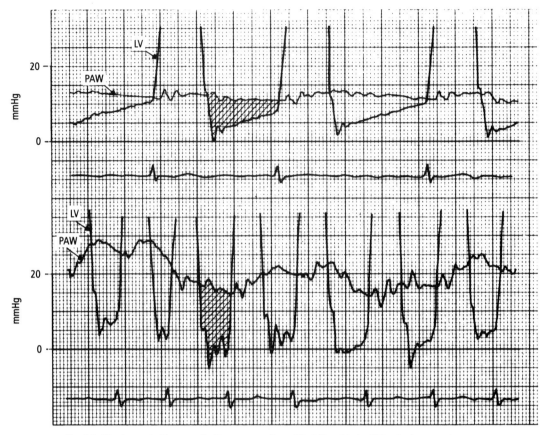

Fig. 9.2 Mitral stenosis. These are simultaneous recordings of the left ventricular (LV) and pulmonary artery wedge (PAW) pressure signals. Recordings at rest are shown above and recordings during exercise below. Note that the diastolic pressure gradient across the mitral valve (shaded area) increases considerably during exercise due to the sharp rise in pulmonary artery wedge pressure. This accounts for the exercise-related dyspnoea that occurs in mitral stenosis.

Clinical manifestations

MS produces orthopnoea and exertional fatigue and dyspnoea in the same way as other causes of left heart failure (page 83). In advanced disease, life-threatening attacks of acute pulmonary oedema occur. Chronic bronchial congestion produces cough and haemoptysis and predisposes towards winter bronchitis. The onset of AF is often associated with abrupt clinical deterioration, which may also occur during the third trimester of pregnancy due to the increase in circulatory volume.

Cyanotic discoloration of the cheeks produces the typical mitral facies. The pulse is commonly irregular, due to AF. Auscultation at the cardiac apex reveals a loud first heart sound and an opening snap in early diastole followed by a low-pitched mid-diastolic murmur; presystolic accentuation of the murmur occurs only in patients who are in sinus rhythm. In advanced MS, the loud first sound and the opening snap become less prominent as the mobility of the thickened valve leaflets becomes progressively restricted; the opening snap also tends to move closer to the second heart sound, as rising left atrial pressure forces open the mitral valve progressively earlier in diastole.

The development of RVF produces peripheral oedema and elevation of the jugular venous pulse (JVP). The dilated right ventricle displaces the apical impulse towards the left axilla and causes a left parasternal systolic thrust. Prominence of the pulmonary component of the second heart sound reflects pulmonary hypertension.

Complications

AF is almost invariable in longstanding disease. Haemostasis in the dilated left atrium leads to thrombosis and commonly results in thromboembolism. Pulmonary hypertension predisposes to chest infections (a common cause of death in MS), and may also lead to RVF. Although endocarditis is rare in pure MS, antibiotic prophylaxis should always be given prior to dental surgery and other non-sterile invasive procedures.

Diagnosis

Left atrial enlargement produces a broad bifid P wave on the ECG before the onset of AF. Evidence of right ventricular hypertrophy occurs if pulmonary hypertension is severe (see Fig. 2.12).

The chest X-ray (CXR) shows signs of left atrial enlargement (see Fig. 3.2) usually with a normal heart size. The heart size may increase with the development of RVF. Prominence of the upper lobe veins is almost invariable and, in advanced cases, pulmonary congestion or frank pulmonary oedema may be present. Calcification of the mitral valve or the left atrial wall is occasionally evident on penetrated or lateral films (Fig. 9.3).

The echocardiogram is diagnostic: thickening and variable rigidity of the valve leaflets is associated with dilatation of the left atrium. The two-dimensional image may show dilatation of the right-sided cardiac chambers but the left ventricle is normal (Fig. 9.4). The transoesophageal technique is particularly useful for identifying thrombus in the left atrial appendage. Doppler studies provide quantitative assessment of the pressure gradient across the mitral valve.

Cardiac catheterization permits measurement of the mitral valve pressure gradient at rest and during exercise (Fig. 9.2). In patients with severe pulmonary hypertension, the effects of inhaling 100% oxygen should be assessed; this usually produces a prompt reduction in pulmonary artery pressure, as oxygen is a potent pulmonary vasodilator, but this does not occur in patients with irreversible pulmonary vascular disease.

Differential diagnosis

Mitral stenosis must be distinguished from left ventricular failure (LVF), which

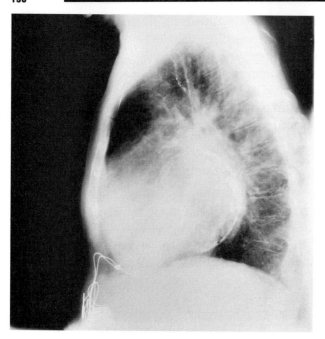

Fig. 9.3 Mitral valve disease—lateral chest X-ray. The patient has a mitral valve prosthesis and also an epicardial pacemaker (see page 219). There is dense calcification in the wall of the left atrium which lies posterior to the prosthetic valve. The left atrium is dilated and there is also right ventricular dilatation with partial obliteration of the retrosternal space.

produces almost identical symptoms. Although a mid-diastolic murmur is not present the third heart sound may cause confusion. Conditions normally associated with a mid-diastolic murmur (e.g. tricuspid stenosis, atrial septal defect) may also cause confusion. However, in all these conditions other auscultatory signs of mitral stenosis are not found and the echocardiogram shows a normal mitral valve.

Treatment

This consists of diuretics to control pulmonary and systemic congestion, digitalis to control the ventricular rate in AF, and anticoagulants to protect against thromboembolism. Anticoagulation with warfarin is mandatory in all patients with mitral stenosis following the onset of AF to protect against thromboembolism. Antibiotic prophylaxis should be given prior to dental procedures.

The major indications for surgery are dyspnoea unresponsive to medical treatment, and RVF. Any patient who has a mitral valve gradient greater than 10 mmHg during exercise is likely to need surgery—either valvotomy, in which the valve cusps are separated along the commissures, or valve replacement. Closed valvotomy without direct visualization of the valve does not require cardiopulmonary bypass but, if the surgeon wishes to inspect the valve, an open operation with full cardiopulmonary bypass is necessary. Valvotomy is the procedure of choice when the valve cusps are pliant and mobile, but valvular calcification or incompetence demands valve replacement. In uncomplicated cases, the mortality risk of mitral valve surgery is < 2% but pulmonary hypertension or heart failure increases the risk to 10% or more.

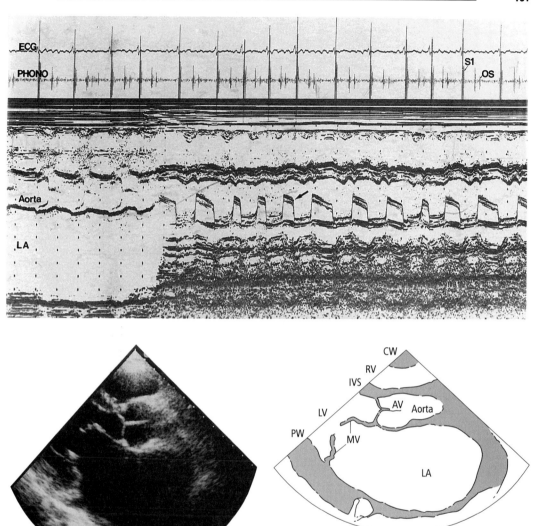

Fig. 9.4 Mitral stenosis—echocardiogram. (a) The M-mode recording shows thickening of the mitral valve (arrowed) with a normal-sized left ventricle. The left atrium lying behind the aorta is considerably dilated. (b) The two-dimensional recording confirms these findings and shows typical doming of the mitral valve leaflets during diastole. The ECG shows atrial fibrillation and the phonocardiogram shows a very loud first heart sound (S1) with an opening snap (OS) following shortly after the second heart sound.

The recent development of mitral balloon valvuloplasty avoids the need for surgery in some patients with non-calcified competent valves. The balloon catheter is advanced from the femoral vein into the right atrium and thence into the left atrium by trans-septal puncture. The balloon is then positioned across the stenosed mitral valve and inflated (Fig. 9.5). This dilates the valve and can

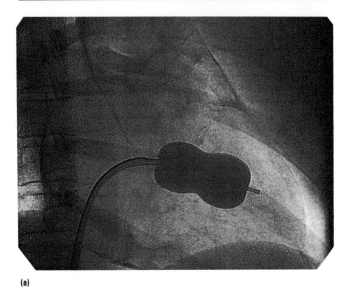

(a)

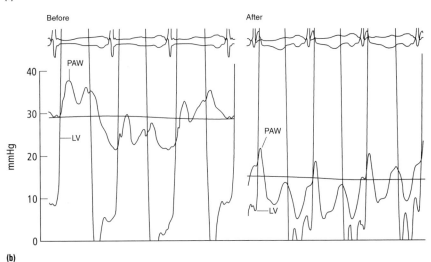

(b)

Fig. 9.5 Mitral balloon valvuloplasty. The cine frame shows the valvuloplasty catheter lying across the atrial septum and passing down into the LV cavity. The balloon is inflated across the mitral valve. Also shown are simultaneous left atrial and LV pressure signals before and after the procedure. Note how the diastolic pressure gradient across the mitral valve is effectively abolished following successful dilatation of the mitral valve.

produce sustained benefit, unlike aortic balloon valvuloplasty in which any improvement is nearly always temporary.

Prognosis

Following rheumatic carditis, the development of symptomatic MS may take up to 20 years although pregnancy, or the early development of AF, often prompts an earlier presentation. Once symptoms are established, progressive deterioration leads to death within 5–10 years, unless the stenosis is relieved by surgery.

Thus, without surgery, death usually occurs in middle age and may be caused by pulmonary oedema, chest infection, endocarditis or thromboembolism.

MITRAL REGURGITATION

Aetiology

Mitral regurgitation (MR) is caused by valve-leaflet disease, subvalvular disease, or dilatation of the left ventricle (Table 9.1).

Mitral valve prolapse

This is a common and usually asymptomatic condition in which one or both of the mitral valve leaflets bulge backwards into the left atrium during systole, producing mitral regurgitation in some cases. Mitral valve prolapse affects about 5% of the population and is particularly common in young women; the cause is unknown but it may be associated with a variety of cardiac and systemic disorders. Most cases are idiopathic, however, and are characterized by myxomatous degeneration of the valve-leaflet tissue. Although patients are usually asymptomatic, some complain of non-specific chest pain, the cause of which is not clear. Others complain of palpitations which are sometimes related to ventricular premature beats or paroxysmal supraventricular tachycardias, although a clear association between mitral valve prolapse and cardiac arrhythmias has yet to be established. The auscultatory signs may vary from day to day but typically there is a mid-systolic click followed by a murmur. Occasionally the murmur is pansystolic, while in other cases only a mid-systolic click is present. The echocardiogram is usually diagnostic, showing posterior displacement of the mitral valve leaflet(s) immediately following the click (Fig. 9.6). For most cases, no treatment is necessary but, in severe MR, valve replacement is occasionally required. Antibiotic prophylaxis, prior to dental surgery and other non-sterile invasive procedures, is recommended only when mitral valve prolapse is associated with a murmur indicating MR.

Table 9.1 Causes of mitral regurgitation.

Valve-leaflet disease	Mitral valve prolapse
	Rheumatic disease
	Infective endocarditis*
Subvalvular disease	Chordal rupture*
	Papillary muscle dysfunction
	Papillary muscle rupture*
Dilating left ventricular disease	'Functional' mitral regurgitation

* These disorders produce acute regurgitation.
Note that the subclassification into valve leaflet and subvalvular disease is to some extent artificial because all the causes of valve leaflet disease are usually associated with subvalvular dysfunction.

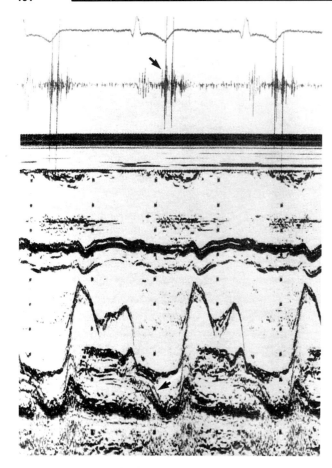

Fig. 9.6 Mitral valve prolapse. The M-mode recording shows typical backward displacement of the posterior leaflet of the mitral valve (arrowed) during systole. The simultaneous phonocardiogram shows a click in mid systole (arrowed) which is followed by two much louder clicks and a systolic murmur.

Chordal rupture

This usually occurs in patients over 50 years of age as an idiopathic degenerative process, but it may be related to endocarditis or rheumatic fever. It produces acute MR, the severity of which relates to the extent of chordal rupture.

Papillary muscle disease

Myocardial ischaemia can lead to dysfunction or rupture of the papillary muscles. Papillary muscle dysfunction is usually well tolerated but, when myocardial infarction (MI) is complicated by papillary muscle rupture, the mitral valve is completely unsupported. Torrential MR and pulmonary oedema then occur and only urgent valve replacement will prevent death.

Pathophysiology

MR volume-loads the left ventricle due to increased filling from the left atrium. In chronic disease, this causes compensatory dilatation and hypertrophy. The lesion is usually well tolerated because the systolic leak of regurgitant blood into the left atrium reduces LV wall tension considerably. The reduction in afterload permits diversion of energy to myocardial shortening, such that forward output is maintained. Moreover, progressive dilatation of the left atrium increases its distensibility (compliance) and prevents marked elevation of atrial pressure during ventricular systole. This protects against pulmonary oedema and the development of pulmonary hypertension. AF commonly supervenes.

Clinical manifestations

MR remains asymptomatic until the left ventricle begins to fail. In acute MR, this often occurs abruptly but in chronic disease it may take several years. Symptoms include orthopnoea and exercise-related fatigue and dyspnoea. Because pulmonary hypertension is unusual in MR, signs of RVF are rarely prominent.

The pulse is commonly irregular, due to AF, but there is no reduction in pulse volume until LVF is advanced. Auscultation reveals an apical pansystolic murmur which radiates into the left axilla. In mitral valve prolapse, the murmur usually occurs later in systole and is preceded by a click (see above). A third heart sound is often present due to rapid filling from the volume-loaded left atrium.

Complications

Patients with MR are prone to thromboembolism from the dilated left atrium, particularly after the onset of AF when anticoagulation is mandatory. There is also a considerable risk of endocarditis, and antibiotic prophylaxis prior to dental surgery and other non-sterile invasive procedures is essential. Although MR is generally well tolerated, in severe cases the chronic volume overload leads inexorably to LVF and irreversible contractile dysfunction. Pulmonary hypertension and RVF, however, are less common than in MS.

Diagnosis

The ECG shows P mitrale before the onset of AF. The CXR shows signs of left atrial dilatation and the heart size is usually increased due to LV dilatation. In rheumatic disease, calcification of the mitral valve is occasionally evident. The lung fields remain normal until the development of LVF.

The echocardiogram confirms left atrial and LV dilatation, although LV contractile function remains well preserved until the development of failure. Diagnostic abnormalities of the valve itself occur in mitral valve prolapse and rheumatic disease, and vegetations can usually be imaged in endocarditis (see Fig. 8.2). Dynamic abnormalities of the valve (e.g. flail leaflet) may be present in chordal or papillary muscle rupture but, in many cases of subvalvular mitral regurgitation, the valve appears normal. Nevertheless, Doppler echocardiography identifies the regurgitant jet in the left atrium and permits assessment of the severity of the lesion (Plate 9.1, opposite p. 244). At cardiac catheterization,

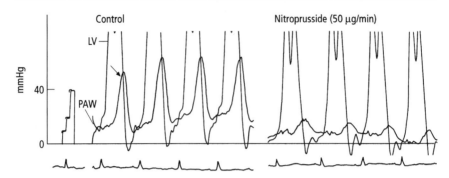

Fig. 9.7 Acute mitral regurgitation. Simultaneous recordings of the left ventricular (LV) and pulmonary artery wedge (PAW) pressure signals are shown before and after nitroprusside infusion. Note that before nitroprusside there is considerable elevation of the left ventricular diastolic and pulmonary artery wedge pressures. A giant 'v' wave is clearly visible (arrowed). Vasodilator therapy with nitroprusside reduces the ventricular filling pressures and also reduces regurgitant flow with disappearance of the 'v' wave.

LV angiography confirms the diagnosis and defines LV contractile function (see Fig. 3.18). In acute MR, the regurgitant jet produces a prominent 'v' wave in the pulmonary artery wedge pressure signal (Fig. 9.7). This occurs less commonly in chronic MR because the dilated left atrium is compliant and the regurgitant jet does not produce such an abrupt rise in pressure.

Differential diagnosis

MR must be distinguished from other conditions causing systolic murmurs. The pansystolic murmur of tricuspid regurgitation is associated with giant 'v' waves in the JVP, augmented by inspiration, and located at the lower left sternal edge without radiation into the left axilla. The pansystolic murmur of ventricular septal defect is also best heard at the lower left sternal edge. Nevertheless, following MI, acute ventricular septal defect may be difficult to distinguish from MR caused by papillary muscle rupture (see Table 5.8). The murmur of aortic stenosis is often clearly audible at the cardiac apex but can be identified by its mid-systolic timing and its association with a slow-rising carotid pulse. In all these situations, echocardiography and Doppler studies are usually diagnostic.

Treatment

Diuretics are often sufficient to control dyspnoea. The development of AF requires digitalis, to prevent a rapid ventricular response, and anticoagulants, to protect against thromboembolism from the dilated left atrium. Antibiotic prophylaxis against endocarditis is essential.

Vasodilators, such as ACE inhibitors, play an important role. As aortic pressure is lowered, forward flow into the aorta increases and regurgitation is reduced. Vasodilators are particularly useful in acute MR, and in papillary muscle rupture complicating MI can be used to stabilize the circulation pending emergency valve replacement (Fig. 9.7). In chronic MR, troublesome symptoms which cannot be controlled medically or evidence of LV contractile dysfunction are indications for valve replacement.

Prognosis

Chronic MR is only slowly progressive and is compatible with a normal life-span. However, if the volume-loaded left ventricle develops contractile failure, the prognosis is considerably worse and death usually occurs within 5–10 years. Prognosis is also influenced by aetiology and the outlook in ischaemic disease (papillary muscle dysfunction), for example, is less favourable than in rheumatic disease.

AORTIC STENOSIS

Aetiology

With the decline in rheumatic fever in developed countries, calcific disease has become the commonest cause of aortic stenosis (AS). Indeed, calcific AS is now the most common of all valve lesions, with the possible exception of mitral valve prolapse. It is a degenerative process affecting congenitally bicuspid valves in the 40–60 age group (see page 325) but may also affect a previously normal valve in the very elderly. Rheumatic AS is now relatively unusual and rarely occurs without associated mitral disease. All the important causes of AS are also causes of aortic regurgitation (AR), and a combination of both defects commonly occurs in the same patient.

Pathophysiology

AS obstructs LV outflow and produces a pressure gradient across the valve during systole (see Fig. 3.22). The left ventricle hypertrophies, enabling it to generate sufficient pressure to maintain normal flow through the diseased valve. Not until the aortic valve area is < 1 cm^2 (about one-quarter its normal valve) is AS regarded as critical. Stenosis of this severity requires a peak systolic pressure gradient of > 50 mmHg to maintain normal flow.

Hypertrophy diminishes LV compliance, such that adequate filling depends upon a high end-diastolic pressure. Vigorous left atrial systole (reflected by a prominent 'a' wave) contributes importantly by boosting ventricular filling and, for this reason, AF is poorly tolerated.

As AS worsens, deterioration in LV contractile function eventually occurs. The pressure gradient across the aortic valve can no longer be sustained and forward flow declines. The heart dilates and frank congestive failure develops.

Clinical manifestations

Dyspnoea, angina and syncope are the principal symptoms but they rarely occur before the valve area is critically reduced.

Elevation of the left atrial pressure causes exertional dyspnoea which is particularly severe following the development of frank LVF. This is a late event in the natural history of AS and, in addition to dyspnoea, produces orthopnoea and exercise-related fatigue.

Angina is caused by the exaggerated oxygen demands of the hypertrophied left ventricle. Although the coronary arteries are often normal, they are unable to deliver sufficient oxygen, particularly when demand is heightened during exertion. Coincidental coronary artery disease makes symptoms worse.

Syncope may occur during exertion because flow through the stenosed aortic valve cannot increase sufficiently to maintain blood pressure as skeletal muscle vasodilates. Vasodilator drugs can produce hypotension and syncope by the same mechanism and must be used with caution in AS. Syncope may also result from paroxysmal ventricular arrhythmias (Stokes–Adams attacks) or, rarely, from the development of complete heart block (see below).

Examination of the carotid pulse reveals a slow upstroke and plateau associated with reduced volume. The apex beat is not usually displaced unless there is associated AR. It is thrusting and may have a double impulse due to vigorous atrial contraction immediately before ventricular systole. Systolic thrills are often palpable over the aortic area and the carotid arteries. Auscultation reveals a medium-pitched mid-systolic murmur, which may be heard all over the left precordium but is usually loudest at the base of the heart, radiating into

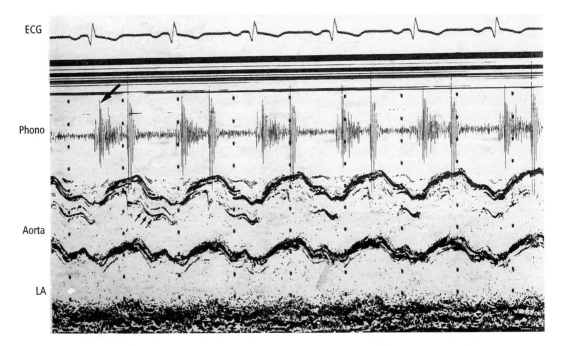

Fig. 9.8 Aortic stenosis—bicuspid aortic valve. In this M-mode echocardiogram the diastolic closure line of the aortic valve (small arrow) lies eccentrically within the aortic root suggesting a bicuspid valve. The valve is normal in other respects. The ejection click (arrowed) and murmur typical of this condition are recorded on the phonocardiogram.

carotids on either side of the neck. It is occasionally preceded by an ejection click if the valve cusps are pliant and not heavily calcified (Fig. 9.8). Other auscultatory findings include a fourth heart sound, reflecting vigorous atrial systole, and reversed splitting of the second heart sound, which may be single—especially when the valve is heavily calcified (see Fig. 1.9).

Complications

Endocarditis is an ever-present risk. Antibiotic prophylaxis prior to dental surgery and other non-sterile invasive procedures is essential. Cardiac arrhythmias are common. AF may produce abrupt clinical deterioration, but more important are ventricular arrhythmias, which are a cause of syncope and sudden death. Heart block requiring pacemaker therapy is an occasional complication of calcific AS and is caused by calcific destruction of the conducting tissue in the adjacent part of the interventricular septum. In advanced AS, the chronic pressure load eventually leads to LVF with irreversible contractile impairment.

Diagnosis

The ECG shows exaggerated voltage deflections, reflecting LV hypertrophy. This may be associated with T-wave inversion in the lateral leads (strain pattern) in advanced cases and, occasionally, left bundle branch block occurs. The CXR shows a normal heart size, unless there is associated AR. Post-stenotic dilatation of the ascending aorta is usually evident and the penetrated film may reveal valvular calcification (Fig. 9.9).

The echocardiogram is diagnostic in most cases. The aortic valve is thickened and rigid. Symmetrical LV hypertrophy is almost invariable (Fig. 9.10). Doppler studies provide a quantitative assessment of the pressure gradient across the valve and may also demonstrate AR. The majority of patients with AS are middle-aged or elderly and many of them have angina. Coronary arteriography is therefore commonly required preoperatively in order that diseased vessels, if present, may be bypassed at the same time as valve replacement. During cardiac catheterization, the pressure gradient across the aortic valve should be measured (see Fig. 3.22). Aortic root angiography permits assessment of associated AR (see Fig. 3.17).

Differential diagnosis

The differential diagnosis of AS includes other causes of hypertrophic LV disease, particularly hypertrophic cardiomyopathy and hypertension. Both conditions may be associated with angina, a mid-systolic ejection murmur and ECG changes similar to AS, but in neither condition is the carotid pulse slow rising, nor does the echocardiogram show a thickened aortic valve.

Innocent systolic murmurs (see page 22) should not be confused with AS. They are usually soft and never produce a slow rising carotid pulse.

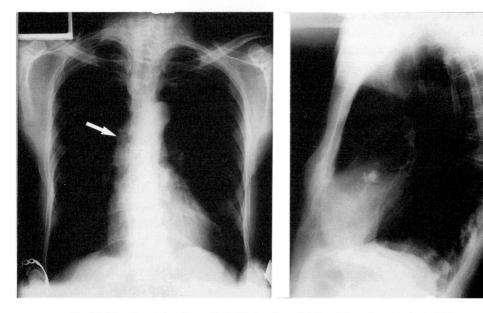

Fig. 9.9 PA and lateral chest X-rays. On the PA chest X-ray dilatation of the aortic root is clearly visible (arrowed) and the calcified valve leaflets can be identified. Note that the heart size is not enlarged because aortic stenosis produces left ventricular hypertrophy without dilatation. On the lateral chest X-ray the calcified valve is more clearly visible.

Treatment

Subcritical AS requires no specific treatment while it remains asymptomatic, although vigorous exertion should be discouraged because of the risk of ventricular arrhythmias. Antibiotic prophylaxis against infective endocarditis is essential.

Surgical treatment is usually by valve replacement. Valvotomy is effective in infants with congenital bicuspid valves but is impossible in adults with calcific disease which prohibits effective division of the commissures. Percutaneous aortic balloon valvuloplasty, now the procedure of choice in infants (see page 326),

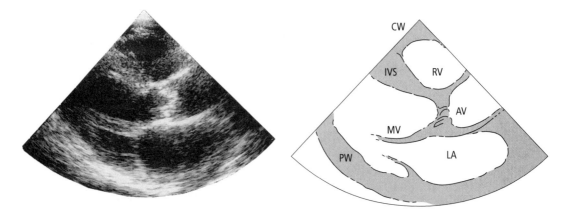

Fig. 9.10 Two-dimensional echocardiogram (long axis view). The aortic valve is grossly thickened and highly echogenic suggestive of calcification. Concentric left ventricular hypertrophy is clearly visible.

is unhelpful in adults for the same reason. Indications for valve surgery in AS are as follows.

- Any symptoms attributable to AS.
- LVF. Regular monitoring of ventricular function by echocardiography or nuclear ventriculography is essential.
- Critical AS (i.e. peak systolic pressure gradient > 50 mmHg). This is usually regarded as an indication for valve replacement even in the asymptomatic patient with well-preserved ventricular function.

Prognosis

AS is well tolerated and most patients are over 60 before they die; following the development of symptoms, however, death usually occurs within 3 years. The outlook is worse in patients with LVF. Valve replacement improves the prognosis for these symptomatic patients considerably.

AORTIC REGURGITATION

Aetiology

Aortic regurgitation (AR) is caused by either disease of the valve cusps or aortic root disease (Table 9.2). In calcific disease AR is usually trivial but in bicuspid valvular disease and rheumatic disease it may be the dominant lesion. Infective endocarditis is an important cause of acute AR, as are deceleration injuries which cause acute AR by traumatic rupture of the valve.

Aortic root disease causes AR by dilatation of the valve annulus. This may occur acutely in aortic dissection but usually it is a chronic process seen in cystic medial necrosis of the aorta (with or without other manifestations of Marfan's syndrome), ankylosing spondylitis and other connective-tissue and rheumatological disorders. Many cases, however, are idiopathic. Syphilis is no longer a common cause of aortic root disease.

Table 9.2 Causes of aortic regurgitation (AR).

Valve-leaflet disease	Congenital bicuspid valve
	Calcific disease
	Rheumatic disease
	Infective endocarditis*
Aortic root dilating disease	Marfan's syndrome
	Ankylosing spondylitis
	Syphilis
	Hypertension
	Aortic dissection*
	Aortic root aneurysm
	Deceleration injury*

* These disorders produce acute AR. In the remainder the course is chronic.

Pathophysiology

Regurgitant flow in AR is greatest immediately following valve closure and declines in mid-diastole as pressure in the aortic root falls. Increments in heart rate reduce the regurgitant volume by shortening diastole.

AR volume-loads the left ventricle. When this occurs acutely the Starling reserve of the ventricle is often exceeded, resulting in pulmonary oedema and low-output failure. In chronic AR, however, LV dilatation and hypertrophy effectively compensate for the volume load. The increase in diastolic filling increases stroke volume (Starling mechanism), such that forward cardiac output is maintained despite the regurgitant flow. LV dilatation is relatively more pronounced than hypertrophy and compliance remains normal or increases. Thus, the volume-loaded left ventricle does not always exhibit significant elevation of end-diastolic pressure. The Starling mechanism and the compliance properties of the ventricle ensure that chronic AR is well tolerated without producing low cardiac output or pulmonary oedema. Nevertheless, the compensatory potential of LV dilatation and hypertrophy is limited (see page 81) and, in advanced disease, contractile function deteriorates—leading to heart failure.

Clinical manifestations

Acute AR may present dramatically with pulmonary oedema and low-output failure. Chronic AR, however, usually remains asymptomatic for several years before the development of exertional fatigue and dyspnoea marks the onset of LVF. Angina affects 50% of cases and is caused by the increased oxygen requirements of the dilated, hypertrophied ventricle (*cf.* aortic stenosis).

The carotid pulse is readily visible in the neck—Corrigan's pulse. It has a rapid upstroke and collapses in early diastole as blood regurgitates into the left ventricle. The pulse pressure is widened, with exaggeration of the systolic peak and the diastolic nadir. During blood-pressure measurement, the Korotkoff sounds often persist to zero so that phase V cannot be identified (see page 13), and phase IV must be used for the diastolic measurement.

The apex beat is displaced towards the left axilla and has a prominent impulse due to LV enlargement. Auscultation at the aortic area reveals a high-pitched early diastolic murmur which radiates down to the left-sternal edge; a mid-systolic murmur due to turbulent forward flow through the aortic valve is usually also present. It relates to increased stroke volume and does not necessarily indicate AS. In severe disease, the regurgitant jet causes preclosure of the anterior leaflet of the mitral valve during diastole. This produces an apical mid-diastolic murmur (Austin–Flint).

Complications

Infective endocarditis is a major complication. In advanced disease, progressive LV dilatation and irreversible contractile dysfunction results in heart failure (Fig. 9.11).

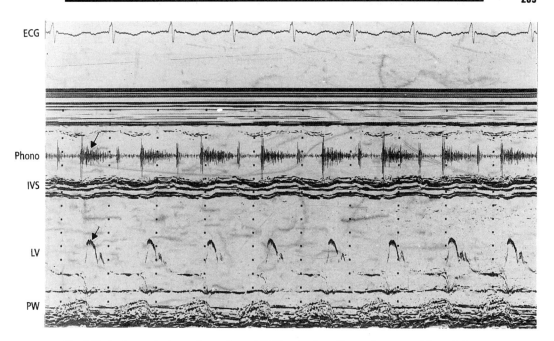

ECG

Phono

IVS

LV

PW

Fig. 9.11 Aortic regurgitation—end-stage disease. This M-mode echocardiogram shows severe left ventricular dilatation with global contractile impairment. Note the fine vibrations on the anterior leaflet of the mitral valve (arrowed) caused by the regurgitant jet. The early diastolic decrescendo murmur has been recorded immediately following the second heart sound (arrowed). The prognosis in this case is very poor, but might have been better if aortic valve replacement earlier in the natural history of the disease had prevented deterioration in left ventricular contractile function.

Diagnosis

The ECG shows evidence of LV hypertrophy. The CXR shows an enlarged heart and dilatation of the ascending aorta. Penetrated films may reveal calcification of the aortic valve.

The echocardiogram may show an abnormally thickened aortic valve. In aortic root disease, however, the valve itself appears normal although the aorta is dilated. The regurgitant jet may produce fine vibrations on the anterior leaflet of the mitral valve and, less commonly, on the interventricular septum. The left ventricle shows variable dilatation and vigorous contractile function until this deteriorates in end-stage disease (Fig. 9.11). Doppler studies identify the regurgitant jet and permit assessment of its severity.

Cardiac catheterization is usually necessary before aortic valve surgery, in order to examine the coronary anatomy. LV and aortic root angiography define contractile function and the severity of AR, respectively (see Fig. 3.17). In patients with associated AS, the valve gradient can be measured.

Differential diagnosis

AR must be distinguished from other conditions associated with an early diastolic murmur. Pulmonary regurgitation is relatively unusual and is nearly always associated with evidence of severe pulmonary hypertension. In patent ductus arteriosus and ruptured sinus of Valsalva aneurysm, the murmurs are continuous but are loudest at end-systole/early diastole. Moreover, these conditions are associated with a wide pulse pressure. Confusion with AR is therefore easy. Echo–Doppler studies, however, can usually confirm the differential diagnosis.

Treatment

In acute AR associated with LVF, valve replacement should not be delayed. In chronic AR, symptoms are rarely obtrusive until the onset of LVF. Mild dyspnoea may respond to diuretic therapy, but vasodilators are often more useful because reductions in peripheral resistance and reflex tachycardia increase forward flow and reduce the regurgitant fraction. Antibiotic prophylaxis against infective endocarditis is essential.

When AR becomes symptomatic, valve replacement is usually indicated, particularly when symptoms are associated with echocardiographic or radionuclide evidence of LV contractile deterioration. If surgery is delayed until LV dysfunction has become irreversible, the results are less satisfactory.

Prognosis

The prognosis is determined principally by the severity of LV dysfunction. Thus, mild AR with normal ventricular function is compatible with a normal life-span but, in more severe cases, LVF often develops in middle age. Thereafter, prognosis is poor and similar to that of other causes of LVF (see page 95). Timely valve replacement improves prognosis considerably.

TRICUSPID STENOSIS

Aetiology

Tricuspid stenosis (TS) is almost invariably rheumatic in origin and is usually associated with mitral valve disease. It is uncommon not only because rheumatic disease tends to spare the right side of the heart but also because the tricuspid valve is very large and can tolerate substantial commissural fusion and leaflet fibrosis before obstruction to flow becomes significant.

Pathophysiology

Obstruction to tricuspid flow causes elevation of the right atrial pressure and establishes a pressure gradient across the valve, increased by inspiration. Vigorous atrial contraction contributes importantly to right ventricular filling and produces a giant 'a' wave in the JVP. As TS increases pulmonary flow decreases. This may produce a paradoxical symptomatic improvement in patients with associated MS by reducing pulmonary-artery and pulmonary-capillary pressures.

Nevertheless, this improvement is at the expense of worsening cardiac output and right heart failure.

Clinical manifestations

TS is usually associated with rheumatic mitral valve disease which tends to dominate the clinical presentation causing dyspnoea. As TS becomes more severe, however, dyspnoea may improve (see above) to be replaced by symptoms of right heart failure including oedema and abdominal discomfort caused by hepatomegaly and ascites. Muscular fatigue caused by low cardiac output is also common.

The examination reveals an elevated JVP with a giant 'a' wave. The 'a' wave disappears with the onset of AF. A low-pitched mid-diastolic murmur, augmented during inspiration, is present at the lower left sternal edge, with presystolic accentuation in sinus rhythm.

Diagnosis

In isolated TS the ECG may show tall peaked P waves indicating right atrial enlargement, but the CXR is usually normal. The two-dimensional echocardiogram confirms thickening and rigidity of the tricuspid valve and right atrial enlargement. Doppler studies permit quantification of the pressure gradient.

Differential diagnosis

TS must be differentiated from other causes of a mid-diastolic murmur and right heart failure, particularly MS and atrial septal defect.

Treatment

In most cases the lesion is mild and haemodynamically unimportant; severe right heart failure, however, requires valve surgery. Valvotomy is rarely satisfactory and valve replacement is the procedure of choice.

TRICUSPID REGURGITATION

Tricuspid regurgitation (TR) is usually functional and secondary to right ventricular dilatation in advanced RVF when it exacerbates the existing haemodynamic derangement. Other causes of TR, including rheumatic disease, infective endocarditis, Ebstein's anomaly and carcinoid disease, are rare.

TR volume-loads the right ventricle and leads to (or, more commonly, exacerbates) symptoms and signs of right heart failure. A pansystolic murmur may be audible at the left sternal edge but this is usually soft; it may be associated with a mid-diastolic tricuspid flow murmur. The regurgitant jet produces pulsatile systolic waves in the jugular veins called giant 'v' waves

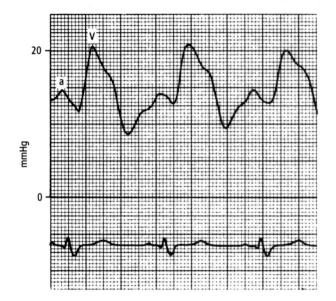

Fig. 9.12 Tricuspid regurgitation. The right atrial pressure recording shows a typical giant 'v' wave caused by the regurgitant jet.

(Fig. 9.12). Sometimes pulsatile expansion of the enlarged liver can be detected. In functional TR signs of pulmonary hypertension are usually present, including a loud pulmonary component to the second heart sound.

TR is essentially a clinical diagnosis based on giant 'v' waves in the JVP. Doppler studies identify the regurgitant jet (see Plate 9.1). The echocardiogram may show a normal tricuspid valve if regurgitation is functional, but there is always dilatation of the right-sided cardiac chambers (Fig. 9.13).

TR is usually well tolerated even when it occurs acutely in endocarditis. Treatment with diuretics controls systemic congestion and reduces right ventric-

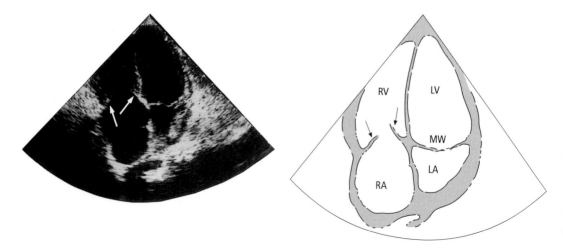

Fig. 9.13 Tricuspid regurgitation—carcinoid. The two-dimensional echocardiogram is a systolic frame (note the mitral valve is closed), but the damaged tricuspid valve leaflets (arrowed) are tethered and remain widely separated allowing tricuspid regurgitation. Thus the right atrium is severely dilated.

ular volume which improves functional regurgitation. Tricuspid valve surgery is only rarely necessary.

PULMONARY VALVE DISEASE

Rheumatic disease of the pulmonary valve is rare. Endocarditis occurs occasionally (usually in intravenous drug abusers) but the most common pulmonary valve defects are congenital valvular stenosis and valvular regurgitation due to pulmonary hypertension. Congenital pulmonary stenosis is discussed in Chapter 15. Pulmonary regurgitation produces an early diastolic murmur at the upper left sternal edge (Graham Steell murmur) which is almost identical to that of AR. Nevertheless in pulmonary regurgitation signs of pulmonary hypertension are usually prominent and the carotid pulse is normal, so differentiation between pulmonary regurgitation and AR should not be difficult. Pulmonary regurgitation is well tolerated, producing negligible haemodynamic embarrassment, and prognosis is determined by the associated pulmonary hypertension.

FURTHER READING

Alpert MA. Mitral valve prolapse. *Br Med J* 1993; 306: 943.

Borow RO. Management of chronic aortic regurgitation. *N Engl J Med* 1994; 331: 736.

Carabello BA, Crawford FA. Therapy for mitral stenosis comes full circle. *N Engl J Med* 1994; 331: 1014.

Collins JJ. The evolution of artificial heart valves. *N Engl J Med* 1991; 324: 624.

Frankl WS. Valvular heart disease: the technologic dilemma. *J Am Coll Cardiol* 1991; 17: 1037.

Rahimtoola SH. Vasodilator therapy in chronic severe aortic regurgitation. *J Am Coll Cardiol* 1990; 16: 430.

Selzer A. Changing aspects of the natural history of valvular aortic stenosis. *N Engl J Med* 1987; 317: 91.

Taggart DP, Wheatley DJ. Mitral valve surgery: to repair or replace? *Br Heart J* 1990; 64: 234.

C H A P T E R   1 0

Conduction Tissue Disease and Pacemakers

CONTENTS

SUMMARY

Idiopathic fibrosis, a condition affecting the elderly, is the most common cause of conduction tissue disease; ischaemic disease and cardiomyopathy are also important. Although the conduction tissue is often diffusely involved, sinoatrial (SA) and atrioventricular (AV) disease are conveniently considered separately.

SA disease. The commonest manifestation is sinus bradycardia which, if the rate fails to increase normally with exercise (chronotropic incompetence), may cause fatigue and dyspnoea. Prolonged sinus pauses lead to dizzy attacks and syncope; in the bradycardia–tachycardia syndrome, paroxysmal tachyarrhythmias (usually atrial fibrillation, AF) cause palpitations and, occasionally, thromboembolism. Because symptoms are typically intermittent, diagnosis may require ambulatory Holter monitoring to document the ECG abnormality. Treatment of bradycardias and sinus pauses is by atrial pacing (dual-chamber pacing for patients with associated AV disease) but is only necessary in patients experiencing symptoms. Associated tachyarrhythmias may require treatment with antiarrhythmic drugs but if these exacerbate SA dysfunction a pacemaker may be necessary to protect against severe bradycardia. AF increases the risk of thromboembolism and prophylactic anticoagulation with warfarin is usually recommended.

AV disease may involve the AV node or the bundle branches. First-degree AV block causes delayed conduction but is asymptomatic because heart rate is unaffected. The ECG shows a prolonged PR interval and no treatment is necessary. In second-degree AV block, failure of conduction is intermittent, and symptoms (fatigue, dizziness) occur only if insufficient sinus impulses are conducted to maintain an adequate ventricular rate. Second-degree block may be within the AV node (Wenckebach) when the PR interval is prolonged and increases progressively, culminating in a dropped beat; the process may then repeat itself. Symptoms are unusual and pacemaker therapy therefore is rarely necessary. When second-degree block affects the bundle branches (Mobitz type II), the ECG usually shows a normal PR interval with bundle branch block, intermittent block in the other bundle branch resulting in dropped beats. Pacing is mandatory because of the risk of prolonged asystole. Third-degree (complete) AV block is characterized by complete AV dissociation with regular P waves (unless the atrium is fibrillating) and regular but slower QRS complexes occurring independently of one another. Block may be at the AV node (congenital block, inferior myocardial infarction) when a reliable junctional escape rhythm usually prevents symptoms, making pacing unnecessary. More often it occurs further down the conduction system in the bundle branches where escape rhythms are slow and unreliable and pacing is mandatory because of the risk of prolonged asystole.

Pacemakers. Ventricular pacing (VVI) is usually only indicated in complete AV block associated with AF when, ideally, a rate responsive unit (VVIR) should be used. Other patients with complete AV block should be offered a dual-chamber (DDD) unit because this re-establishes AV synchrony and allows the sinus node to control the heart rate which increases normally with exercise. In SA disease, atrial pacing (AAI) is the method of choice, although patients with chronotropic incompetence require a rate-responsive unit (AAIR); DDD pacing is required in patients with associated AV block.

INTRODUCTION

Disease of the cardiac conduction tissues can occur at any level from the sinus node, through the sinoatrial junction, the atrioventricular (AV) node and the bundle of His, to the bundle branches and Purkinje system (Fig. 10.1).

SINOATRIAL DISEASE

Aetiology

Causes of sinoatrial (SA) disease are shown in Table 10.1. The most common is idiopathic fibrosis which affects the conduction tissue at any level and occurs particularly in the elderly.

Pathophysiology

The sinus node, the conduction tissue with the highest intrinsic firing rate, is the

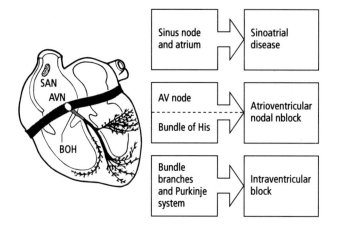

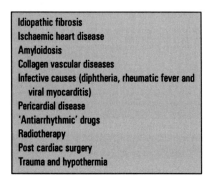

Fig. 10.1 Classification of conduction tissue disease. SAN, sinoatrial node; AVN, atrioventricular node; BOH, bundle of His.

pacemaker of the normal heart. The spontaneous discharge of the sinus node is influenced by a variety of neurohumoral factors, particularly vagal and sympathetic stimulation which, respectively, slow and speed the sinus rate. The normal sinus rate varies with activity and with age. A rate of 40 beats per minute is often normal during sleep and rates up to 200 beats per minute may be achieved during exertion. Sinus arrhythmia (in which the rate increases during inspiration and decreases during expiration) is common in the young but tends to disappear with advancing age. Progressive slowing of the sinus rate occurs after the age of 55–60.

Sinus node discharge can be recorded endocardially using special electrodes. It is not, however, visible on the surface ECG although the atrial depolarization it initiates produces the P wave. Sinus node discharge may be suppressed by drugs or disease, or it may be blocked and fail to activate the atrium. Under these circumstances pacemaker function can be assumed by 'escape' foci in atrial tissue, the AV node, His–Purkinje tissue or the ventricular myocardium. The intrinsic rates of all these escape pacemakers are slower than the normal sinus rate and usually decrease progressively down the conduction system (Fig. 10.2).

Table 10.1 Causes of sinoatrial disease.

Idiopathic fibrosis
Ischaemic heart disease
Amyloidosis
Collagen vascular diseases
Infective causes (diphtheria, rheumatic fever and
    viral myocarditis)
Pericardial disease
'Antiarrhythmic' drugs
Radiotherapy
Post cardiac surgery
Trauma and hypothermia

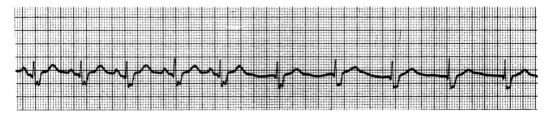

Fig. 10.2 Junctional escape rhythm. Sinus rhythm ceases abruptly after the fifth beat and a junctional (AV node/bundle of His) focus takes over. Because ventricular depolarization proceeds by normal pathways, the QRS complexes of the escape rhythm are identical to the sinus complexes. However, P waves are not seen and the rate is slower.

Clinical manifestations

SA disease is often asymptomatic. Presentation is usually with episodes of dizziness or syncope caused by severe bradycardia or prolonged sinus pauses without an effective escape rhythm. Pauses longer than 3 or 4 seconds are usually necessary to produce symptoms, although the elderly may be more susceptible. Additional complaints may include exertional fatigue and dyspnoea due to the failure of a physiological increase in heart rate (chronotropic incompetence). Patients may complain of palpitations due to associated tachycardias, and thromboembolic events may also occur.

Complications

Paroxysmal atrial or junctional tachycardias (usually atrial fibrillation, AF) often occur in association with bradyarrhythmias. This is known as the bradycardia–tachycardia syndrome (see below). More important is thromboembolism, which is particularly common in patients with paroxysmal tachycardias.

Diagnosis

Arrhythmia detection (see page 37)

ECG documentation is essential for accurate diagnosis but the resting recording is rarely helpful in SA disease. Ambulatory ECG monitoring is usually required, but symptoms are often infrequent and documentation of the arrhythmia may be impossible without repeated Holter recordings. Although patient-activated recorders are preferable, symptoms are often transitory, and a device with a loop facility should be chosen which, when triggered manually by the patient, provides a record of the ECG in the seconds leading up to the episode. Electrophysiological studies are rarely helpful because measurements of SA function are very insensitive, often yielding false-negative results in patients with SA disease.

Electrocardiographic diagnosis

Sinus bradycardia

This may be defined as a resting sinus rate below 50 beats per minute. Like other bradycardias it may be associated with atrial, junctional (Fig. 10.2) or ventricular escape rhythms. Sinus bradycardia is physiological during sleep and in trained athletes, but in other circumstances may reflect SA disease, particularly when associated with chronotrophic incompetence (see page 211).

Sinus pauses

Sinus pauses may be caused by SA block or sinus arrest. In SA block a normal sinus impulse occurs but its exit to the atria is blocked and the P wave is absent. In sinus arrest the pause is caused by intermittent failure of sinus node discharge. SA block can sometimes be distinguished from sinus arrest if the pause is a precise multiple of preceding PP intervals. However, this is not reliable, and in practical and prognostic terms there is little point in attempting to distinguish between the different causes of sinus pauses (Fig. 10.3).

Bradycardia–tachycardia syndrome

Paroxysmal atrial or junctional tachyarrhythmias often occur in patients with SA disease. The tachycardias may be escape rhythms after pauses or may occur during periods of normal SA function. AF (Fig. 10.4) is one of the more common

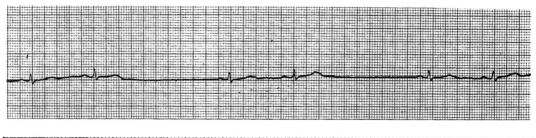

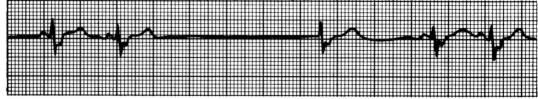

Fig. 10.3 Sinus pauses. Upper panel: intermittent sinoatrial block (after the second and fourth complexes) which has prevented sinus impulses from depolarizing the atrium. No P waves are seen but because the sinus discharge continues uninterrupted, the pauses are each a precise multiple of the preceding P–P interval. Lower panel: sinus arrest with junctional escape. This occurs after the second sinus beat when there is a long pause terminated by a junctional escape beat (no P wave). Thereafter sinus rhythm becomes re-established.

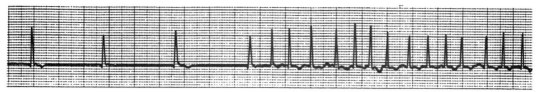

Fig. 10.4 Bradycardia–tachycardia syndrome. A very slow junctional rhythm gives way to rapid atrial fibrillation.

arrhythmias and the main cause of thromboembolic events associated with this condition.

Differential diagnosis

SA disease must be distinguished from other cardiac and non-cardiac causes of dizzy attacks and syncope (see page 5).

Carotid sinus syndrome is caused by carotid sinus hypersensitivity. As a diagnostic test, pressure over the carotid sinus may cause sinus bradycardia, sinus arrest or AV block as well as vasodilatation (Fig. 10.5)—care must be taken first to ensure by auscultation and gentle palpation that the carotids are normal. Patients may complain of syncope although, paradoxically, this is rarely caused by actual pressure on the carotid bodies. Carotid sinus massage is usually diagnostic (see page 40). Pacing corrects bradycardias in the carotid sinus syndrome. The vasodilator component, however, may be difficult to treat and is often exacerbated if VVI rather than dual-chamber pacing is used (see below).

Malignant vasovagal syndrome also has bradycardic and vasodilator elements caused usually by exaggerated vagal responses to emotional or painful stimuli. Diagnosis is by tilt testing (see page 39). Repeated syncopal attacks may become very disabling and require dual-chamber pacing. However, there is often a strong (or even predominant) vasodepressor element, which can be almost impossible to overcome.

Treatment

Most asymptomatic patients with sinus bradycardia or sinus pauses require no specific treatment. Drugs such as beta-blockers which suppress the sinus node should be avoided. Patients who have symptomatic bradycardias or pauses require pacemaker therapy to maintain the heart rate and prevent syncope. Atrial pacing is preferred because, unlike ventricular pacing, it reduces the risk of thrombo-

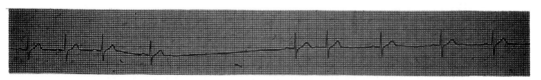

Fig. 10.5 Carotid sinus hypersensitivity. The beginning of the trace shows normal sinus rhythm. Carotid sinus massage produces a long sinus pause which continues until massage is stopped.

embolism. It also maintains normal cardiac activation and heart rate, improves exercise tolerance and often prevents associated tachyarrhythmias. If abnormalities of AV conduction are manifest or suspected, it is normal practice to provide additional ventricular pacing using a dual-chamber pacemaker (see below).

Associated tachyarrhythmias may require treatment with antiarrhythmic agents but most drugs of this type will exacerbate SA dysfunction, when a pacemaker is necessary to protect against severe bradycardia. AF increases the risk of thromboembolism and anticoagulation with warfarin is required. In patients under 50, the risk is lower, but warfarin remains recommended, low-dose aspirin (75–300 mg/day) being considerably less effective in protecting against embolic events.

In malignant vasovagal syndrome, bradycardia can be treated with a pacemaker, but treatment of symptoms caused by vasodilatation can be very difficult. Beta-blockers, disopyramide for its anticholinergic properties, and fludrocortisone have all been used, with little by way of consistent success.

Prognosis

The prognosis of SA disease depends mainly on the underlying cause and on the thromboembolic risk. Death is rarely a direct consequence of sinus bradyarrhythmias.

ATRIOVENTRICULAR BLOCK

Aetiology (Table 10.2)

The commonest cause of AV block in the western world is idiopathic fibrosis of the bundle branches, particularly in the elderly. Ischaemic heart disease and

Idiopathic fibrosis (Lenegre's disease/Lev's disease)
Ischaemic heart disease
Calcific aortic stenosis
Congenital AV block (isolated or associated with other congenital malformations)
Cardiomyopathy (including Chagas' disease)
Infection (tuberculosis, diphtheria, syphilis)
Sarcoidosis
Myeloma and other tumours (including Hodgkin's disease)
Connective tissue disease (ankylosing spondylitis, rheumatoid disease)
Myxoedema
Muscular dystrophies
'Antiarrhythmic' drugs
Radiotherapy
Trauma
Hypothermia

Table 10.2 Causes of atrioventricular (AV) block.

cardiomyopathy are also important. Chagas' disease is the most common cause in Central and South America.

Pathophysiology

AV block can occur in either the AV node or the His–Purkinje system. When conduction is merely delayed (e.g. first-degree AV block, bundle branch block) the heart rate is unaffected. When conduction is completely interrupted, however, the rate may slow and cause symptoms. In second-degree AV block, failure of conduction is intermittent, and if sufficient sinus impulses are conducted to maintain an adequate ventricular rate symptoms do not occur. In third-degree AV block, there is complete failure of conduction and continuing ventricular activity depends on the emergence of an escape rhythm; the higher the level in the conduction system at which block occurs, the faster the escape rhythm. If block is within the AV node the escape rhythm is often, but not always, fast enough to prevent major syncope. If both bundle branches are blocked the ventricular escape rhythm may be very slow and unreliable and lead to syncope and death.

Clinical manifestations

First-degree AV block is asymptomatic and can only be diagnosed from the ECG. In second-degree AV block, symptoms depend on the number of conducted impulses and although patients are often asymptomatic, fatigue and dyspnoea commonly occur. The development of higher degrees of block may cause syncope.

In third-degree (complete) AV block, the symptoms depend on the level in the conduction system at which block occurs. In congenital AV block and acute inferior myocardial infarction, block is usually at the level of the AV node and a reliable junctional escape rhythm is common. However, in most other cases, block occurs further down the conduction system in the bundle branches where escape rhythms are slow and unreliable. Exertional fatigue and dyspnoea are common and frank heart failure may occur, particularly in patients with associated valvular or myocardial disease. Very slow rates and prolonged pauses cause dizziness and syncope (Stokes–Adams attacks).

Examination in third-degree AV block reveals a slow regular pulse, usually less than 50 beats per minute. The atrial and ventricular rhythms are dissociated and, if the sinus node is functioning normally, intermittent cannon 'a' waves in the JVP (Fig. 10.6) and beat-to-beat variation in the intensity of the first heart sound are present. If the atrium is fibrillating, however, these signs are absent.

Diagnosis

Detection of AV block

All forms of AV block may be persistent or intermittent. If persistent, they are easily diagnosed from the resting ECG. If they are intermittent, ambulatory

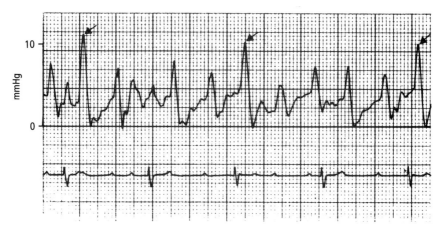

Fig. 10.6 Cannon 'a' waves in congenital complete heart block. The ECG shows complete dissociation of atrial and ventricular activity. The random coincidence of atrial and ventricular systole (occurring shortly after the QRS complex) produces intermittent cannon 'a' waves (arrowed) on the right atrial pressure recording.

monitoring is usually required (see page 38). Abnormalities on the resting ECG (e.g. prolonged PR interval or bundle branch block with axis deviation) pointing to underlying conduction abnormalities must be interpreted cautiously because, in the absence of symptoms, they are often clinically unimportant and even in patients with syncope, paroxysmal ventricular tachycardia is as likely to be responsible as intermittent complete heart block.

Electrophysiological study (see page 40) is more useful for diagnosing intermittent complete AV block than SA disease, but the predictive accuracy remains low and ambulatory monitoring techniques are preferred.

First-degree AV block (Fig. 10.7)

Delayed AV conduction causes a prolonged PR interval (> 0.2 seconds) on the ECG. Ventricular depolarization, however, usually occurs rapidly using normal His–Purkinje pathways. Thus the QRS complexes are narrow and of normal duration unless there is associated bundle branch block.

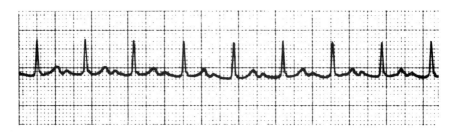

Fig. 10.7 First-degree AV block. Note the prolongation of the PR interval (0.28 seconds).

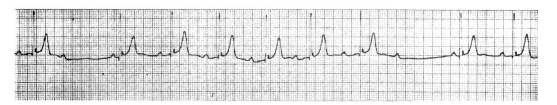

Fig. 10.8 Second-degree AV block—Wenckebach type. The PR interval shows progressive prolongation until failure of AV conduction occurs and a beat is dropped.

Second-degree AV block—Wenckebach type I (Fig. 10.8)

This is also called Mobitz type I block and occurs within the AV node. Successive sinus beats find the AV node increasingly refractory until failure of conduction occurs. The delay permits recovery of nodal function and the process may then repeat itself. The ECG often shows a prolonged PR interval which increases progressively, culminating in a dropped beat. The QRS complexes are usually narrow and of normal duration.

Second-degree AV block—Mobitz type II (Fig. 10.9)

This usually indicates advanced conduction tissue disease affecting the bundle branches. There is usually bundle branch block, intermittent block in the other bundle branch resulting in complete failure of AV conduction and dropped beats. The PR interval in conducted beats is constant and often normal.

Patients with 2 : 1 AV block may have Wenckebach or Mobitz type II block. The precise level of the block can be difficult to determine in these cases but generally if there is a prolonged PR interval in the conducted beat and normal QRS complexes then the block is more likely to be of the Wenckebach type, with AV nodal disease. If the conducted PR interval is normal but there is bundle branch block, it is more likely to be Mobitz type II block, with His–Purkinje disease.

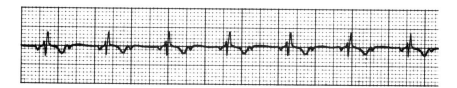

Fig. 10.9 Second-degree AV block—Mobitz type II. The ECG shows 2 : 1 AV block in which every second sinus discharge fails to penetrate the ventricular conduction system. Note that in those beats that are conducted normally, the QRS complex shows a bundle branch block pattern and the PR interval is normal—both typical features of Mobitz type II AV block.

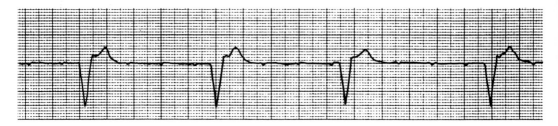

Fig. 10.10 Third-degree AV block below the bundle of His. There is complete dissociation of atrial and ventricular activity. The ventricular escape rhythm arises distally in the ventricular conduction system and has a broad QRS complex. Compare with Figs 5.22 and 10.6 in which block is at the level of the AV node.

Third-degree—complete AV block (Fig. 10.10)

Complete failure of AV conduction produces dissociated atrial and ventricular rhythms. The ECG shows regular P waves (unless the atria are fibrillating) and regular but slower QRS complexes occurring independently of one another. When block is within the AV node a junctional escape rhythm often occurs, with a narrow QRS complex and a reliable rate of 40–60 beats per minute. When block is within the bundle branches the ventricular escape rhythm is generally slow and unreliable with broad QRS complexes. Complete AV block may be misdiagnosed as 2 : 1 AV block when the atrial rate is approximately twice the ventricular rate and only a short rhythm strip is examined.

Right bundle branch block (see Fig. 2.11)

This may be a congenital defect, occurring as an isolated phenomenon. However, it is more commonly the result of organic conduction tissue disease which may be idiopathic or associated with other cardiac disorders, notably coronary disease. Right ventricular depolarization is delayed and this results in a broad QRS complexes with an rSR pattern in lead V1 and a prominent S wave in leads I and V6.

Left bundle branch block (see Fig. 2.11)

Although this may occur as an isolated finding it usually indicates organic conduction tissue disease which, like right bundle branch block, may be idiopathic or associated with other cardiac disorders. Left ventricular depolarization is delayed and there is a broad QRS complex with a large slurred or notched R wave in leads I and V6. Block may be confined to the anterior or posterior divisions of the left bundle (hemiblock) when it is associated with left or right axis deviation, respectively, on the ECG.

Treatment

All patients with complete AV block require a permanent pacemaker unless block is likely to be temporary (acute myocardial infarction, drug effect). A pacemaker is also required if the risk of developing complete AV block is high, e.g. in Mobitz type II block, and selected patients with trifascicular block (prolonged PR interval, right bundle branch block and left axis deviation) in whom AV conduction is dependent on the remaining division of the left bundle branch. Pacing relieves symptoms and, importantly, prevents prolonged asystole and sudden death. Only in congenital AV block are the indications for pacemaker therapy less well defined. These patients often remain asymptomatic for prolonged periods and the usual recommendation has been for pacing only in the event of symptoms. However, elective early pacing is favoured by some cardiologists because it may prevent the later development of irreversible cardiomegaly.

Temporary pacemakers

Temporary pacemakers are used predominantly for the treatment of bradycardias (very occasionally for tachycardias) when the conduction disturbance is temporary and reversible or when pacing is required as a 'bridge' to a permanent device. Transvenous, endocardial pacing catheters are used most commonly. The catheter is inserted through either a central (usually subclavian or internal jugular) or a peripheral vein and positioned within the right ventricle; temporary right atrial pacing can also be performed. Temporary epicardial pacing is reserved for patients who have undergone heart surgery: epicardial wires, placed perioperatively, are used to protect against bradycardia during the recovery period.

Endocardial temporary pacing catheters are usually bipolar with the two electrodes mounted at the distal end (cathode at the tip, anode about 1 cm more proximally). The electrodes are connected to an external pulse generator which consists of electronic circuitry and a battery power source. Complications, less common in experienced hands, include haemorrhage due to venous puncture, pneumothorax if the subclavian approach is used, infection, and cardiac perforation.

Permanent pacemakers

A permanent pacemaker consists of a hermetically sealed pulse generator driven by a lithium/lithium iodide cell. It is inserted under local anaesthetic into a subcutaneous 'pocket' (usually in the left prepectoral position) and attached to one, or often two, pacing catheters using a special connector block. The pacing catheters are introduced transvenously either through the cephalic vein or, failing this, by direct subclavian puncture and are positioned in the right side of the heart (Fig. 10.11). Modern pacemaker pulse generators weigh about 25 g, are about 6 mm thick and last approximately 8 years before the battery expires. They are all programmable using an external radiofrequency programmer which allows performance to be optimized by controlling the pacing rate, voltage output, sensitivity and a variety of other more sophisticated variables. In general the lowest output compatible with reliable pacing should be selected in order to

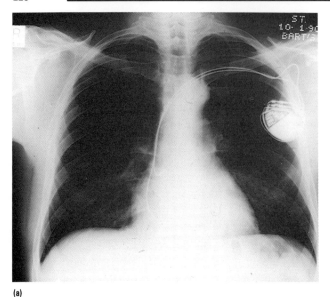

(a)

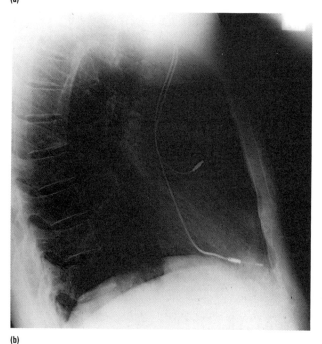

(b)

Fig. 10.11 Permanent dual-chamber pacemaker. The PA and lateral chest X-rays (panels A and B, respectively) show a modern dual-chamber pacemaker in the left prepectoral position attached to right atrial and ventricular pacemaker electrodes.

prolong battery life. The choice of rate depends on the indication for pacing. Modern pacemakers are usually bipolar, with the anode and cathode mounted at the distal end of the pacing catheter, closely applied to the endocardium; some older pacemakers are unipolar, with the cathode at the distal end of the pacing catheter and the anode provided by the metal casing of the pulse generator.

Pacing catheters are usually coaxially wound insulated coils connected to the pulse generator and terminating within the heart in a pair of platinum or carbon

Table 10.3 Methods of pacing: five-letter code.

Chamber paced	Chamber sensed	Response to sensing	Programming and rate responsiveness	Anti-tachycardia capability
0 = None	0 = None	0 = None	0 = None	0 = None
A = Atrium	A = Atrium	T = Triggered	P = Simple	P = Pacing
V = Ventricle	V = Ventricle	I = Inhibited	M = Multiprogrammable	S = Shock
D = Dual (A + V)	D = Dual (A + V)	D = Dual (T + I)	C = Communicating	P = Dual (P + S)
			R = Rate-responsive	

electrodes. The distal cathodal electrode is specially treated to reduce electrical resistance. This in turn reduces the pacing 'threshold' and permits the voltage output to be programmed to a low level. A fixation device at the catheter tip, usually fine tines or a retractable screw, helps anchor it within the heart and prevent catheter displacement (Fig. 10.11). Atrial pacing catheters usually have a J-shaped tip to facilitate positioning within the right atrial appendage.

An international five-letter code describes the various methods of pacing (Table 10.3). For practical purposes, however, only the first three letters are usually used, describing the chamber paced, the chamber sensed and the mode of response to sensing. The fourth letter R is applied when the unit is rate responsive, permitting a physiological increase in heart rate with exercise; the fifth letter is rarely used. The most widely used pacing methods are AAI, VVI, DDD and DDI. Any of these may be rate responsive, when R is added.

VVI pacing (Fig. 10.12)

This is still the most commonly used method of pacing even though it is no longer the method of choice for the majority of cases. The right ventricle is paced at a preselected rate, programmed into the pulse generator, which depends on the indication for pacing. Spontaneous ventricular beats, whether normally

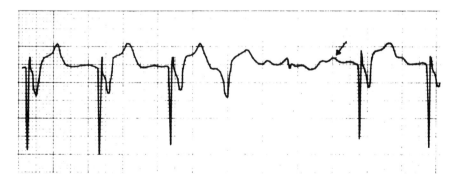

Fig. 10.12 VVI pacing. The first three complexes are paced and are preceded by a pacing artefact. A spontaneous ventricular premature beat then inhibits the pacemaker and is followed with a sinus beat conducted with delay (prolonged PR interval). The next sinus impulse (arrowed) is not conducted and the ventricular pacemaker takes over again.

conducted or ectopic, are sensed and inhibit the pulse generator. This prevents competitive 'fixed-rate' pacing (VOO) in which delivery of electrical pulses during the vulnerable period of the cardiac cycle may initiate potentially lethal tachyarrhythmias. Thus the pacemaker is only activated when the spontaneous ventricular rate falls below the preselected pacing rate. If the pacemaker is prophylactic against occasional sinus pauses a slow rate (perhaps 50/minute) is sufficient to guard against syncopal attacks but in complete AV block, in which the escape rhythm is slow and unreliable, a faster pacing rate is necessary. A function called 'hysteresis' can also be selected which allows the sensed rate at which the pacemaker is activated to be lower than the pacing rate. Hysteresis is useful for intermittent conduction disturbances because it ensures that the pacemaker is not activated unnecessarily often.

VVI pacing is simple, no doubt accounting for its continued use. However, it is not the optimal pacing method for either SA disease or AV block. AV dissociation is an inevitable consequence of VVI pacing because it fails to maintain the normal physiological conduction sequence of atrial followed by ventricular activation. This may cause 'pacemaker syndrome' where atrial and ventricular depolarizations occur simultaneously, with adverse haemodynamic effects. Moreover, because this is a ventricular pacing method, normal atrial contraction is lost and in patients with SA disease this can increase the risk of thromboembolism. In addition, VVI pacing does not permit a physiological increase in heart rate with exercise, unless a rate-responsive (VVIR) unit is chosen. Perhaps the only major indication for VVI pacing is AV block associated with AF in which synchronous atrial activation can never be restored. A VVIR unit should usually be selected in these cases (see below).

AAI pacing (Fig. 10.13)

This is an atrial pacing method in which the pacing electrode is positioned in the right atrial appendage. The atrium is sensed and spontaneous contractions inhibit the pulse generator. Thus pacing only occurs during atrial stand-still to prevent prolonged asystolic pauses. Clearly, AAI pacing cannot be used in patients with AV block. However, it is the method of choice in patients with isolated SA disease in whom AV conduction is normal. In patients with chronotrophic incompetence the rate-responsive variant (AAIR) ensures a normal heart-rate response to exercise.

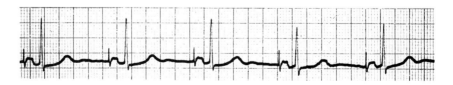

Fig. 10.13 AAI pacing. The atrial pacing artefacts are seen followed by a P wave and then a normally conducted QRS complex.

DDD pacing (Fig. 10.14)

This is a dual-chamber pacing method using two bipolar pacing catheters, one positioned in the right atrium and the other in the right ventricle. If SA and AV function is normal and the patient is in stable sinus rhythm at a satisfactory rate, the pacemaker remains quiescent (Fig. 10.14a). Reductions in atrial rate caused by sinus arrest or bradycardia are sensed by the atrial pacer which is then activated to maintain the rate above a preselected level (Fig. 10.14b). AV delay is monitored and so long as the atrial beats (spontaneous or paced) are conducted promptly to the ventricle, initiating depolarization, the ventricular pacer remains

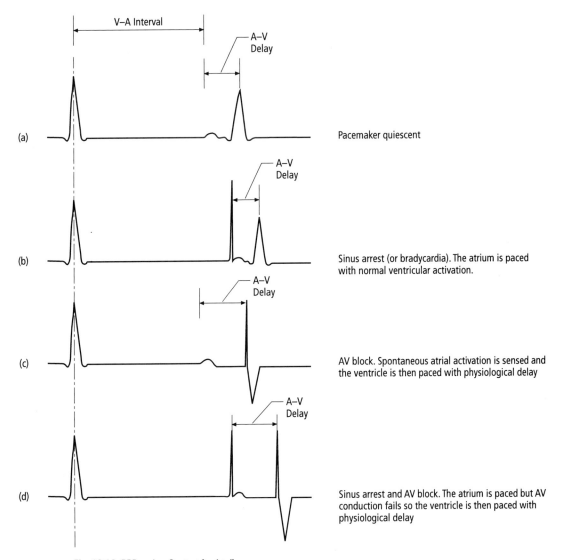

Fig. 10.14 DDD pacing. See text for details.

inhibited; ectopic beats also inhibit the ventricular pacer. However, if ventricular depolarization fails to occur, the ventricle is paced (Fig. 10.14c), and if neither atrial nor ventricular depolarizations occur spontaneously, both chambers are paced sequentially (Fig. 10.14d). Thus neither, either or both chambers of the heart may be paced with this form of pacemaker. If AV block is present, but the sinus node is functioning normally with a physiological response to exercise, the ventricular rate will follow the atrial rate during exercise in a synchronized manner. This mode therefore re-establishes AV synchrony and allows the sinus node to control the heart rate. It can be combined with rate-responsive mode (DDDR) if there is chronotropic incompetence.

DDD pacing comes closest to restoring normal physiology in patients with AV block, with or without associated SA disease, and is the method of choice in this group. However, it depends upon an intact atrial rhythm and cannot be used in AF, although reprogramming to other pacing modes is possible should AF develop after the system has been implanted. The major complication of DDD pacing is endless loop tachycardia. It occurs in the minority of patients who retain normal ventriculoatrial conduction, despite anterograde AV block. In these patients, ventricular pacing, following either a spontaneous or a paced P wave, can cause retrograde and premature activation of the atrium which in turn triggers ventricular pacing (after the appropriate AV delay), completing the circuit and providing the substrate for endless loop tachycardia. Modern pacemakers have many safeguards which protect against endless loop tachycardia, but if they are not effective, DDI pacing provides an alternative method.

DDI pacing

This is a dual-chamber pacing method similar to DDD. Both the atria and the ventricles are sensed and both can be paced. However, an increase in atrial rate above a preselected level does not trigger a further increase in ventricular rate. This prevents endless loop tachycardia and is useful when conduction disturbance is only intermittent, particularly in patients with malignant vasovagal and carotid sinus syndromes (see page 213). The disadvantage of DDI pacing is that an exertional increase in the atrial rate will not trigger a similar increase in the ventricular rate but this can be overcome by incorporation of rate responsiveness (DDIR).

Rate-responsive pacing

DDD pacemakers are rate responsive if the atrial rhythm is intact and increases normally with exercise. However, they cannot be used in patients with AF or other atrial arrhythmias. Rate-responsive pacemakers are now available which sense a specific physiological response to exertion and then trigger an appropriate increase in either atrial or ventricular rate (or both) depending on the type of unit. The most widely used device senses physical activity from vibration and muscle noise. Others sense minute ventilation, body acceleration, temperature, or adrenergic activity as reflected by the QT interval. Some pacemakers now have dual sensors, one a rapid onset sensor (e.g. activity) and the other a more physiological one such as minute ventilation.

Rate-responsive pacing improves exercise tolerance and patient well-being. The DDD pacemaker comes closest to normal physiology and for most patients with AV block is the rate-responsive device of choice. However, patients with isolated SA disease benefit from AAIR units and patients with AV block in whom the atrium is fibrillating benefit from VVIR units (see above).

Complications of pacemakers

Infection. This may be localized to the pacemaker pocket or be more generalized and is often difficult to eradicate without removing the pacing system; endocarditis is rare. Erosion through the skin of the pulse generator or its connecting electrodes is less common than in the past when devices were much larger.

Battery failure. This is the usual, and ultimately inevitable, cause of pacemaker failure. In older pacemakers, impending failure was signalled by incremental reductions in the pacing rate which occurred in a predictable fashion. In modern pacemakers, the rate remains constant and battery depletion is monitored by measurement of battery impedance using telemetry. Premature battery failure is usually caused by a component failure within the pacemaker that results in an internal short circuit. This is now uncommon, however, because quality control has reduced the rate of premature failure to $< 1 : 10\,000$ devices.

Pulse generator. Problems with the sensing device are seen occasionally. Undersensing, in which the pacemaker fails to sense spontaneous cardiac activity, leads to inappropriate pacing. The competition between spontaneous and paced beats causes uncomfortable palpitations and may be dangerous if ventricular arrhythmias are triggered. Oversensing, when electrical noise is sensed and pacing is inappropriately inhibited, can cause syncopal attacks. A special form of oversensing may occur during vigorous exertion in patients with unipolar systems (see page 220) when pectoral muscle myopotentials inhibit the pacemaker (Fig. 10.15). Similarly, inappropriate stimulation of the pectoral muscles may

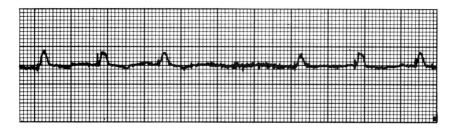

Fig. 10.15 Myopotential inhibition. After the third paced complex, random myopotentials caused by increased muscular activity inhibit the pacemaker producing a prolonged pause on the ECG. As the myopotentials decrease, normal pacemaker function becomes re-established.

cause troublesome twitching. However, these problems have largely disappeared with the use of bipolar pacemakers in which the electrical circuit is confined to the terminal portion of the pacing wire, far removed from the pectoral muscles.

Pacing electrode. Displacement can occur early after implantation, but this is now rare because active fixation electrodes secure the tip of the wire against the endocardium. Myocardial perforation has also become a rare complication since the introduction of modern flexible electrodes. Fracture of the pacing catheter is an occasional cause of premature pacemaker failure.

Exit block. The pacing threshold (voltage output necessary to initiate depolarization) normally shows a small rise early after implantation but in some patients the rise is exaggerated, leading to loss of capture. This is called exit block and is the result of fibrous infiltration into the tip of the electrode, a problem that has become less common with improvements in materials used in tip manufacture, and with tiny doses of corticosteroids that are incorporated into the tips of most modern electrodes.

Other complications. Thrombosis affecting the subclavian vein or superior vena cava is occasionally troublesome, although thromboembolism is unusual. Other complications such as pacemaker syndrome and endless loop tachycardia have been described above.

Pacemaker follow-up

Pacemaker patients should be seen every 6 months for clinical assessment. Careful analysis of the ECG and manipulation of settings using the programmer permit accurate diagnosis and correction of most pacemaker problems and malfunctions. At each visit, the pacing threshold should be checked and the voltage output programmed down to the lowest level compatible with safe pacing in order to prolong battery life. The extent of battery depletion should be monitored by impedance measurement (see above); prophylactic replacement of the pulse generator is recommended when 1 year's life remains. Patients require hospital admission (often as a day case) for the replacement procedure at which the old generator is excised and the new one attached to the existing pacing electrodes.

Prognosis

First-degree block poses no direct threat to the patient and prognosis relates to the aetiology of the underlying conduction tissue disorder. Nevertheless, the ECG and 24-hour Holter recordings should be monitored at regular intervals because progression to higher degrees of AV block is not uncommon. Isolated bundle branch block also poses no threat, although when right bundle branch block is associatedwith left axis deviation and prolongation of the PR interval (trifascicular block) the risk of progression to complete AV block is particularly high and prophylactic pacing is often recommended. Wenckebach AV block is benign in most cases, occurring in some normal individuals, and pacing is not usually necessary. In Mobitz type II and third-degree AV block the risk of prolonged asystole and sudden death demands pacing, even if block is transient, unless the conduction disturbance is clearly a temporary response to drug therapy or acute myocardial infarction. Following pacemaker insertion, the risk of asystole and sudden death is removed and prognosis relates to the aetiology of the underlying conduction tissue disorder. In idiopathic fibrosis of the conduction system, for example, prognosis is excellent but in ischaemic heart disease it is much worse.

FURTHER READING

Furman S. Rate-modulated pacing. *Circulation* 1990; 82: 1081.
Kusumoto FM, Goldschlager NG. Cardiac pacing. *N Engl J Med* 1996; 334: 89.
Nathan AW, Davies DW. Is VVI pacing outmoded? *Br Heart J* 1992; 67: 205.
Petch MC. Who needs dual chamber pacing? *Br Med J* 1993; 307: 215.
Working Party of the British Pacing and Electrophysiology Group. Recommendations for pacemaker prescription for symptomatic bradycardia. *Br Heart J* 1991; 66: 185.

C H A P T E R 1 1

Cardiac Arrhythmias

C O N T E N T S

SUMMARY

Cardiac arrhythmias (atrial, junctional or ventricular) are usually caused by a re-entry mechanism, less commonly by enhanced automaticity. Symptoms (palpitations, angina, dyspnoea and syncope) are determined less by the origin of the arrhythmia, more by the ventricular rate and the presence and severity of underlying heart disease. Atrial arrhythmias and most junctional arrhythmias are conducted by the atrioventricular (AV) node, producing a narrow, morphologically normal, QRS complex. Occasionally, rate-related (or pre-existing) bundle branch block produces a broad-complex tachycardia, difficult to distinguish from ventricular tachycardia (VT). Nevertheless, differential diagnosis is nearly always possible from scrutiny of the ECG.

Atrial arrhythmias. Atrial premature beats have an early bizarre P wave, usually followed by a normal QRS complex. In atrial fibrillation (AF), P waves are replaced by irregular fibrillatory waves (rate 400–600/minute), only a proportion of which are conducted to produce an irregular ventricular rate of 130–200 beats/minute. Atrial flutter produces sawtooth flutter waves, rate 300 beats/minute, which are usually conducted with 2 : 1 block to give a ventricular rate of 150 beats/minute.

Junctional arrhythmias. These re-entrant arrhythmias are caused by either an abnormal atrionodal pathway or an accessory AV pathway. Atrionodal pathways are the substrate for AV nodal re-entrant tachycardias (AVNRT, rate 140–250 beats/minute). The accessory AV pathway in Wolff–Parkinson–White (WPW) syndrome pre-excites the ventricles during sinus rhythm, producing a short PR interval and slurring of the initial QRS deflexion (delta wave). It provides the substrate for re-entrant tachycardias which are usually 'orthodromic' (conduction anterogradely by the AV node, retrogradely by the accessory pathway) with a narrow QRS complex. These are known as atrioventricular re-entrant tachycardias (AVRT). Occasionally the re-entrant circuit is in the opposite direction ('antidromic'), causing pre-excitation with a broad-complex tachycardia. Atrial fibrillation may be dangerous if the accessory pathway permits rapid conduction of the fibrillatory impulses resulting in an uncontrolled ventricular response (> 300 beats/minute) which may degenerate into ventricular fibrillation (VF).

Ventricular arrhythmias. Ventricular premature beats produce an early, broad QRS complex and are usually benign in themselves, requiring no treatment. VT, on the other hand, often indicates important heart disease and requires urgent treatment. In the differential diagnosis of broad-complex tachycardias, ECG findings suggesting VT include a very broad QRS (> 140 milliseconds), extreme axis deviation, evidence of AV dissociation (P waves 'marching through' the tachycardia), capture or fusion beats, concordant QRS deflexions in V1–V6, and an RSr' complex in V1 or a QS complex in V6. VF, characterized by irregular fibrillatory waves with no discernible QRS complexes, demands urgent DC cardioversion or death is inevitable.

Treatment. Primary aims are termination of sustained arrhythmias and prevention of paroxysmal arrhythmias; in refractory atrial arrhythmias treatment is aimed at controlling the ventricular rate. An empirical approach is satisfactory for benign atrial or junctional arrhythmias: AV nodal blockers (digoxin, beta-blockers, verapamil) for rate control in AF; intravenous verapamil or adenosine for terminating AVNRT or AVRT; and drugs from Vaughan Williams classes 1A (disopyramide), 1C (flecainide) or III (amiodarone) for termination and prevention of most other supraventricular arrhythmias. For ventricular arrhythmias, Class 1B drugs (lignocaine, mexiletine) are also effective but in VT (or dangerous variants of WPW syndrome), there is no role for empirical measures, and the efficacy of treatment must be confirmed by provocative testing. Non-pharmacological antiarrhythmic therapy is playing an increasing role. Anti-tachycardia pacing terminates most re-entrant arrhythmias acutely, but catheter ablation of accessory pathways and arrhythmogenic foci in the atria or ventricles provides a better long-term solution. Where this fails surgical treatment is often successful. Direct current (DC) shock remains the treatment of choice for terminating life-threatening arrhythmias; implantable defibrillators are now available for patients with refractory VT or VF not amenable to catheter ablation or arrhythmia surgery.

CARDIAC ARRHYTHMIAS

Introduction

Cardiac arrhythmias may originate anywhere in the atrial, junctional or ventricular conduction tissue, requiring only a pathological 'substrate' and a 'trigger
mechanism'. Cardiac causes include congenital abnormalities, such as accessory
atrioventricular (AV) pathways in patients with junctional arrhythmias; and
organic disease, particularly ischaemia and cardiomyopathy. Arrhythmias may
also be caused by a variety of non-cardiac disorders including metabolic disorders, electrolyte imbalance and drug toxicity.

Pathophysiology

Major mechanisms responsible for most tachyarrhythmias are re-entry and
enhanced automaticity.

Re-entry (Fig. 11.1)

Re-entry may occur within the atria or the ventricles, or may involve the AV
junction via an accessory pathway. The substrate is provided by two or more
non-homogeneous conduction pathways with different electrical characteristics.
The trigger is usually provided by a premature beat which causes transient
unidirectional block in one of the pathways. A typical re-entry circuit is seen in
the Wolff–Parkinson–White (WPW) syndrome involving the AV node (slow
conductor) and an accessory AV pathway (fast conductor). The sinus impulse is
conducted slowly through the AV node but more rapidly through the accessory
pathway, pre-exciting the ventricles (Fig. 11.1a). An atrial premature beat,
however, may find the accessory pathway refractory, particularly if it occurs very
early after the previous sinus beat (Fig. 11.1b). Thus the premature beat is

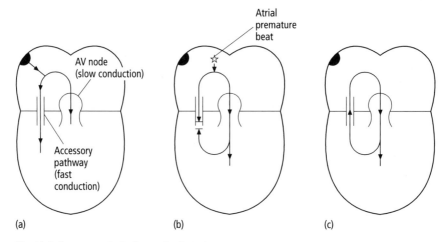

Fig. 11.1 A re-entrant circuit. See text for discussion.

conducted slowly by the AV node into the His–Purkinje system, depolarizing the ventricles without pre-excitation. By this time the accessory pathway has recovered, and can conduct the impulse retrogradely into the atria, thereby completing the circuit and initiating self-sustaining re-entry arrhythmia (Fig. 11.1c). The anatomical distribution of the re-entry circuit is large in the WPW syndrome, but when re-entry occurs in the atria or ventricles it is much smaller, often consisting of only a few myocardial cells which together constitute a microcircuit with slow and fast conducting limbs.

Enhanced automaticity

Automaticity (or spontaneous depolarization) is a property common to all the specialized conducting tissues. The automatic discharge of the sinus node normally proceeds at a faster rate than that of the remainder of the conducting tissues, which remain suppressed. Nevertheless, a variety of stimuli including ischaemia, drug toxicity and trauma can enhance the automaticity of an ectopic focus within the atria or ventricles allowing it to depolarize more rapidly than the sinus node. This produces a premature beat. Repeated automatic discharge at a rate in excess of the sinus node results in sustained atrial or ventricular tachyarrhythmias.

Clinical manifestations

Tachyarrhythmias may be entirely asymptomatic. Symptoms, when they do occur, are determined by the ventricular rate and also by the presence and severity of underlying heart disease.

Palpitations are the most common symptom caused by tachyarrhythmias. They are usually regular and, in patients with paroxysmal attacks, start and terminate abruptly. Irregular palpitations occur in atrial fibrillation (AF) and also in patients with ectopic beats due to the compensatory pauses or the forceful beats that follow.

Angina may occur if the rapid ventricular rate causes oxygen demand to exceed supply and, although troublesome in patients with coronary artery disease, may also occur in the presence of normal coronary arteries.

Dyspnoea due to heart failure commonly occurs in patients with rapid tachyarrhythmias, particularly when there is associated left ventricular or valvular disease. Arrhythmias are an important treatable cause of heart failure.

Syncopal episodes (Stokes–Adams attacks) occur when paroxysmal tachyarrhythmias produce abrupt reductions in cardiac output associated with cerebral hypoperfusion. Paroxysmal ventricular arrhythmias are usually responsible and, if sustained, may be fatal. Sudden death is an inevitable consequence of sustained ventricular fibrillation (VF).

Complications

Myocardial ischaemia, heart failure and death are the major complications.

Thromboembolism may occur, particularly in patients with AF who are not anticoagulated with warfarin.

Arrhythmia detection (see page 37)

ECG documentation of the arrhythmia is essential for accurate diagnosis. This may require ambulatory ECG monitoring for paroxysmal arrhythmias, but in patients presenting with a sustained arrhythmia, a full 12-lead ECG should always be obtained. This is particularly important for patients with broad-complex tachycardias because it helps determine whether the arrhythmia is atrial or ventricular in origin. Availability of a 12-lead ECG also helps interpret the clinical significance of arrhythmias induced during provocative testing. Simple provocative tests such as exercise testing have a role in patients with exertional symptoms, but electrophysiological study (EPS) is usually more help-ful, particularly for diagnosing junctional and ventricular arrhythmias and assessing responses to therapy. During EPS, premature stimuli are delivered to the atria or ventricles with the aim of stimulating re-entry arrhythmias (AV junctional re-entrant tachycardia, ventricular tachycardia (VT)). In the normal heart, sustained arrhythmias of this type cannot usually be provoked. Arrhyth-mia provocation during programmed stimulation is often diagnostic, particularly when the arrhythmia reproduces symptoms or is morphologically identical to the spontaneous arrhythmia recorded previously. The test can be repeated after administration of antiarrhythmic drugs to assess the efficacy of treatment.

Atrial arrhythmias

Atrial arrhythmias commonly occur without overt heart disease. However, they may be associated with a variety of cardiac disorders including pericardial, rheumatic, coronary and cardiomyopathic disease. Non-cardiac disorders associ-ated with atrial arrhythmias are pulmonary disease, thyrotoxicosis, phaeo-chromocytoma, hypothermia, hypoxia, acidosis, electrolyte imbalance (notably hypokalaemia and hypomagnesaemia) and toxic stimuli such as caffeine, alcohol, anaesthetic agents, digoxin and other antiarrhythmic drugs. Patients recovering from major surgery, particularly cardiac procedures, are also susceptible to atrial arrhythmias.

Atrial arrhythmias are conducted by the AV node and ventricular depolariza-tion therefore is by normal His–Purkinje pathways. This usually results in a narrow (morphologically normal) QRS complex. However, rate-related (or pre-existing) bundle branch block produces a broad complex (> 0.12 seconds) which may be difficult to distinguish from VT (see below). Atrial arrhythmias in the WPW syndrome may also be associated with a broad QRS complex if rapid AV conduction through the accessory pathway pre-excites the ventricles.

Atrial arrhythmias are often asymptomatic and are not usually dangerous. Nevertheless, they may predispose to thromboembolism and, like any arrhyth-

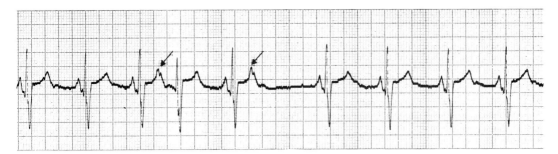

Fig. 11.2 Atrial premature beats. After the third sinus beat, the premature discharge of an ectopic atrial focus produces an early P wave (arrowed) distorting the T wave. It is conducted with delay, producing a morphologically normal QRS complex with a long PR interval. After the next sinus beat, the ectopic focus discharges again, and an early P wave (arrowed) is seen distorting the P wave. On this occasion, however, it finds the AV node refractory and the ectopic beat is not conducted. Thereafter stable sinus rhythm resumes.

mia, may precipitate heart failure or ischaemia if the rate is very rapid or if there is underlying valvular, myocardial or coronary disease.

Atrial premature beats (Fig. 11.2)

Atrial premature beats (APBs) are caused by the premature discharge of an ectopic atrial focus. This produces an early P wave, morphologically distinct from the normal sinus P waves, which is essential for the diagnosis. The premature impulse usually enters and depolarizes the sinus node, such that a partially compensatory pause occurs before the next sinus beat. Because the atrial discharge is premature the AV node is often partially refractory and conduction is slow, resulting in a prolonged PR interval. If one or other of the bundle branches is also refractory, a broad QRS complex may occur. Very premature beats sometimes find the AV node completely refractory and are blocked, producing a pause on the ECG; this may be misdiagnosed as a sinus pause if the premature P wave is not identified. Atrial premature beats do not usually require treatment unless they cause troublesome palpitations or are responsible for initiating other arrhythmias.

Prevention: flecainide, disopyramide, amiodarone.

Atrial tachycardia (Fig. 11.3)

This is a relatively uncommon arrhythmia, although in the past the term 'paroxysmal atrial tachycardia' (PAT) has often been misused to describe AV junctional (nodal) re-entrant tachycardias (see below). Most cases are re-entrant,

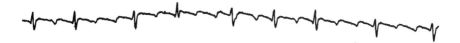

Fig. 11.3 Atrial tachycardia with 3 : 1 block.

234

but it may also be caused by enhanced automaticity, particularly in digoxin toxicity. The atrial rate varies between 120 and 240 beats/minute, and with rapid rates there is often variable AV block.

Termination: flecainide, disopyramide, amiodarone, direct current (DC) cardioversion, anti-tachycardia pacing.

Rate control: digoxin, verapamil or diltiazem, beta-blockers.

Prevention: flecainide, disopyramide, amiodarone.

Atrial flutter (Fig. 11.4)

This is a re-entrant arrhythmia with an atrial rate of approximately 300 beats/minute. There is usually 2 : 1 AV block giving a ventricular rate of 150 beats/minute. Higher degrees of block may occur, and some patients show variable block due to Wenckebach periodicity within the AV node. The ECG characteristically shows a sawtooth flutter wave which may not be evident in all leads, but should be looked for whenever a narrow-complex tachycardia is associated with a ventricular rate of 150. Sometimes block can be increased transiently by vagal manoeuvres (e.g. carotid sinus pressure) allowing the flutter waves to become apparent. Atrial flutter may degenerate into AF or develop from it. Anticoagulation to prevent thromboembolic complications is usually recommended but treatment of the arrhythmia has often been difficult. However, it is now known that it is a macro-re-entrant arrhythmia, usually taking a counter-clockwise movement around the right atrium. Catheter ablation is very effective in providing a long-term cure, and is achieved by creating an insulating line between the tricuspid annulus and the inferior vena cava.

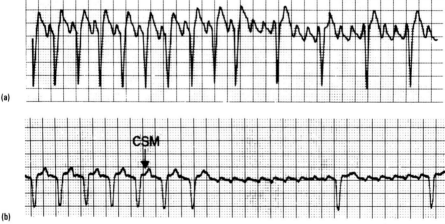

(a)

(b)

Fig. 11.4 Atrial flutter. (a) Typical 'sawtooth' flutter waves, initially with 2 : 1 conduction. Later block increases abruptly and conduction becomes 4 : 1. The flutter rate is a little faster than 300/minute. (b) The ventricular rate of this tachycardia is 150 which is strongly suggestive of atrial flutter with 2 : 1 block. Not until AV block is increased by carotid sinus massage (CSM) do the flutter waves become apparent. In this example the flutter rate is exactly 300/minute.

Termination: flecainide, disopyramide plus verapamil, amiodarone; DC cardioversion, anti-tachycardia pacing.

Rate control: digoxin, verapamil or diltiazem, beta-blockers; catheter ablation to block AV nodal conduction has a minor role (see below).

Prevention: flecainide, disopyramide, amiodarone, beta-blockers; catheter ablation to cure the arrhythmia now has a major role.

Atrial fibrillation (see Figs 1.4 and 9.4)

In AF atrial activity is chaotic and mechanically ineffective. P waves are therefore absent and are replaced by irregular fibrillatory waves (rate 400–600/minute). Only a proportion of the atrial impulses are conducted through the slowly conducting AV node to produce an irregular ventricular rate of 130–200 beats/minute. In the presence of a rapidly conducting accessory pathway in the WPW syndrome, ventricular rates of more than 300 beats/minute may occur. Anticoagulation with warfarin is indicated in most patients with AF, whether chronic or paroxysmal, to prevent embolic complications. Aspirin is a less effective alternative. Catheter ablation techniques to cure AF are being developed, although at present ablation of the AV node (such that the fibrillatory impulses are no longer conducted) is the only clinically available procedure; permanent pacing is necessary after the ablation procedure.

Termination: flecainide, disopyramide plus verapamil, amiodarone; DC cardioversion.

Rate control: digoxin, verapamil or diltiazem, beta-blockers; catheter ablation to block AV nodal conduction in refractory cases.

Prevention: flecainide, disopyramide, amiodarone, beta-blockers.

Multifocal atrial tachycardia (Fig. 11.5)

This is not uncommon in the elderly, and can be caused by chest infection or digitalis toxicity. Competing atrial–ectopic foci result in a rapid and somewhat irregular rhythm with multiform P waves usually associated with narrow QRS complexes. Correction of the arrhythmia is often difficult and treatment should be directed at the underlying cause.

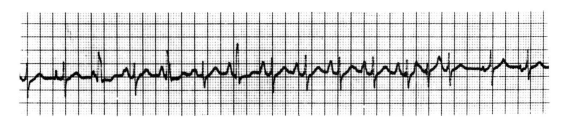

Fig. 11.5 Multifocal atrial tachycardia. The arrhythmia is somewhat irregular, but each QRS complex is preceded by a P wave. P-wave morphology, however, is very variable and at least four different configurations are apparent in this example.

Junctional arrhythmias

Junctional arrhythmias are the commonest supraventricular tachycardias (SVTs) and are usually paroxysmal without obvious cardiac or extrinsic causes. They are re-entrant arrhythmias caused by either an abnormal pathway between the atrium and the AV node (atrionodal pathway) or an accessory AV pathway (bundle of Kent) as seen in WPW syndrome.

AV junctional (nodal) re-entrant tachycardia (AVNRT) (Fig. 11.6)

The substrate for this arrhythmia is a slow atrionodal pathway, not dual AV nodal pathways as previously thought. This abnormal pathway provides the basis for a small re-entrant circuit (see page 230). In sinus rhythm the ECG is usually normal, although occasionally there is a short PR interval which, in association with AVNRT, is called the Lown–Ganong–Levine (LGL) syndrome, even though the short PR interval has nothing to do with the tachycardia, and persists after successful ablation. During tachycardia the heart rate is 140–250 beats/minute. P waves are usually very early after the QRS complexes in 1 : 1 ratio but are not always visible; rarely AV or VA block alters the ratio. Because AV conduction is by normal His–Purkinje pathways, QRS morphology is typically normal though, as in atrial arrhythmias, rate-related (or pre-existing) bundle branch block produces a broad complex which may be difficult to distinguish from VT (see below).

Termination: vagal manoeuvres; adenosine or verapamil (by rapid intravenous (IV) injection); anti-tachycardia pacing; DC cardioversion.

Prevention: flecainide, disopyramide, verapamil, beta-blockers, amiodarone; catheter ablation or surgery to destroy the slow atrionodal connection.

Wolff–Parkinson–White syndrome

Wolff–Parkinson–White (WPW) syndrome is common, affecting approximately 0.12% of the population. It is a congenital disorder in which there is an accessory pathway (bundle of Kent) between the atria and ventricles (Fig. 11.7). During sinus rhythm, atrial impulses conduct more rapidly through the accessory pathway than through the AV node. Thus, the initial phase of ventricular

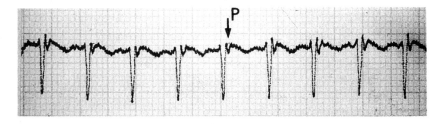

Fig. 11.6 AV junctional re-entrant tachycardia (AVNRT). Note the very early retrograde P wave (arrowed).

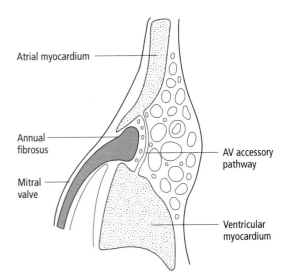

Fig. 11.7 Wolff–Parkinson–White syndrome—the AV accessory pathway (in longitudinal section) connecting the atrium and ventricle.

depolarization occurs early through the accessory pathway (pre-excitation) and spreads slowly through the myocardium (Fig. 11.8). The PR interval is therefore short and the initial deflexion of the QRS complex is slurred, producing a 'delta wave'. The remainder of ventricular depolarization, however, is rapid because the delayed arrival of the impulse conducted through the AV node completes ventricular depolarization by normal His–Purkinje pathways. The vector of the delta wave on the 12-lead ECG (Fig. 11.9) indicates the approximate location of the accessory pathway within the heart, but this is of practical importance only for the surgeon or cardiologist who is operating upon or ablating the pathway.

Cardiac tachyarrhythmias affect about 60% of patients with WPW syndrome and are usually re-entrant (rate 140–250 beats/minute), triggered by a premature beat. In most patients the re-entrant tachycardias are 'orthodromic' with anterograde conduction through the AV node, and retrograde conduction through the accessory pathway (Fig. 11.10). Because anterograde conduction is

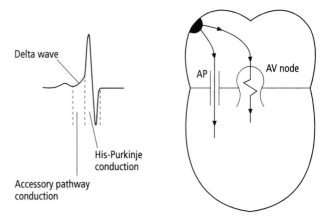

Fig. 11.8 Wolff–Parkinson–White syndrome—ECG abnormalities caused by pre-excitation. AP, accessory pathway.

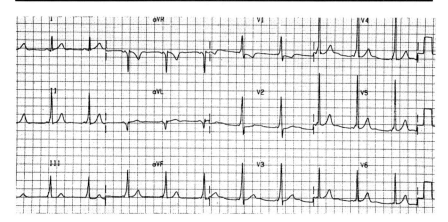

Fig. 11.9 Wolff–Parkinson–White syndrome—12-lead ECG. Note the short PR interval. A positive delta wave is clearly visible, particularly in the inferior leads (II, III and aVF). The patient has Wolff–Parkinson–White syndrome type A with a left lateral accessory pathway.

through the AV node, the QRS complexes are narrow, without pre-excitation, unless there is rate-related (or pre-existing) bundle branch block. Occasionally the re-entrant circuit is in the opposite direction ('antidromic'), causing a very broad, pre-excited, tachycardia.

Termination: vagal manoeuvres; adenosine or verapamil (by rapid IV injection); anti-tachycardia pacing; DC cardioversion.

Prevention: flecainide, disopyramide, verapamil, amiodarone, beta-blockers; catheter ablation or surgery to destroy the accessory pathway.

Patients with the WPW syndrome are more prone to AF than the general population. This is of little consequence if the accessory pathway is incapable of rapid conduction. In a minority of patients, however, the fibrillatory impulses are conducted very rapidly through the accessory pathway, producing an uncontrolled ventricular response with a rate > 300 beats/minute (Fig. 11.11). This may degenerate into VF, resulting in sudden death.

Termination: IV flecainide, disopyramide, amiodarone; DC cardioversion.

Prevention: flecainide, disopyramide, amiodarone, beta-blockers; catheter ablation of accessory pathway (digoxin is contraindicated because it enhances conduction in the accessory pathway).

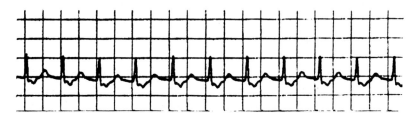

Fig. 11.10 Wolff–Parkinson–White syndrome—AV re-entrant tachycardia. This is an orthodromic tachycardia with anterograde conduction by the AV node. Thus the complexes are narrow and a P wave (inverted) follows early after each QRS complex.

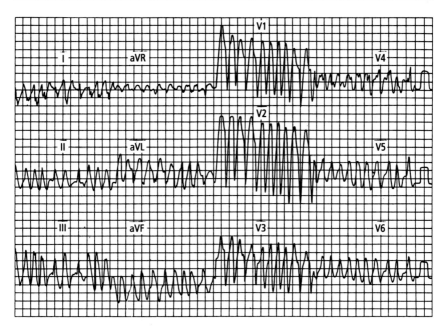

Fig. 11.11 Wolff–Parkinson–White syndrome—12-lead ECG showing rapid, pre-excited atrial fibrillation. This patient is at risk of sudden death if not adequately treated.

Concealed accessory pathways

In some patients with accessory pathways, anterograde conduction through the pathway cannot occur. Thus, in sinus rhythm, impulses are conducted normally by the AV node resulting in a narrow QRS complex without pre-excitation. The ECG, therefore, is normal and the accessory pathway 'concealed'. However, the pathway can conduct retrogradely providing the substrate for orthodromic re-entrant tachycardia. Clearly, AF poses no threat to the patient because the pathway will not conduct anterogradely. Treatment is the same as in the WPW syndrome.

Ventricular arrhythmias

Ventricular arrhythmias, particularly ectopic beats, may be benign and occur without overt heart disease. They are commonly triggered by toxic stimuli such as caffeine, or sympathomimetic drugs. Nevertheless, ventricular arrhythmias may also reflect important underlying heart disease (Table 11.1) and are an important cause of sudden death.

Because of the arrhythmias originate in the ventricular myocardium, depolarization is by abnormal pathways producing a broad QRS complex, usually > 0.12 seconds in duration. Retrograde VA conduction may result in a P wave early after the QRS complex, but penetration of the sinus node is unusual and for this reason ventricular ectopic beats are usually followed by a fully compensatory pause before the next sinus beat. In VT, however, retrograde VA conduction does

Myocardial infarction (acute or chronic)
Dilated cardiomyopathies
Hypertrophic cardiomyopathy
Other cardiomyopathies
Valvular heart disease (especially mitral prolapse and
    aortic stenosis)
Hypertensive heart disease
Congenital heart disease
Long QT syndrome
Cardiac tumours
Various metabolic disorders
Antiarrhythmic drugs

Table 11.1 Substrates for ventricular arrhythmias.

not usually occur, and this results in 'dissociated' atrial and ventricular rhythms in which the atrial rhythm continues uninterrupted, though at a slower rate than the VT, producing cannon 'a' waves in the jugular venous pulse (JVP) (see page 14).

Ventricular premature beats (see Fig. 6.4)

Ventricular premature beats (VPBs) are caused by the premature discharge of a ventricular ectopic focus which produces an early, broad QRS complex. There is usually a fully compensatory pause before the next sinus beat. Treatment is not indicated on prognostic grounds, and indeed may unpredictably produce more serious arrhythmias. If symptoms are intolerable (which is rare), Class I or III antiarrhythmic drugs can be used, cautiously.

Accelerated idioventricular rhythm (see Fig. 5.19)

This usually occurs as a complication of myocardial infarction (MI) and is discussed in Chapter 5.

Ventricular tachycardia (Fig. 11.12)

Ventricular tachycardia (VT) is defined as three or more consecutive ventricular beats at a rate above 100/minute. It usually reflects important underlying heart disease but may occur in an apparently normal heart. VT is usually regular and monomorphic (constant QRS morphology) except when it complicates acute MI when it is commonly irregular and polymorphic (variable QRS morphology). The tachycardia originates from a single ventricular site and depolarization of the ventricular myocardium is by slow, muscle-to-muscle conduction resulting in a broad-complex tachycardia. This distinguishes it from most supraventricular tachycardias in which the QRS complexes are narrow. However, differential diagnosis may be more difficult for supraventricular tachycardia with a broad complex due to rate-related (or pre-existing) bundle branch block. Symptoms are unhelpful because they depend on heart rate and underlying ventricular func-

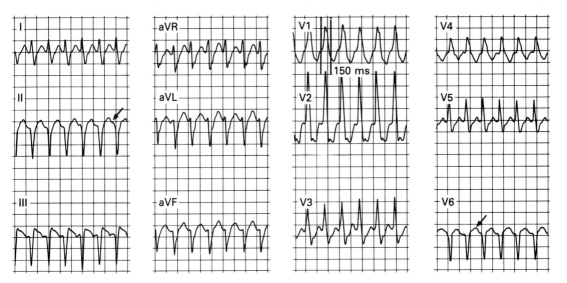

Fig. 11.12 Ventricular tachycardia—12-lead ECG. Features which point to the ventricular origin of the tachycardia include the very broad QRS complex (150 milliseconds) with an indeterminate axis, dissociated P waves (arrowed), an RSr′ complex in V1 and a QS complex in V6.

tion, not the origin of the tachycardia. Clinical circumstance may provide a guide: early after MI, for example, broad-complex tachycardia is more likely to be ventricular in origin. In most cases, however, the differential diagnosis of broad-complex tachycardias depends on careful scrutiny of the ECG (Fig. 11.12). Findings that support a diagnosis of VT include:

1 Very broad QRS complex (> 140 ms).

2 Extreme left or right axis deviation.

3 AV dissociation evidenced by P waves, at a slower rate than the QRS complexes, 'marching through' the tachycardia (Fig. 11.13).

4 Ventricular capture and/or fusion beats, in which the dissociated atrial rhythm penetrates the ventricle by conduction through the AV node and interrupts the tachycardia, producing either a normal ventricular complex (capture) or a broad

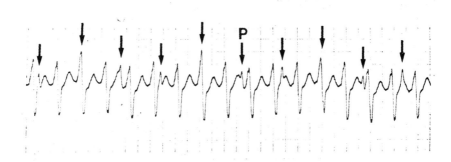

Fig. 11.13 Ventricular tachycardia—AV dissociation. The independent P waves are arrowed 'marching through' the tachycardia, confirming its ventricular origin.

hybrid complex (fusion) that is part-sinus and part-ventricular in origin (Fig. 11.14).

5 Concordance of the QRS deflexions in V1–V6, either all positive or all negative.

6 Configurational features of the QRS complex, including an RSr' complex in V1 ('left rabbit ear') and a QS complex in V6 (Fig. 11.12). Comparison with the ECG during sinus rhythm may be helpful.

VT nearly always needs urgent treatment with either IV antiarrhythmic drugs, anti-tachycardia pacing or, most effectively, DC shock. Prognosis is often poor and, in patients with recurrent attacks, the efficacy of preventative therapy should be confirmed by exercise testing and Holter monitoring. Serial EPS may be needed to find an effective drug. Patients refractory to antiarrhythmic drugs should be considered for an implantable cardioverter defibrillator (ICD) or antiarrhythmic surgery.

Termination: IV lignocaine, disopyramide, flecainide, amiodarone; anti-tachy-
    cardia pacing, DC cardioversion (external or ICD).

Prevention: Mexiletine, disopyramide, flecainide, amiodarone; antiarrhythmic
    surgery.

Long QT syndrome and torsades de pointes

Abnormalities of ventricular repolarization may produce the long QT syndrome, characterized by an abnormally long QT interval on the ECG. This is inherited as an autosomal dominant trait in the Romano–Ward syndrome and as an autosomal recessive trait in the Lange–Nielsen syndrome (when it is associated with congenital deafness). It may also be caused by drugs (e.g. disopyramide, phenothiazines) and hypokalaemia. Patients with the syndrome are at risk of sudden death due to complex ventricular arrhythmias, particularly torsades de pointes, so called because of their changing wavefronts (Fig. 11.15). In the idiopathic forms of long QT syndrome, treatment is aimed at preventing life-threatening

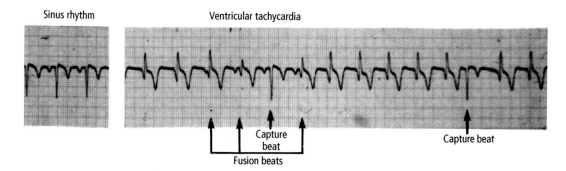

Sinus rhythm   Ventricular tachycardia

Capture beat

Capture beat

Fusion beats

Fig. 11.14 Ventricular tachycardia—capture and fusion beats. The panel on the left shows the patient in sinus rhythm. The panel on the right shows a broad-complex tachycardia: after the first two complexes two fusion beats followed by a capture beat (normal QRS morphology) are seen. Another capture beat is seen towards the end of the strip. The presence of fusion and capture beats confirms the ventricular origin of the tachycardia.

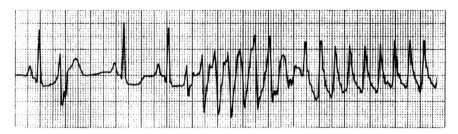

Fig. 11.15 Long QT syndrome with *torsades de pointes*. The second complex is a ventricular premature beat interrupting sinus rhythm (note the long QT interval). A second ventricular premature beat triggers a broad complex tachycardia with changing wavefronts (first negative, later positive) confirming the ventricular origin of the tachycardia.

arrhythmias with beta-blockers (with or without atrial pacing), or left stellate ganglionectomy in refractory cases. Drug-induced torsades de pointes should be treated by drug withdrawal, electrolyte correction if necessary, and atrial pacing.

Ventricular fibrillation (Fig. 11.16)

Ventricular fibrillation (VF) may be a primary arrhythmia or may degenerate from VT. It is characterized by irregular fibrillatory waves with no discernible QRS complexes. There is no cardiac output and death is inevitable unless resuscitation is instituted rapidly. VF in the first 24–48 hours after acute MI does not usually warrant long-term prophylactic therapy after resuscitation, but in all other circumstances the risk of recurrence is high and therapy should be instituted as for VT.

Termination: DC cardioversion (external or ICD).

Prevention: Mexiletine, disopyramide, flecainide, amiodarone; antiarrhythmic surgery.

Treatment

The aims of treatment are to correct symptoms and also to improve prognosis in those patients at risk of major morbidity or sudden death. These aims are usually

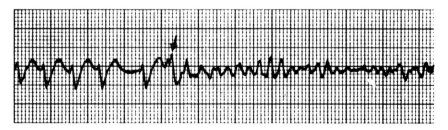

Fig. 11.16 Ventricular fibrillation. The first five complexes are atrial fibrillation but a very early ventricular premature beat (arrowed) triggers ventricular fibrillation.

met by preventing paroxysmal arrhythmias and terminating sustained arrhythmias, although in patients with refractory atrial arrhythmias (particularly AF), treatment must be directed at controlling the rate of the ventricular response, and reducing the risk of thromboembolism.

ECG documentation of the arrhythmia is essential before treatment is started. In the patient with a relatively benign atrial or junctional arrhythmia treatment is usually chosen empirically, with more sophisticated testing reserved for cases refractory to this approach. However, in the patient with a dangerous WPW syndrome or VT, there is no role for empirical measures, and treatment must be guided by appropriate tests to confirm its efficacy. This will usually involve provocative testing to ensure effective suppression of the arrhythmia. In all cases, other cardiac or non-cardiac disorders must be treated, particularly myocardial ischaemia, heart failure, metabolic and electrolyte disturbance and drug intoxication.

Antiarrhythmic drugs

Table 11.2 shows the Vaughan Williams classification of antiarrhythmic drugs. All these drugs, however, may themselves exacerbate cardiac arrhythmias due to proarrhythmic side-effects. This may account for the recent demonstration that patients with ectopic beats after MI randomized to treatment with type I

Table 11.2 The Vaughan Williams classification of antiarrhythmic drugs.

Vaughan Williams classification	Intravenous bolus dose	Chronic oral therapy—daily dose (mg)	Therapeutic plasma level (mg/l)
Class IA			
Disopyramide	2 mg/kg*	400–600	2–5
Procainamide	Up to 1000 mg	3000–4500	4–8
Quinidine	N/A	500–1000	3–6
Class IB			
Lignocaine	2 mg/kg*	N/A	2–5
Mexiletine	2 mg/kg*	400–720	0.6–2
Class IC			
Flecainide	2 mg/kg*	200	0.2–0.8
Propafenone	N/A	450–900	—
Class II			
Metoprolol	5 mg	50–200	
Propranolol	1–10 mg	40–320	0.05–0.1
Class III			
Amiodarone	300 mg	100–400	1–2
Sotalol	0.4–1 mg/kg	80–480	—
Class IV			
Diltiazem	N/A	180–360	—
Verapamil	0.15 mg/kg	120–360	0.1–0.2

* Maximum dose 150 mg.

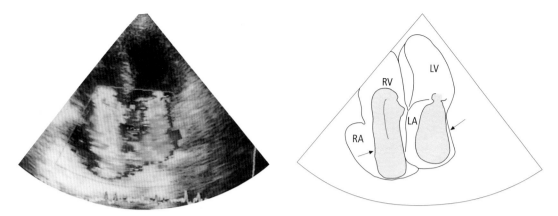

Plate 9.1 Mitral and tricuspid regurgitation. The colour Doppler study shows large regurgitant jets extending back through both valves into the left and right atrial cavities.

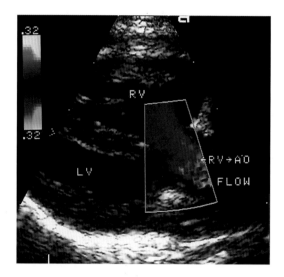

Plate 15.1 Subaortic ventricular septal defect in a neonate with tetralogy of Fallot. Colour flow Doppler confirms flow from right ventricle to aorta in systole.

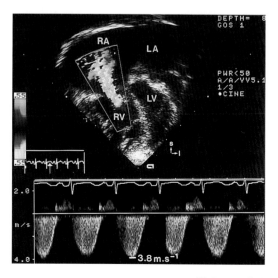

Plate 15.2 Neonantal critical pulmonary stenosis. Right ventricular systolic pressure, estimated from the peak velocity of the tricuspid regurgitant jet, is approximately 70 mmHg.

[facing page 244]

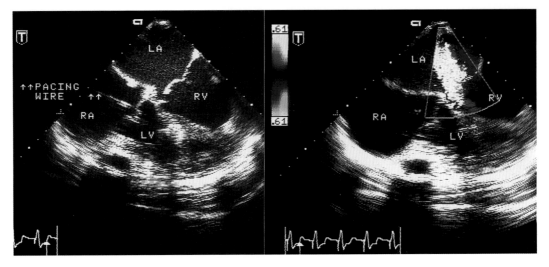

Plate 15.3 Transoesophageal echocardiographic view in the mid-oesophageal transverse plane in a young adult with atrioventricular and ventriculoarterial discordance (congenitally corrected transposition of the great arteries). There is left atrioventricular valve regurgitation (morphological tricuspid valve), and an endocardial pacing wire, inserted because of complete heart block.

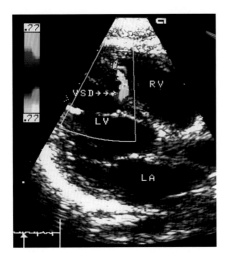

Plate 15.4 Flow through a small muscular ventricular septal defect (VSD) is clearly demonstrated by colour flow Doppler. There is allso a fibrous band within the left ventricular cavity.

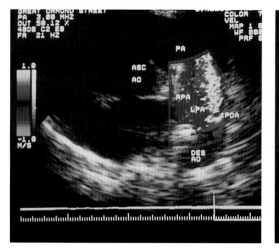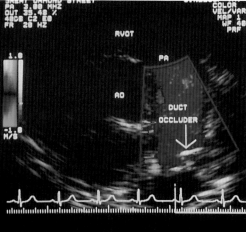

Plate 15.5 (left) Colour flow Doppler signal of ductal flow is (right) abolished following transcatheter occlusion of the duct using a double umbrella device.

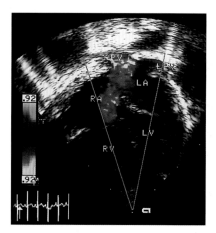

Plate 15.6 Secundum atrial septal defect with left atrial to right atrial flow confirmed by colour flow Doppler.

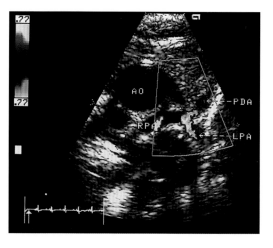

Plate 15.7 Duct-dependent pulmonary blood flow in a newborn infant with tetralogy of Fallot and pulmonary atresia, right aortic arch and left duct. The duct perfuses hypoplastic central pulmonary arteries.

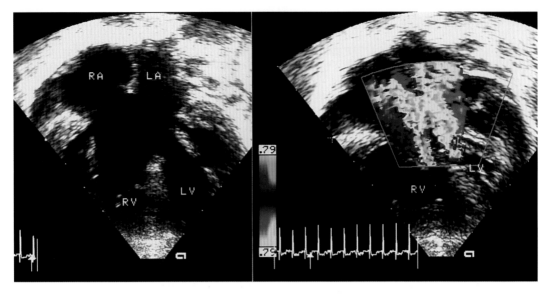

Plate 15.8 (Left) Atrioventricular septal defect with common atrioventricular valve orifice in diastole. (Right) In systole the common atrioventricular valve is severely regurgitant, with two separate jets of regurgitant flow.

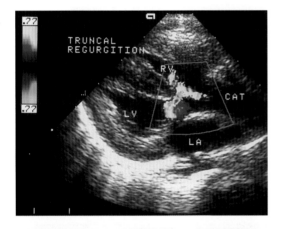

Plate 15.9 Common arterial trunk. The truncal valve regurgitant flow impinges on the crest of the trabecular septum.

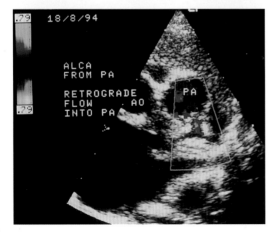

Plate 15.10 Retrograde flow from left coronary artery into the pulmonary trunk in an infant with anomalous origin of the left coronary artery from the pulmonary artery.

Box 11.1 CAST: The Cardiac Arrhythmia Suppression Trial	
Study design Randomized, double-blind, placebo-controlled, multicentre.	**Randomization** Group 1: encainide vs placebo; group 2: flecainide vs placebo.
Inclusion Ventricular ectopy 6 days–2 years after acute myocardial infarction, which could be suppressed by one of the study drugs (flecainide, encainide).	**End points** Death or cardiac arrest with resuscitation.
Patients 1498: encainide 432, placebo 425; flecainide 323, placebo 318.	**Results** After 10 months, 89 patients had died: 59 arrhythmic deaths, 43 receiving drug, 16 receiving placebo ($P = 0.0004$); 22 non-arrhythmic cardiac deaths, 17 receiving drug, 5 receiving placebo ($P = 0.01$); 8 non-cardiac deaths, 3 receiving drug, 5 receiving placebo (NS).
Conclusions Findings suggest that the administration of type 1 antiarrhythmic drugs to patients with ectopy recovering from myocardial infarction has an adverse effect on arrhythmic and non-arrhythmic cardiac deaths.	

Echt DS (1991) Mortality and morbidity in patients receiving encainide, flecainide, or placebo: The Cardiac Arrhythmia Suppression Trial (CAST). *N Engl J Med*; **324**: 781–8.

antiarrhythmic drugs (see below) are at greater risk of death than patients randomized to placebo (Box 11.1). Thus, a cautious and rational approach to treatment should be adopted. ECG documentation of the arrhythmia is essential before starting treatment. Because the therapeutic range for most drugs is very narrow, regular measurements of plasma concentrations should, if possible, be obtained, particularly during early treatment and, if the arrhythmia persists despite therapeutic levels, an alternative drug from a different class should be substituted. A partial response might justify the addition of a second agent but combination regimens of this type should, if possible, be avoided because of the risk of drug interactions and exaggerated side-effects. Class III and Class IA drugs, for example, both prolong the QT interval and their combination can induce the long QT syndrome which is associated with severe ventricular arrhythmias. Class II and Class IV agents both slow conduction through the AV node. The combination is generally safe if the drugs are given orally but IV use of one with concomitant use of the other must be avoided, because of the risk of complete heart block and asystole.

Class I drugs

These are the local anaesthetic or sodium-blocking drugs and slow phase 0 of the action potential (see page 25). Effects on repolarization are variable and provide the basis for a subclassification into groups A, B and C which prolong, shorten and have little effect on the QT interval, respectively.

Class IA drugs are effective against atrial and ventricular arrhythmias. Quinidine is the prototype but is not often used because of well-documented proarrhythmias and gastrointestinal side-effects. Disopyramide is effective against atrial and ventricular arrhythmias but is moderately proarrhythmic and has marked negative inotropic properties demanding caution in patients with heart failure. Anticholinergic side-effects include blurred vision, dry mouth and urinary retention. Procainamide is less negatively inotropic but is also proarrhythmic and can cause the lupus syndrome with long-term use.

Lignocaine and mexiletine are the most widely used Class IB drugs, mainly useful against ventricular arrhythmias. Lignocaine has its major role in the treatment of ventricular arrhythmias complicating acute MI but is not very effective in other circumstances. IV administration is always necessary because of first-pass metabolism in the liver. Major side-effects include bradycardia, hypotension, drowsiness and convulsions, particularly if the drug is administered too rapidly. Negative inotropic effects are minimal. Mexiletine is in all respects similar but can be given orally. Gastrointestinal side-effects, especially nausea, may be troublesome. Flecainide and propafenone are potent Class IC agents, useful for atrial, junctional and ventricular arrhythmias. Both are moderately negatively inotropic but are well tolerated although therapeutic margins are narrow. Proarrhythmic effects are well documented.

Class II drugs

These are the beta-blockers that protect the heart against excessive adrenergic stimulation. They are useful in combination with digoxin for controlling the ventricular rate in AF but their antiarrhythmic effects are generally weak except in thyrotoxicosis. They are occasionally useful in junctional arrhythmias, although large doses are necessary which are often not tolerated. They also have a special role for long-term therapy after MI when they increase the fibrillation threshold and reduce the incidence of arrhythmic death. Propranolol is usually chosen for IV use, but for long-term oral use there is little to choose between beta-blockers in terms of their antiarrhythmic efficacy.

Class III drugs

Amiodarone is the most important drug in this class although sotalol, a beta-blocker, also has Class III activity. Amiodarone prolongs the action potential increasing the effective refractory period throughout the conduction system. It has unusual pharmacokinetics with a plasma half-life of 7–8 weeks and it may take several months to achieve steady state. Amiodarone is effective against a wide range of arrhythmias and may be used intravenously, although it is toxic to vascular endothelium and should be given into a central vein. It may be proarrhythmic, though not as frequently as Class IA or IC drugs, and has only minor negative inotropic effects. Chronic therapy is associated with a variety of side-effects including photosensitivity rash, skin discoloration, corneal infiltrates, thyrotoxicosis or hypothyroidism, pulmonary infiltrates, hepatic dysfunction, neuropathies, myopathies and encephalitis. For this reason amiodarone should rarely be used as a first-line agent.

Class IV drugs

These drugs are calcium antagonists. Verapamil has been the most important drug in this class although diltiazam is also useful. Selective blockade of the slow calcium channel decreases depolarization and slows conduction through the AV node. Thus Class IV drugs have an important role for controlling the ventricular rate in AF, particularly in combination with digoxin. Given intravenously they are useful for terminating junctional arrhythmias, and they can also be used prophylactically, although in WPW they shorten the refractory period of the accessory pathway, increasing the ventricular rate in AF. Verapamil and diltiazem are negatively inotropic and should be used with caution in heart failure.

Digoxin

Digoxin, the most commonly used cardiac glycocide, defies classification by Vaughan Williams' criteria. In addition to its mild positive inotropic properties the drug slows conduction through the AV node by a direct effect on depolarization and by its vagotonic action. In AF it is the drug of choice for slowing the ventricular rate, except in WPW syndrome when it is contraindicated; it is only rarely useful for prophylaxis against paroxysmal attacks. It has almost no other role for the treatment of arrhythmias. Digoxin can be given by slow IV infusion for loading purposes, but is most commonly used orally. The therapeutic range is narrow and dose increases may need to be titrated against plasma concentrations. It is excreted by the kidneys, and in patients with renal failure the dose must be reduced. Other factors which increase the risk of digoxin toxicity include old age, hypokalaemia and hypomagnesaemia. Important side-effects are loss of appetite, nausea, vomiting, visual disturbances and bradyarrhythmias. Digoxin may also cause a variety of tachyarrhythmias by enhancing automaticity. Digoxin therapy produces important ECG changes, including prolongation of the PR interval and sagging of the ST segment with T-wave inversion. These abnormalities do not necessarily indicate toxicity.

Adenosine

Adenosine, like digoxin, defies classification by Vaughan Williams' criteria. Its short half-life of < 10 seconds requires it to be given by very rapid IV injection followed by a large bolus of saline flush. It is a potent AV nodal blocker and a dose of 0.1 or 0.2 mg/kg will nearly always terminate junctional arrhythmias; even if complete AV block occurs its short half-life ensures almost immediate recovery. Other side-effects (flushing, nausea, hypotension) are similarly evanescent. Thus adenosine is safe and is particularly useful in the critically ill, haemodynamically compromised patient, although in many other situations IV verapamil remains the drug of first choice for terminating junctional arrhythmias. It is contraindicated in asthmatics as it can provoke acute bronchospasm.

Non-pharmacological treatment

Autonomic manoeuvres

The reflex vagotonic response to carotid sinus pressure and the Valsalva manoeuvre slow AV conduction and may terminate junctional re-entrant arrhythmias. These manoeuvres also facilitate the diagnosis of atrial arrhythmias (see Fig. 11.4).

Anti-tachycardia pacing

Re-entrant arrhythmias can always be terminated by anti-tachycardia pacing using either a temporary pacing catheter or a permanent anti-tachycardia pacemaker. Carefully timed single or double premature stimuli (Fig. 11.17), or a longer burst of overdrive pacing are usually effective. Occasionally, however, this causes unpredictable and potentially dangerous acceleration of the tachycardia—in the atrium to AF and in the ventricle to rapid VT or VF. Although pacing continues to be used as a temporary measure for termination of re-entrant tachycardias, permanent anti-tachycardia pacemakers have become virtually redundant in the current era of catheter ablation. They are now rarely used for atrial or junctional arrhythmias but continue to have a role in the treatment of paroxysmal VT, although the risk of VF demands that they are incorporated into an implantable cardioverter defibrillator (see below).

Catheter ablation

Electrode catheters attached to an energy source may be placed strategically within the heart and used to cause selective damage to the conduction system. DC electrical energy from a defibrillator or radiofrequency energy (similar to surgical diathermy) are used most commonly. The technique was used originally for ablation of the AV node in patients with troublesome atrial arrhythmias (particularly paroxysmal or sustained AF) resistant to conventional drug therapy (Fig. 11.18). It results in complete AV block which prevents conduction of the arrhythmia to the ventricles, thereby abolishing palpitations and other conse-

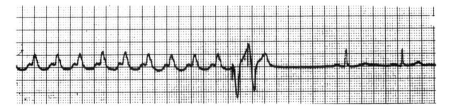

Fig. 11.17 Anti-tachycardia pacing—the broad-complex tachycardia is terminated by two intracardiac electrical stimuli which break the re-entrant circuit and allow sinus rhythm to become re-established.

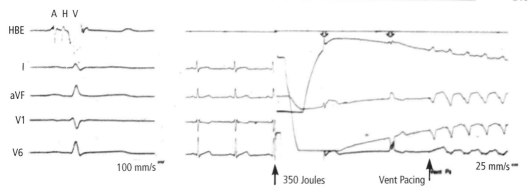

Fig. 11.18 Catheter ablation of the AV node. The patient, with troublesome paroxysmal atrial fibrillation, was in sinus rhythm at the time of the ablation procedure. The His bundle electrogram (HBE) is seen in the His bundle channel. The His bundle electrode is disconnected and attached to a defibrillator. Following the shock, successful ablation is achieved resulting in complete AV heart block requiring ventricular pacing.

quences of a rapid ventricular response (see page 231). Following the procedure, permanent ventricular pacing is required, ideally with a rate-responsive unit (VVIR).

The role of catheter ablation has been extended, however, and it now finds its major application in the management of junctional arrhythmias (Fig. 11.19). Skilled operators, using radiofrequency energy, are able to ablate accessory pathways in virtually any part of the heart. The technique is new but results are excellent and produce complete correction of re-entrant tachycardias in patients with atrial–nodal pathways and WPW syndrome.

Arrhythmia surgery

This was once restricted to the induction of complete AV block in patients with intractable atrial arrhythmias, but catheter ablation has now rendered the procedure obsolete. Current indications for arrhythmia surgery are the WPW syndrome and life-threatening, drug-refractory, ventricular arrhythmias. Surgery in WPW syndrome is reserved for those rare patients in whom catheter ablation fails. It involves close collaboration between the cardiologist who maps the

Fig. 11.19 Catheter ablation of the accessory pathway in Wolff–Parkinson–White syndrome. The patient with obvious pre-excitation (note the delta wave) undergoes radiofrequency ablation (RFA) of the pathway after the third beat. After a further two beats the accessory pathway is successfully destroyed and pre-excitation is lost, never to return.

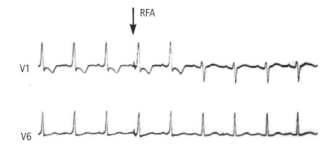

position of the accessory pathway, and the cardiac surgeon who either resects it or destroys it with a cryoprobe. Surgery for ventricular arrhythmias also requires preoperative mapping of the arrhythmogenic focus prior to its resection. Most ventricular arrhythmias originate from the endocardial surface and limited endocardial resection, leaving the rest of the muscle intact, preserves left ventricular function and prevents further arrhythmias. The operative mortality is approximately 10–15% and is higher in those with very poor left ventricular function or recent MI.

External direct current countershock (Fig. 11.20)

Electrode paddles placed against the chest wall permit the delivery of a high-energy DC shock across the heart. Anaesthesia is necessary if the patient is conscious. This technique corrects the majority of acute onset atrial, junctional and ventricular arrhythmias by completely depolarizing the heart and allowing the sinus node to re-establish itself. The rapid, almost instantaneous, response makes DC shock the treatment of choice in emergency cases. The shock is always synchronized with the QRS complex (except in VF) to reduce proarrhythmic effects. A low-energy shock (50 joules) will usually terminate atrial tachycardia, flutter, junctional arrhythmias and monomorphic VT. However, higher energy (up to 360 joules) is required for AF, polymorphic or very rapid VT, and VF. In patients undergoing elective cardioversion of chronic AF, anticoagulation reduces the risk of thromboembolism. Digoxin does not contraindicate DC shock, but it should not be used in digoxin toxicity (except in emergency) because it may induce asystole or severe ventricular arrhythmias.

Implantable cardioverter defibrillator

An implantable cardioverter defibrillator (ICD) device can detect and treat most sustained ventricular arrhythmias. It is indicated in refractory VT or VF, when ablation or arrhythmia surgery is inappropriate. Initially, implantation required a thoracotomy to sew the defibrillator patches directly onto the heart, but defibrillator coil electrodes are now used for transvenous insertion. The defibrillator itself (smaller than a pack of cards) is implanted in the subpectoral area. The ICD

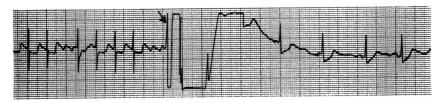

Fig. 11.20 External DC countershock. Atrial flutter is terminated by a DC shock (arrowed) allowing sinus rhythm to become re-established.

monitors heart rate and automatically delivers a DC shock when an abrupt rate increase indicates VT or VF (Fig. 11.21). The number of shocks that can be delivered is limited by the battery life of the defibrillator. However, most ICDs now have anti-tachycardia pacing capability and only use shocks if this fails to terminate VT, or if VF occurs.

The ICD is palliative and does not prevent arrhythmias from occurring. Nevertheless it has been shown to improve survival considerably in this high-risk group of patients and has become the gold standard against which other treatments for ventricular arrhythmias are measured.

Cardiac transplantation

Some patients with severe ventricular arrhythmias and very poor left ventricular function are best treated by cardiac transplantation.

Prognosis

The prognosis in patients with cardiac arrhythmias depends on the nature of the arrhythmia and the underlying cause. Atrial arrhythmias are commonly associated with a normal life expectancy although, when caused by ischaemia, mitral valve disease or heart failure, the prognosis is less good. Most patients with junctional arrhythmias have a normal prognosis, with the important exception of WPW syndrome associated with a rapidly conducting accessory pathway when the risk of sudden death is high unless the patient is adequately treated. Ventricular arrhythmias are more sinister and, although premature beats may occur in normal individuals, more complex arrhythmias are usually associated with severe underlying heart disease when the prognosis is poor.

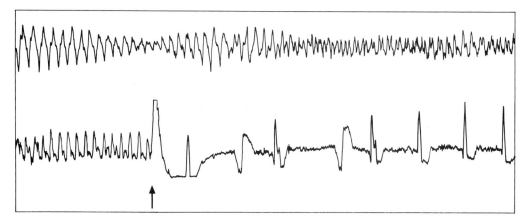

Fig. 11.21 Implantable cardioverter defibrillator (ICD). Ventricular fibrillation is terminated by a DC shock (arrowed) from an ICD.

CARDIAC ARREST

Aetiology

Cardiac arrest is usually caused by VF or asystole but may also be caused by rapid VT. These arrhythmias are usually the result of severe myocardial ischaemia or infarction but may also complicate hypoxia, electrolyte imbalance and a variety of drug interventions. Autonomic reflexes in response to endotracheal intubation or urethral catheterization occasionally cause cardiac arrest.

Clinical manifestations

In cardiac arrest, there is no effective cardiac output. The diagnosis is made clinically by loss of the arterial pulse followed rapidly by unconsciousness, apnoea and dilatation of the pupils. Irreversible brain damage usually occurs if the circulation is not re-established within 3–4 minutes, though factors such as hypothermia may prolong this time.

Treatment

A firm thump over the sternum occasionally converts VT or fibrillation to sinus rhythm; if this fails, full cardiopulmonary resuscitation should be instituted. The patient is placed supine on a firm surface with the neck extended. The airway must be cleared, and positive-pressure ventilation and external cardiac massage can then be started. These should be continued uninterrupted until adequate spontaneous circulatory and respiratory function are restored. All drugs during resuscitation should be given into a central vein but if this is impossible double doses of adrenaline, lignocaine and atropine can be given by the endotracheal tube. Acidosis commonly develops in a prolonged resuscitation and may be corrected by IV sodium bicarbonate (50 ml of an 8.4% solution), though ideally requirements should be titrated against arterial gas analysis.

Positive-pressure ventilation

The lungs should be inflated about 12 times/minute. Adequate oxygenation of the blood can usually be achieved by hand ventilation, using a face mask, or by mouth-to-mouth techniques. Endotracheal intubation, however, should not be delayed because this not only improves alveolar ventilation but also protects the airway against regurgitated gastric contents.

External cardiac massage

This is applied by sharp compression of the lower end of the sternum about 60 times/minute. As soon as possible, the patient should be attached to an ECG monitor in order to determine the cardiac rhythm. Further management is directed at restoring an effective spontaneous cardiac output.

Ventricular fibrillation

This is treated with DC shock using 200 joules first which, if unsuccessful, may be repeated once before higher energy (360 joules) is resorted to. Patients resistant to cardioversion should be given adrenaline (1 mg) before DC shock is tried again, with repeat injections every 5 minutes as necessary. This produces a coarser fibrillatory pattern that is often more susceptible to cardioversion. Antiarrhythmic drugs such as lignocaine (100 mg given slowly intravenously) may make resistant VF more responsive to DC cardioversion.

Asystole

Successful treatment is difficult. Inotropic drive is provided by adrenaline (1 mg) repeated every 5 minutes as necessary. Patients unresponsive to the first dose of adrenaline should be given atropine (2 mg). If asystole persists it is always worth trying DC shock. When available, external or transoesophageal pacing may help, or a pacemaker catheter can be introduced into the right ventricle. A paced rhythm can usually be established by these means, but electromechanical dissociation often prevents restoration of effective cardiac output. Calcium chloride (10 ml in 10% solution) should only be used if the patient is hyperkalaemic, hypocalcaemic or known to be on calcium antagonists.

If these measures succeed in restoring spontaneous circulatory function, further management is directed towards the maintenance of a stable cardiac rhythm and oxygenation of the blood. Prophylactic antiarrhythmic drugs are often necessary and many patients require mechanical ventilation.

Prognosis

Following resuscitation, prognosis depends upon the cause of arrest and the resultant ischaemic cerebral damage. Prompt resuscitation prevents neurological sequelae and in those cases caused by drugs and other toxic insults, life expectancy may be normal. In the majority of cases, however, cardiac arrest reflects severe underlying heart disease and prognosis is usually poor. An important exception is primary VF in acute MI, when prognosis following resuscitation is only a little worse than for other survivors.

FURTHER READING

Camm AJ, Garratt CJ. Drug therapy: adenosine and supraventricular tachycardia. *N Engl J Med* 1991; 325: 1621.
Chesebro JH, Fuster V, Halperin JL. Atrial fibrillation—risk marker for stroke. *N Engl J Med* 1990; 323: 1556.

Cunningham D, Rowland E. Endocavitary ablation of atrioventricular conduction. *Br Heart J* 1990; 64: 231.

Florin D. Decisions about cardiopulmonary resuscitation. *Br Med J* 1994; 308: 1653.

Ganz LI, Friedman PL. Supraventricular tachycardia. *N Engl J Med* 1996; 332: 162.

Garratt C, Ward DE, Camm AJ. Lessons from the cardiac arrhythmia suppression trial. *Br Med J* 1989; 299: 805.

Kastor JA. Multifocal atrial tachycardia. *N Engl J Med* 1990; 322: 1713.

Niemann JT. Cardiopulmonary resuscitation. *N Engl J Med* 1992; 327: 1075.

Plum F. Vulnerability of the brain and heart after cardiac arrest. *N Engl J Med* 1991; 324: 1278.

Pritchett ELC. Management of atrial fibrillation. *N Engl J Med* 1992; 326: 1264.

Roden DM. Risks and benefits of antiarrhythmic therapy. *N Engl J Med* 1994; 331: 785.

Ruskin J. Catheter ablation for SVT. *N Engl J Med* 1991; 324: 1660–2.

Singer DE. Randomized trials of warfarin for atrial fibrillation. *N Engl J Med* 1992; 327: 1451.

Ward DE, Camm AJ. Dangerous cardiac arrhythmias—can we predict drug efficacy? *N Engl J Med* 1993; 329: 498.

Wardrope J, Morris F. European guidelines on resuscitation. *Br Med J* 1993; 306: 1555.

Wellins HJJ. Atrial fibrillation—the last big hurdle for treating SVT. *N Engl J Med* 1994; 331: 944.

White HD. Aspirin or warfarin for nonrheumatic atrial fibrillation. *Lancet* 1994; 343: 683.

Hypertension

SUMMARY

Hypertension, defined as abnormal elevation of the blood pressure, is nearly always the result of increased peripheral vascular resistance. It is an important and potentially treatable cause of cardiovascular disease and death. In about 10% of cases hypertension is secondary to renal or endocrine disorders, but in the remainder the aetiology is unknown (*essential hypertension*) although evidence points to a complex interaction of hereditary and environmental factors. The hypertensive patient is usually asymptomatic but examination may reveal a fourth heart sound, reflecting left ventricular hypertrophy, and signs of hypertensive retinopathy. The major complications are heart disease (coronary atherosclerosis and left ventricular failure), stroke and renal failure. Diagnosis is by sphygmomanometry, but additional investigations are necessary to assess damage to the heart (ECG, chest X-ray, echocardiogram) and kidneys (urinalysis and simple renal function tests). Special investigations to identify causes of secondary hypertension are only necessary when clinical suspicion is high, particularly in young patients with no family history of hypertension. Treatment is directed at lowering the blood pressure to protect against end-organ damage, particularly stroke and ongoing renal disease. General measures, particularly weight reduction and restriction of salt and alcohol intake are helpful but the majority of patients require additional drug treatment with either diuretics, beta-blockers, calcium antagonists, ACE inhibitors, alpha-blockers or angiotensin receptor antagonists. Treatment should be tailored to the individual patient, and if a single agent fails to control the blood pressure others should be added.

Definition

It is now well established, from life-insurance actuarial analysis, that the risk of morbid complications rises in approximately linear relation to both systolic and diastolic blood pressure measurements. Indeed, levels of blood pressure commonly accepted as at the upper end of the 'normal' range are usually associated with a significant increase in eventual cardiovascular mortality. Attempts to define normal blood pressure are further confounded by its diurnal and random variability and the effects of age, sex and race.

Diurnal and random variability

Continuous recording of blood pressure, with an indwelling arterial canula, shows a clear diurnal variability—with peak levels occurring during the day (usually in the early morning) and trough levels at night during sleep. Superimposed on this are the effects of anxiety and exertion, both of which cause a variable increase in blood pressure.

Age

Blood pressure tends to rise with age and there is a corresponding rise in the prevalence of hypertension. Nevertheless, this does not appear to be a truly physiological phenomenon, because it is largely confined to western cultures and is more marked in urban than rural societies.

Sex

Blood pressure is usually higher in men than in women, particularly in childhood and early adulthood. Nevertheless, the age-related rise in blood pressure tends to be steeper in women so that, by middle age, blood-pressure measurements in both sexes are similar.

Racial groups

People of African origin living in western cultures have, on average, higher blood pressures than white people. It is difficult, however, to attribute this entirely to genetic effects because rural populations in Africa usually have low measurements. Other population comparisons confirm that genetic and environmental factors show a complex interaction; environmental factors of major importance to immigrant populations include psychosocial effects and changes in diet and body-weight (see below).

All this means that any definition of hypertension must be arbitrary. Nevertheless, it is important that levels of 'normality' are defined—in order that decisions can be taken to investigate and treat. Thus, for practical purposes, hypertension in adults may be defined as follows:

Mild hypertension:	140/90–160/100 mmHg
Moderate hypertension:	160/100–180/115 mmHg
Severe hypertension:	> 180/115 mmHg

Mechanisms of hypertension

Blood pressure is determined by cardiac output and systemic vascular resistance. Although increments in cardiac output may make an early contribution to the pathogenesis of hypertension, in established disease it is nearly always elevated systemic vascular resistance that plays the major role. This may be due to increased arteriolar tone, thickening of the arteriolar wall, or both, but in the majority of patients the underlying mechanisms are unknown. Enhanced secretion, or sensitivity to, arteriolar vasoconstrictors, particularly angiotensin II, may be important and, although blood levels are not usually elevated, there is evidence of hyperactivity of 'tissue-bound' converting enzyme within the arteriolar wall which increases angiotensin II concentrations locally.

Abnormalities of sodium balance have been the basis of many theories of the mechanism of hypertension. One proposal is that reduced renal excretion of sodium leads to salt and water retention which increases cardiac output, leading to peripheral arteriolar constriction—an autoregulatory phenomenon which prevents overperfusion. Thus blood pressure rises and, as afterload increases, cardiac output falls into the normal range again.

Recently attention has been focused on the handling of sodium at cell-membrane level, which is often abnormal in hypertension. Evidence exists for a circulatory inhibitor of the sodium pump (produced in response to subtle expansion of the extracellular fluid volume) which leads to increased intracellular sodium concentration. It has been suggested that this stimulates sodium–calcium exchange in arteriolar smooth muscle, increasing the availability of calcium for vasoconstriction.

At present these remain hypotheses. Hypertension is almost certainly multifactorial in origin and caused by a breakdown of the control mechanisms that regulate cardiac output, blood volume, sodium balance and systemic vascular resistance.

Aetiology

In the majority of hypertensive patients, no specific aetiological factor can be identified *(essential hypertension)*. This must be distinguished from secondary hypertension in which a specific cause can be identified.

Essential hypertension

This accounts for 85–90% of all cases. By definition, the cause is unknown but evidence points to an interaction between hereditary and environmental factors.

Hereditary factors

The familial incidence of hypertension is due, at least in part, to hereditary factors, although these are often difficult to separate from environmental influences. Thus, concordance for hypertension is greater between monozygotic than dizygotic twins and between natural than adoptive siblings. Nevertheless, the tendency for spouses to have similar blood pressures reflects the associated importance of the environment in determining the familial incidence of hypertension.

Environmental factors

The importance of this is emphasized by population studies in which migrants from rural to industrialized societies often show an increase in blood pressure to a level characteristic of the indigenous population. Diet plays an important role, particularly when obesity results: several studies have shown a close correlation between body fat and blood pressure. Specific dietary factors have been more difficult to identify, but recent work has shown an important relation with both salt and alcohol consumption. Thus, an increase in sodium intake of 100 mmol/ 24 hours is associated with an average rise in blood pressure ranging from 5 mmHg at age 15–19 years to 10 mmHg at age 60–69. Excessive alcohol consumption also has an adverse effect on blood pressure, systolic blood pressure being almost 10 mmHg higher in men drinking 6–8 drinks daily than in abstainers. Importantly, reductions in body weight, salt or alcohol consumption cause parallel reductions in the blood pressure.

The role of stress and other psychosocial factors is difficult to define. Acute stress produces a variable rise in blood pressure which, if exaggerated, may account for the phenomenon of 'white-coat' hypertension prompted by a visit to the doctor. Recent evidence indicates that white-coat hypertension may have adverse prognostic implications, although it is not normally regarded as an indication for specific treatment. If stress becomes chronic, hypertension may be sustained. Thus job loss, bereavement, divorce and other life-events of this type are all associated with a greater than expected incidence of hypertension.

Secondary hypertension

In most cases, secondary hypertension is the result of renal disease or hormonal disorders (Table 12.1). Renal causes include both vascular and parenchymal disease in which activation of the renin–angiotensin system and plasma volume excess (respectively) are seen. Hormonal disorders are responsible for hypertension in primary aldosteronism and Cushing's syndrome (due to excessive mineralocorticoid activity resulting in sodium retention) and also in phaeochromocytoma (due to catecholamine stimulation). The cause of hypertension in acromegaly is not certain. The most common hormonal cause of hypertension, however, is the oral contraceptive which almost invariably produces an increase

Table 12.1 Causes of secondary hypertension.

Renal parenchymal disease
Glomerulonephritis
Pyelonephritis
Polycystic disease
Diabetic nephropathy
Connective tissue disease
Hydronephrosis

Renal artery stenosis
Atherosclerosis
Fibromuscular hyperplasia
Congenital

Endocrine disease
Adrenal cortex—Cushing's syndrome, Conn's
  syndrome
Adrenal medulla—phaeochromocytoma
Acromegaly
Iatrogenic—contraceptive pill, oestrogen
replacement therapy, corticosteroids,
  sympathomimetic agents

Miscellaneous
Coarctation
Pregnancy—pre-eclampsia, eclampsia
Acute porphyria
Increased intracranial pressure

in blood pressure. Nevertheless, the increase is usually small and reverses promptly on stopping the drug; activation of the renin–angiotensin system is probably responsible. Other iatrogenic causes of hypertension include oestrogen replacement and corticosteroid therapy and treatment with liquorice derivatives.

Pathophysiology

Hypertension is an important risk factor for atherosclerosis, especially in the coronary, cerebral and renal circulations. It may also cause direct vascular damage independently of atherosclerosis, resulting in aortic dissection or haemorrhagic stroke.

The heart

Hypertension is a major risk factor for coronary artery disease and predisposes to myocardial ischaemia, infarction and sudden death. Left ventricular (LV) hypertrophy (probably driven by the local effects of angiotensin II secreted in response to tissue-bound converting enzyme) occurs to compensate for the increase in afterload, and in longstanding disease irreversible deterioration in systolic and diastolic function may develop, leading to heart failure. The reduction in cardiac output often normalizes the blood pressure and the condition may become clinically indistinguishable from dilated cardiomyopathy.

The brain

Hypertension is an even more potent risk factor for cerebrovascular disease. The principal lesions are accelerated atherosclerosis in the larger cerebral vessels and mechanical dilatation of the small vessels and arterioles resulting in micro-aneurysms. Stroke may result from thrombotic occlusion of atherosclerotic vessels or from intracerebral haemorrhage caused by vascular rupture. Although intracerebral haemorrhage is potentially more devastating in its consequences, the rupture of a microaneurysm may be clinically silent resulting in a typical lacunar infarct. Multiple lacunar infarcts, however, may combine to cause subtle defects of cerebral function manifested by intellectual deterioration.

Hypertension also predisposes to subarachnoid haemorrhage and transient ischaemic attacks which precede major stroke in a significant proportion of cases.

The eye

Fundoscopy provides a unique opportunity to examine the retinal vascular changes in hypertension which presumably reflect similar changes in small vessels elsewhere in the central nervous system. These are discussed later.

The kidney

Hypertension is probably the most common cause of chronic renal failure. Nevertheless, because hypertension may also be the result of renal disease, the precise cause-and-effect relationship is often difficult to establish. Hypertension leads to vascular changes in the renal arterioles and glomerular tufts, which produce tubular dysfunction and lower glomerular filtration rate. Proteinuria and haematuria occur and a 'vicious cycle' of worsening renal function and increasing hypertension may develop.

Peripheral vascular disease

Accelerated atherosclerosis in the peripheral vessels predisposes to ischaemic symptoms—particularly in the legs—and also to aneurysm and dissection of the aorta.

Clinical manifestations

Uncomplicated hypertension is usually asymptomatic, although individual patients may complain of occipital headaches (particularly on waking in the morning) or epistaxis. The onset of symptoms usually signals the development of major complications. Angina due to coronary atherosclerosis, LV hypertrophy or a combination of the two is common and, in end-stage disease, left ventricular failure (LVF) with fatigue and dyspnoea may develop. Retinal haemorrhages and exudates produce blurring of vision and field defects while cerebrovascular disease may lead to transient ischaemic episodes or major stroke.

Examination confirms elevated blood pressure. The cardiac apex is not usually displaced (before LVF supervenes) but it has a thrusting quality and a double impulse due to a palpable fourth heart sound. Auscultation confirms the fourth sound and may also reveal accentuation of the aortic component of the second sound. A soft mid-systolic murmur at the aortic area is common, due to forceful ejection by the hypertrophied LV. Aortic root dilatation occasionally causes mild aortic regurgitation with an early diastolic murmur.

Examination of the optic fundus permits direct inspection of the small blood vessels. Four grades of hypertensive retinopathy are recognized:

Grade 1. Narrowing and increased tortuosity of the retinal arteries.

Grade 2. Accentuation of the arterial changes and compression of the retinal veins at arteriovenous crossings.

Grade 3. Vascular changes associated with haemorrhages and exudates. The haemorrhages are typically flame-shaped and the exudates have a soft 'cotton-wool' appearance.

Grade 4. Previous grades with papilloedema. The optic cup is obliterated and the disk is pink with blurred edges.

Complications

The major complications of hypertension are heart disease, stroke, retinal damage, renal failure and peripheral vascular disease. These have been discussed previously.

Diagnosis

Hypertension is diagnosed by sphygmomanometry (see page 12). Blood pressure may show considerable variation in an individual and, if it is found to be elevated, further measurements should be taken after a brief rest and again at a subsequent clinic visit before the patient is committed to lifelong treatment. In cases where anxiety-related fluctuations in blood pressure cause diagnostic difficulties, devices are available for self-measurement of blood pressure in the more relaxed home environment. Alternatively, ambulatory blood pressure recorders may be used to provide measurements over a 24-hour period. Once the diagnosis is established, further investigation is directed at assessing end-organ damage and determining the aetiological diagnosis.

Assessment of end-organ damage

Routine investigations for all hypertensive patients should include an ECG (Fig. 12.1) and a chest X-ray for assessment of LV hypertrophy and heart failure, respectively. An echocardiogram permits direct inspection of LV wall thickness and contractile function (Fig. 12.2). Renal status is evaluated by analysis of the

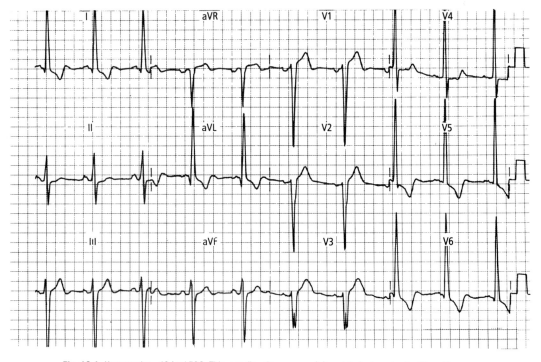

Fig. 12.1 Hypertension—12-lead ECG. This recording shows severe left ventricular hypertrophy. The voltage deflexions are exaggerated and there is T-wave inversion in leads I, aVL and V5 and V6 (strain pattern). Note also the broad notched P waves indicating associated left atrial enlargement.

urine for blood and protein and measurement of blood creatinine. A blood-potassium level is needed as a baseline prior to starting diuretic therapy, and also provides a simple screening test for primary aldosteronism.

Aetiological diagnosis

Because the large majority of patients have essential hypertension, special investigations to screen for primary renal disease and hormonal disorders are only indicated when the clinical findings suggest that hypertension is secondary. This is more important in hypertensive patients aged under 35—particularly when there is no family history—because in this group the incidence of secondary hypertension is relatively high.

Renovascular hypertension

Renal artery stenosis should be suspected in young patients with hypertension (when it is often the result of fibromuscular dysplasia), and in older patients who show an abrupt deterioration in renal function. In the latter age-group, atherosclerosis is the usual case and may be associated with bruits over the renal arteries. Definitive diagnosis requires renal arteriography but intravenous urography and the radionuclide Hippuran renogram are suggestive if they show

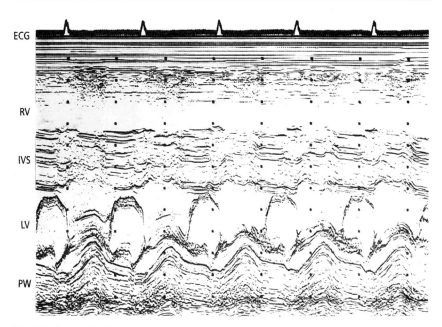

ECG

RV

IVS

LV

PW

Fig. 12.2 Hypertension. M-mode echocardiogram. There is severe concentric thickening of the left ventricle involving the interventricular septum (IVS) and posterior wall (PW). The vertical dots are a 1-cm scale.

delayed opacification of the affected kidney or a delayed rate of rise of radiotracer in the kidney, respectively.

Renal parenchymal disease

The diagnosis of acute nephritis is suggested by hypertension, oedema and haematuria following a recent throat infection. In chronic renal parenchymal disease, the aetiological diagnosis is often more difficult and it may be unclear whether the renal disease is the cause or the effect of hypertension. Renal biopsy may be helpful because, in a number of cases, specific treatment will be available to halt the progression of disease, e.g. minimal-change nephritis, systemic lupus erythematosus. In end-stage disease, however, when ultrasound examination shows severe reduction in renal size, establishment of the renal diagnosis is less likely to influence treatment which aims to control uraemia and correct blood pressure.

Hormonal disorders

Hypokalaemia is essential for the diagnosis of *primary hyperaldosteronism* (Conn's syndrome) and often causes muscular weakness. Confirmation of hyperaldosteronism first requires correction of hypokalaemia by replacement therapy. Following this, stimuli for renin secretion are given (e.g. intravenous frusemide 40 mg followed by 30 minutes upright posture) which invariably show an attenuated response. *Cushing's syndrome* is suspected in patients with typical physical findings including central obesity, moon facies, hirsutism, striae, proximal myopathy and osteoporosis. The diagnosis is confirmed if the dexamethasone suppression test fails to suppress blood-cortisol levels and urinary excretion of 17-hydroxycorticoids. Up to half of all patients with *phaeochromocytoma* have sustained hypertension, although the classical presentation is with fluctuating blood pressure in which the hypertensive episodes may be associated with headache, flushing and anxiety. Diagnosis is by demonstration of elevated levels of catecholamines in the blood or urine. In all the adrenal causes of secondary hypertension, computed tomography will often identify the adrenal hyperplasia or tumour. Nevertheless, failure to image the tumour does not rule out the diagnosis if biochemical tests are conclusive.

Treatment

Only a small minority of patients have hypertension amenable to surgical correction. This includes those with adrenal disease, renal artery stenosis, unilateral renal parenchymal disease and coarctation. Even so, medical therapy is sometimes preferable, with surgery being reserved for resistant cases. This is particularly true of primary aldosteronism if a discrete adrenal tumour cannot be identified, and unilateral renal parenchymal disease in which nephrectomy is the only surgical option.

Aims of treatment

Treatment is aimed at lowering the blood pressure in order to reduce the incidence of major complications. The efficacy of treatment for preventing stroke is well established (Box 12.1). It has also been possible to demonstrate a reduced incidence of renal failure, but effects on coronary artery disease and myocardial infarction are disappointingly small. Nevertheless, the overall mortality of treated hypertensives is lower than untreated. In severe hypertension, the mortality reduction during long-term follow-up exceeds 50%.

Whom to treat?

Large-scale studies have failed to show that the treatment of mild hypertension (up to 160/100 mmHg) produces an appreciable benefit in terms of long-term mortality, although variable improvements in morbidity, particularly stroke, have been found (Box 12.1). The benefits of treating moderate and severe hypertension, however, are well established. One large study showed that, in patients with diastolic blood pressure above 115 mmHg (severe hypertension), active treatment reduced the risk of complications from 55% to 18%, and more than halved the number of deaths.

There is no evidence that different treatment policies are required in particular racial, sex or age-groups. Thus beta-blockers and angiotensin-converting enzyme (ACE) inhibitors remain useful in black people even though they tend to

Box 12.1 Medical Research Council (MRC) 'Young Hypertensives'

Study design Randomized, single-blind, parallel-group, placebo-controlled, multicentre.

Randomization Bendrofluazide, 10 mg/day; or propranolol, maximum 240 mg/day; or placebo. Additional antihypertensive drugs were allowed if blood pressure did not respond satisfactorily to the above treatments.

Inclusion Mild hypertension.

End points Mortality, stroke, blood pressure response, coronary events.

Patients 354 (4297 bendrofluazide; 4403 propranolol; 8654 placebo), aged 35–64 years with diastolic blood pressure 90–109 mmHg.

Results At 1 year, diastolic blood pressure < 90 mmHg was achieved in 66%, 60% and 38% of men in the bendrofluazide, propranolol and placebo groups, respectively. Corresponding figures for women were 71%, 64% and 42%. At 5 years, diastolic blood pressure < 90 mmHg was achieved in 72%, 71% and 43% of men in the bendrofluazide, propranolol and placebo groups, respectively. Corresponding figures for women were 78%, 76% and 50%. Active treatment did not significantly influence overall mortality (248 active treatment vs 253 placebo) nor overall coronary events (222 active treatment vs 234 placebo). However, the incidence of cardiovascular events was reduced by active treatment compared with placebo (286 vs. 352; $P < 0.05$); the incidence of stroke was also reduced (60% vs 109; $P < 0.01$).

Conclusions Findings suggest that, in terms of blood-pressure control, propranolol and thiazide diuretics have similar efficacy. Treatment reduces the risk of stroke and cardiovascular events, but does not influence mortality in young patients with mild hypertension.

Anonymous (1985) MRC trial of treatment of mild hypertension: principal results. *B Med J*; **291**: 97–104.

respond less vigorously to these drugs than white people. Although the elderly (> 70 years) are often less able to tolerate antihypertensive drugs, they are most at risk of stroke and benefit from treatment as much as, if not more than, younger hypertensives.

Non-pharmacological measures

Hypertension is not a medical emergency and in many cases can be improved (or even corrected) without drug treatment. Women on the contraceptive pill should, where possible, use an alternative method of contraception. The obese patient should be encouraged to lose weight because this often produces a significant reduction in blood pressure. Moderation of alcohol consumption is beneficial, particularly in the heavy drinker. Patients should be advised not to add extra salt to their food. Relief of stress, though difficult to achieve, is beneficial in some patients. A variety of relaxation and meditation techniques have been shown to lower blood pressure, at least in the short term. Undoubtedly the most important general measure, however, is the avoidance or correction of other risk factors for arterial disease, particularly smoking and hypercholesterolaemia. In the majority of clinical trials, smoking has emerged as a more important predictor of both myocardial infarction and stroke than a moderate increase in blood pressure.

Drug therapy (Table 12.2)

Despite the importance of non-pharmacological methods to control hypertension, many patients will require treatment with antihypertensive drugs and, because this must continue indefinitely, its acceptability in terms of side-effects and dosage frequency must always be a major consideration. Indeed, poor compliance with the treatment regimen is the usual reason for inadequate control of blood pressure. From the wide range of drugs available, six groups of agents come closest to fulfilling the combined requirement for efficacy and acceptability. These are diuretics, beta-blockers, calcium antagonists, ACE inhibitors, angiotensin receptor blockers and alpha-blockers.

Previously, beta-blockers and thiazide diuretics have been recommended as the first-line agents in moderate and severe hypertension because their benefits for mortality reduction have been best documented. However, many of the more recently introduced agents are better tolerated and there is growing consensus that the choice of antihypertensive treatment should be tailored to the individual. In young patients an ACE inhibitor or alpha-blocker is often preferred because side-effects are rarely obtrusive and impotence, in particular, is seldom a problem. In addition, these drugs do not have unfavourable effects on glucose or

Table 12.2 Drugs for the treatment of hypertension

Drug	Dose (mg)
Diuretics	
Bendrofluazide	2.5 mg daily
Cyclopenthiazide	0.5–1.0 mg daily
Beta-blockers	
Atenolol	50–200 mg daily
Bisoprolol	5–20 mg daily
Calcium antagonists	
Nifedipine (long acting)	30 mg daily
Verapamil	240 mg daily (slow-release preparation)
Amlodipine	5–10 mg daily
Angiotensin-converting enzyme inhibitors	
Captopril	12.5–50 mg twice daily
Enalapril	5–40 mg daily
Lisinopril	2.5–40 mg daily
Quinapril	10–40 mg daily
Alpha-blockers	
Doxazosin	1–16 mg daily
Angiotensin receptor blockers	
Losartan	50–100 mg daily
Valsartan	40–160 mg daily

lipid metabolism and, on theoretical grounds, may protect against development of arterial disease in later life. The elderly are sometimes unwilling to take vasodilators because of postural hypotension and often find a low dose of diuretic more acceptable. Beta-blockers have a useful role in patients with exaggerated tachycardia, an anxiety component to their hypertension or associated angina, while for many patients calcium antagonists or angiotensin receptor blockers are the best-tolerated drugs. For patients unable to tolerate ACE inhibitors (dry cough is the usual reason for this), angiotensin receptor blockers are a useful alternative. If a single agent provides inadequate blood-pressure control a second can be added—ideally as a combined preparation for ease of administration and better compliance. Persistent hypertension requires the addition of a third agent and in the most severe cases, four or more different drugs may be necessary.

Diuretics

Salt and water excretion lowers blood pressure by reducing plasma volume and cardiac output. Nevertheless, these changes are short-lived and the mechanisms responsible for the long-term antihypertensive efficacy of diuretics are unknown. Although thiazides and loop diuretics are equally effective, thiazides are usually preferred because they produce a less vigorous diuresis. They should be used in combination with a potassium-sparing diuretic (or ACE inhibitor) to prevent hypokalaemia. Impotence may affect up to 15% of patients treated with thiazide diuretics which are therefore best avoided in younger sexually active patients. Thiazides cause modest elevations of blood sugar and triglycerides and there is a theoretical risk of long-term cardiovascular complications in young patients. At present, however, there is no evidence that the metabolic side-effects of thiazides increase cardiovascular morbidity.

Beta-blockers

These drugs tend to lower cardiac output through their effect on heart rate and contractility; they also inhibit sympathetically mediated renin release from the kidney, reducing angiotensin II synthesis. Nevertheless, it is unlikely that these properties account fully for the antihypertensive efficacy of beta-blockers, the mechanism of which remains uncertain.

Beta-blockers are effective in all degrees of hypertension. They may be used as monotherapy but are particularly useful in combination with thiazides or calcium antagonists, both of which tend to increase renin release—an unwanted effect which is modified by beta-blockers. In addition, beta-blockers prevent reflex tachycardia caused by the vasodilator effects of calcium antagonists and alpha-blockers. The choice of beta-blocker depends principally on patient acceptability, atenolol usually being preferred because it is long-acting and cardioselective and does not cross the blood–brain barrier (see page 116). The more recently available bisoprolol has similar properties but is longer acting and more cardioselective and has a neutral effect on blood lipids. Other beta-blockers may cause a small rise in blood cholesterol though whether this affects the risk of developing arterial disease is not known.

Calcium antagonists

These drugs relax vascular smooth muscle, producing arteriolar dilatation and reduction in systemic vascular resistance, and are effective in all degrees of hypertension. Nifedipine is best given in combination with a beta-blocker to prevent reflex tachycardia. Verapamil and diltiazem cause less reflex tachycardia and can be used as monotherapy. Although these drugs are relatively short acting and require to be given three times daily, slow-release preparations are now available for once-daily dosage which improves patient compliance. The newer long-acting calcium antagonists for once-daily administration, such as amlodipine and lacidipine, already have a useful role in the long-term management of hypertension.

Angiotensin-converting enzyme inhibitors

These drugs produce arteriolar dilatation and reduction in systemic vascular resistance by blocking the synthesis of angiotensin II—a potent vasoconstrictor. They are effective in all degrees of hypertension and are now being used increasingly because side-effects are rarely troublesome and quality of life is often well preserved. A troublesome dry cough develops in up to 10% of patients and may require discontinuation of treatment. Impotence and drowsiness, however, seldom occur. ACE inhibitors do not have adverse effects on lipid profiles and in many cases cause small reductions in blood cholesterol, though whether this protects against arterial disease during long-term treatment is unknown. A wide variety of different agents are now available but long-acting drugs for once daily administration (e.g. lisinopril, quinapril) are usually preferred in the management of hypertension.

Alpha-blockers

Doxazosin, a postsynaptic alpha-adrenoceptor-blocker for once-daily administration, is now widely used in the treatment of hypertension. It is effective and well tolerated and, like ACE inhibitors, may cause concomitant small reductions in blood cholesterol levels. Side-effects related to vasodilatation (headache, dizziness) are rarely troublesome and, as with ACE inhibitors, the incidence of impotence is low.

Angiotensin receptor blockers

Losartan was the first orally active drug in this class; also available is valsartan. These drugs displace angiotensin II from its type-1 receptor subtype and antagonize its actions, including smooth-muscle contraction and aldosterone release. Once-daily administration is effective and well tolerated. Angiotensin receptor blockers are lipid neutral, have no adverse effect on glucose tolerance and, unlike ACE inhibitors, do not cause a cough.

Prognosis

When hypertension is untreated, 50% of patients die of heart disease, 30% of strokes and 15% of renal failure. The extent of end-organ damage relates principally to the duration of hypertension and its severity: thus by detecting hypertension at an early stage and treating it effectively prognosis can be improved. Prognosis is also affected by the age, race and sex of the patient, with young black men being at greatest risk of premature death. The outlook is worse in those patients with associated risk factors for arterial disease, particularly hypercholesterolaemia and smoking.

Accelerated hypertension

This affects about 1% of all hypertensive patients and occurs in both essential and secondary hypertension. Cigarette smoking is a predisposing factor. Severe elevation of the blood pressure (often > 200/140 mmHg) may be associated with encephalopathy characterized by headache, nausea, clouding of consciousness and convulsions. The marked increase in afterload commonly causes LVF and pulmonary oedema. Grade IV retinopathy is invariable. Impairment of renal function usually occurs and, if treatment is not instituted rapidly, oliguric renal failure develops.

Accelerated hypertension is a medical emergency. Treatment is aimed at reducing the diastolic blood pressure to between 90 and 110 mmHg. Blood-pressure reduction should be smooth and controlled because there is risk of cerebral infarction if it drops abruptly to very low levels. For this reason bolus injections of diazoxide or hydralazine are no longer recommended because the blood-pressure response is unpredictable and difficult to control. Sublingual nifedipine or captopril should be avoided for the same reason. Intravenous infusion of labetalol is preferred because a graded reduction in blood pressure can be achieved with an incremental dosage regimen (1 mg/minute with increments every 30 minutes). Labetalol has a short half-life and potentially dangerous falls in blood pressure are reversed by temporarily stopping the infusion. Following control of the blood pressure, oral antihypertensive drugs should be prescribed to prevent recurrence of the hypertensive crisis.

FURTHER READING

Alderman MH. Non-pharmacological treatment of hypertension. Lancet 1994; 344: 307.
Bennet NE. Hypertension in the elderly. *Lancet* 1994; 344: 447.
Calhoun DA, Oparil S. Hypertensive crisis since FDR—a partial victory. *N Engl J Med* 1995; 332: 1029.

Chambers J. Left ventricular hypertrophy: an under-appreciated coronary risk factor. *Br Med J* 1995; 311: 273.

Fletcher AE, Bulpitt CJ. How far should blood pressure be lowered? *N Engl J Med* 1992; 326: 251.

Frohlich ED, Apstein C, Chobanian AV, *et al.* Heart in hypertension. *N Engl J Med* 1992; 327: 998.

Frohlich ED. Cardiac hypertrophy in hypertension. *N Engl J Med* 1987; 317: 831.

Harrap SB. Hypertension: genes versus environment. *Lancet* 1994; 344: 169.

Law MR, Frost CD and Wald NJ. By how much does dietary salt reduction lower blood pressure? *Br Med J* 1991; 302: 811.

McGrath BP. Is white-coat hypertension innocent? *Lancet* 1996; 348: 630.

Oparil S. Antihypertensive therapy—efficacy and quality of life. *N Engl J Med* 1993; 328: 1167.

Pickering TG. Blood pressure measurement and detection of hypertension. *Lancet* 1994; 344: 31.

Saunders JB. Alcohol: an important cause of hypertension. *Br Med J* 1987; 294: 1045.

Setaro JF, Black HR. Refractory hypertension. *N Engl J Med* 1992; 327: 1075.

Simon JA. Treating hypertension: the evidence from clinical trials. *Br Med J* 1996 ;313: 437.

Swales JD. Pharmacological treatment of hypertension. *Lancet* 1994; 344: 380.

Victor RG, Hansen J. Alcohol and blood pressure—a drink a day . . . . *N Engl J Med* 1995; 332: 1782.

Whelton PK. Epidemiology of hypertension. *Lancet* 1944; 344: 101.

CHAPTER 13

Aortic Aneurysm and Dissection

SUMMARY

Aortic aneurysms are usually abdominal, caused by atherosclerotic disease of the arterial wall. Aneurysms of the ascending aorta may also be atherosclerotic but more commonly are the result of cystic medial necrosis, seen typically in Marfan's syndrome. Most aneurysms are asymptomatic, though local pressure may cause pain in the lumbar or thoracic spine. Abdominal aneurysms may be palpated as a pulsatile mass in the abdomen but thoracic aneurysms produce no physical signs unless they involve the aortic valve ring when the early diastolic murmur of aortic regurgitation may be audible. The other principal complication is rupture, unusual in thoracic aneurysms but more common in abdominal aneurysms, particularly those > 6 cm in diameter. If the aneurysm is calcified, it is often visible on the plain chest or abdominal X-ray, but ultrasound, computed tomography or magnetic resonance imaging is required for more precise diagnosis. Blood-pressure control is essential, and surgical resection is indicated for abdominal aneurysms > 6 cm or for the correction of complications.

Aortic dissection is a medical emergency caused by a tear in the intima of the ascending aorta or the aortic arch. The high-pressure arterial blood creates a false lumen through the media which may either re-enter the true lumen more distally or rupture externally, usually into the pericardial or left pleural spaces. The dissection may partially or completely occlude any of the branch arteries arising from the aorta and, if proximal, may disrupt the aortic valve ring causing aortic regurgitation. Presentation is with severe chest pain and examination may reveal reduced or absent pulses; coronary occlusion may cause myocardial infarction. Aortic regurgitation is common in proximal dissection and rupture externally may be associated with signs of tamponade or hypovolaemic shock. Diagnosis requires demonstration of the intimal flap separating true and false aortic lumens. The echocardiogram is helpful (particularly by the transoesophageal approach) but computed tomography is more usually diagnostic. In most cases, however, urgent aortic root angiography is necessary to demonstrate the origin and extent of dissection. For proximal dissections, surgical repair improves prognosis and is treatment of choice. Distal dissections arising in the aortic arch are best treated medically with beta-blockers to lower blood pressure.

AORTIC ANEURYSM

Aetiology

Aortic aneurysms occur most commonly in the abdominal aorta where they are usually the result of atherosclerosis. Aneurysms of the descending thoracic aorta are also atherosclerotic in most cases, but in the ascending aorta Marfan's syndrome and other causes of cystic medial necrosis have replaced syphilis as the usual cause.

Pathophysiology

Risk factors are the same as for atherosclerotic disease elsewhere in the body. Thus, patients at greatest risk are middle-aged or elderly men, particularly when there is a history of cigarette smoking, hypertension or hypercholesterolaemia.

The wall tension in a blood vessel is determined by the product of intravascular pressure and diameter (law of Laplace). The aorta is the largest artery in the body and its walls therefore are under considerable tension. Disease of the aortic wall causes destruction of the elastic fibres in the media which allows the vessel to dilate. This increases wall tension and a vicious circle becomes established.

Most aortic aneurysms are fusiform, involving the total circumference of a segment of the vessel wall. Occasionally, they are sacular and consist of an outpouching of the vessel wall. Sacular aneurysms are often the result of syphilis or other infections (mycotic aneurysm) and are particularly prone to rupture.

About 76% of aortic aneurysms occur in the abdominal aorta below the renal arteries where the risk of rupture is greatest and closely related to the size of the aneurysm. When the diameter is < 6 cm the incidence of rupture within 1 year is 20%, but the incidence approaches 50% for larger aneurysms.

Clinical manifestations

Aortic aneurysms are usually asymptomatic. When they are located in the abdominal aorta, low back pain may occur (due to pressure over the lumbar spine) but in many cases aortic rupture is the first manifestation. Examination reveals an expansile pulsating mass in the abdomen, and a bruit is often audible due to turbulent flow through the aneurysm.

Thoracic aortic aneurysms are more likely to be symptomatic although rupture is unusual: large aneurysms often cause an aching chest discomfort which may be associated with pain in the back due to pressure over the thoracic spine. Other symptoms caused by compression of adjacent structures include dysphagia, cough and hoarseness. They rarely produce physical signs unless they involve the aortic root when the early diastolic murmur of aortic regurgitation may be audible. This is particularly common in Marfan's syndrome and other causes of cystic medial necrosis.

Complications

Rupture is the principal complication; it is a surgical emergency and often rapidly fatal. Abdominal aortic aneurysms are most prone to rupture—usually into the retroperitoneal space. Patients who survive the acute episode present in hypovolaemic shock with severe pain in the abdomen and the back, often extending into the iliac fossae; emergency surgery saves about 50% of these patients. Occasionally, rupture is into the duodenum or the inferior vena cava causing massive gastrointestinal haemorrhage and arteriovenous fistula, respectively.

Unusual complications include thromboembolism, due to thrombosis within the aneurysmal sac; and infection which produces a syndrome similar to endocarditis. Aneurysm of the ascending aorta is particularly common in Marfan's syndrome and commonly causes aortic regurgitation.

Diagnosis

Abdominal aortic aneurysms are identified by clinical examination and, if calcified, can usually be seen on the plain abdominal X-ray. The diagnosis is confirmed by ultrasonography which permits accurate assessment of the size of the aneurysm; computed tomography (CT) or magnetic resonance imaging (MRI) provide alternative means for identification of abdominal aortic aneurysms.

Thoracic aortic aneurysms are nearly always visible on the chest X-ray (Fig. 13.1). Echocardiography identifies aortic root aneurysms (see Fig. 16.1), and the transoesophageal technique permits examination of the aortic arch. For most purposes, however, thoracic aortic aneurysms are best examined by CT, MRI or aortography.

Differential diagnosis

Abdominal aortic aneurysms must be differentiated from other masses, particularly those that overlie the aorta and transmit pulsation; non-aneurysmal masses, however, are never expansile. Ultrasound examination is usually suffi-

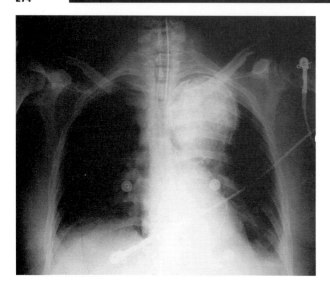

Fig. 13.1 Thoracic aortic aneurysm. The chest X-ray shows a large calcified mass in the left upper mediastinum. The calcification extends downwards behind the heart in the wall of the aorta, confirming that the mass is an aortic aneurysm.

cient to resolve the differential diagnosis. Thoracic aortic aneurysms require differentiation from other causes of a mediastinal mass.

Treatment

Specific treatment is usually unnecessary although blood-pressure control is important. Surgical resection is indicated when symptoms or complications (e.g. aortic regurgitation) cannot be controlled or when rupture threatens (abdominal aneurysms > 6 cm in diameter or those that show rapid radiographic enlargement on serial examinations).

Prognosis

Patients with atherosclerotic aortic aneurysms nearly always have coronary artery disease and this, together with the size of the aneurysm, has an important influence on prognosis. Thus 5-year survival is only 20% in patients with symptomatic ischaemic heart disease, but this rises to 50% in the absence of ischaemic heart disease. The size is also important, abdominal aneurysms > 6 cm in diameter being at greatest risk of potentially fatal rupture. Aortic root aneurysms in Marfan's syndrome may cause severe aortic regurgitation and ultimately death if surgical replacement of the aortic root is delayed.

Sinus of Valsalva aneurysm

Sinus of Valsalva aneurysm may be mycotic, occurring as a complication of infective endocarditis. More commonly, however, it is congenital when it usually affects the right coronary sinus, particularly in men. The fusion between the aortic media and the fibrous ring of the aortic valve is weakened or absent, so

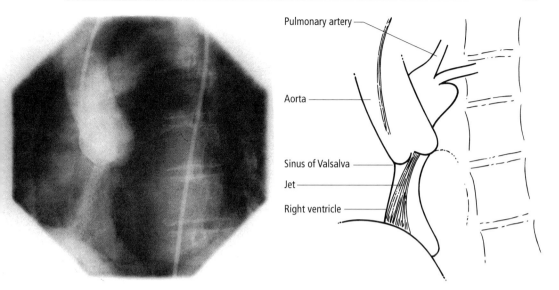

Fig. 13.2 Aortogram of ruptured sinus of Valsalva aneurysm. A jet of contrast material highlights the communication between the sinus of Valsalva and the right ventricle. The right ventricle and the pulmonary artery are opacified.

that progressive aneurysmal bulging of the affected area occurs. This usually remains asymptomatic until adulthood, when rupture of the aneurysm into a right-sided cardiac chamber (usually the right ventricle) produces an arteriovenous shunt. This volume-loads both sides of the heart resulting in biventricular failure, and may cause sudden death although, more commonly, the patient presents with chest pain associated with shortness of breath.

Examination reveals early diastolic collapse of the carotid pulse and a precordial continuous murmur which is audible throughout the cardiac cycle. The diagnosis is confirmed by ascending thoracic aortography which demonstrates prompt opacification of the right-sided cardiac chambers due to shunting through the ruptured aneurysm (Fig. 13.2). Treatment is by surgical repair of the defect.

AORTIC DISSECTION

Aetiology

Like aortic aneurysm, dissection is caused by disease of the aortic media, usually atherosclerosis. Marfan's syndrome and other causes of cystic medial necrosis also predispose to aortic dissection. Patients are often hypertensive, particularly when the dissection arises in the aortic arch.

Pathophysiology

Dissection nearly always arises in the ascending or arch aorta. The development of a tear in the aortic intima causes the high-pressure aortic blood to create a false lumen for a variable distance through the diseased media. The tear is usually proximal just above the sinus of Valsalva, but in about 25% of cases it is distal and located within the aortic arch close to the origin of the left subclavian artery. The dissection can partially or completely occlude any of the branch arteries arising from the aorta and, if proximal, may disrupt the aortic valve ring producing aortic regurgitation. The false lumen may rupture externally (usually into the pericardial sac or left pleural space) or re-enter the true lumen of the aorta more distally.

Clinical manifestations

Presentation is with abrupt-onset severe tearing chest pain which may be experienced in the front or the back of the chest. Pain is maximal at the outset, unlike in acute myocardial infarction (MI), in which the pain has a crescendo quality. The patient is cold and sweaty and may be shocked if the aneurysm ruptures externally, causing tamponade or hypovolaemia. Examination commonly reveals an asymmetrical pulse deficit due to involvement of the carotid or subclavian arteries arising from the aorta. Pulses may be either absent or reduced so that a difference between the blood pressures in the arms is detectable. The early diastolic murmur of aortic regurgitation is commonly present in proximal dissection.

Complications

Branch artery occlusions may cause MI, stroke, intestinal infarction, renal failure or limb ischaemia; vertebral artery occlusion may result in paraplegia. Because occlusion of the left main coronary artery is almost invariably fatal, MI in survivors of aortic dissection is usually located inferiorly and is caused by right coronary occlusion.

When aortic dissection is complicated by external rupture, presentation is with hypovolaemic shock although rupture into the pericardial sac causes tamponade. In either case, the outcome is usually fatal.

Proximal aortic dissection may disrupt the aortic valve ring, producing aortic regurgitation. Its severity is variable, but resuspension or replacement of the aortic valve is often necessary during surgical repair of the dissection.

Diagnosis

ECG changes are non-specific, but may show acute MI if the dissection occludes a coronary ostium. The chest X-ray shows dilatation of the aorta, often with widening of the entire mediastinum (Fig. 13.3). External rupture into the pericardial or pleural spaces causes cardiac enlargement or left pleural effusion, respectively. Definitive diagnosis requires an imaging technique showing the intimal flap separating true and false aortic lumens. The echocardiogram has been widely used (Fig. 13.4), but requires the transoesophageal technique for

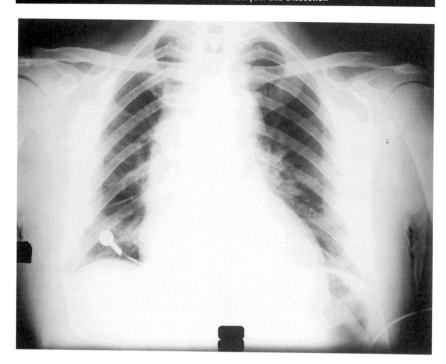

Fig. 13.3 Aortic dissection. The chest X-ray shows widening of the entire mediastinum. In the patient with chest pain this is strongly suggestive of aortic dissection.

complete examination of the ascending aorta and the arch (Fig. 13.5). Indeed, transoesophageal echocardiography is now regarded as the imaging technique of choice for aortic dissection, although CT continues to be widely used (Fig. 13.6). MRI has also found application for this purpose (see Fig. 3.16) in those centres

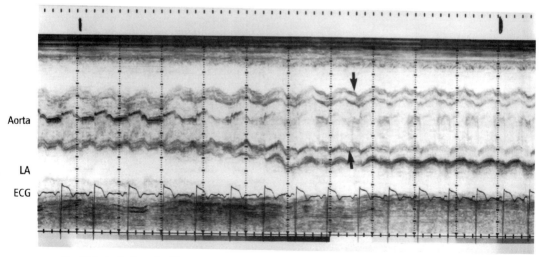

Fig. 13.4 Aortic dissection: M-mode echocardiogram. This is a scan from the sinuses of Valsalva up the ascending aorta. Just above the sinuses of Valsalva the aorta widens considerably and a false lumen (arrowed) becomes apparent in its wall.

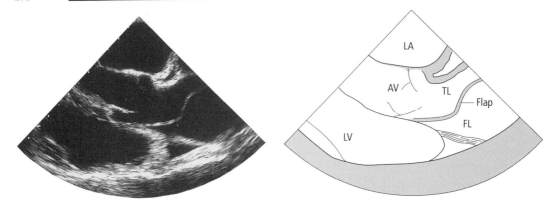

Fig. 13.5 Aortic dissection—transoesophageal echocardiogram. The flap separating true (TL) and false (FL) aortic lumens is clearly visible in the ascending aorta, just above the aortic valve leaflets (AV).

where this technology is available. In most cases, the surgeon will also require aortic angiography to define the origin and the extent of the dissection (Fig. 13.7).

Differential diagnosis

This is from other causes of acute-onset chest pain, particularly MI. The history is helpful (abrupt vs. crescendo onset of pain) and serial-ECG and enzyme studies indicate acute infarction if the typical evolution of changes occurs. It must be remembered, however, that these differential diagnoses are not necessarily mutually exclusive.

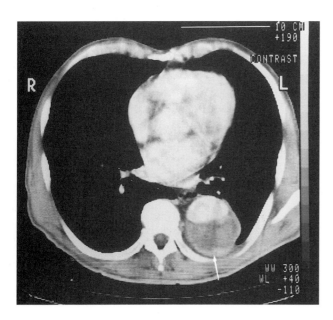

Fig. 13.6 Aortic dissection—computed tomography. The descending thoracic aorta (arrowed) is grossly dilated. Contrast enhancement of the blood pool reveals two columns within the aorta separated by an intimal flap. This confirms the diagnosis of dissection.

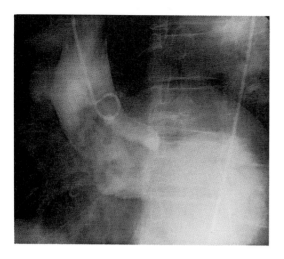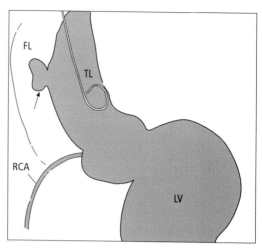

Fig. 13.7 Aortic dissection—aortic root angiography. Contrast injection into the ascending aorta shows the tear in the aortic wall (arrowed) 2 cm above the right coronary artery (RCA) with contrast passing from the true (TL) into the false (FL) aortic lumen. Note the aortic regurgitation evidenced by opacification of the left ventricle (LV) caused by backflow of contrast across the disrupted aortic valve.

Treatment

The emergency management requires blood-pressure reduction to reduce the risk of rupture. If rapid control cannot be achieved with oral beta-blockers or calcium antagonists, labetolol should be infused (see page 269) to maintain the systolic blood pressure at no more than 100 mmHg. Transfer to a cardiothoracic centre for aortography must be arranged as soon as possible. If the dissection involves the ascending aorta (whether from a proximal tear or from proximal extension of a distal dissection) the risk of rupture into the pericardial sac and aortic regurgitation is very high. Expeditious surgical repair reduces the risk and is the treatment of choice. In uncomplicated distal dissection, surgery has not been shown to affect prognosis, but strict control of the blood pressure is essential. Beta-blockers are the drugs of choice for maintenance therapy because they reduce the pulse pressure and the systolic pressure.

Prognosis

Untreated proximal dissection involving the ascending aorta is usually fatal within a month of presentation, although successful surgical treatment ensures a better outcome. Patients with distal dissection fare little better (regardless of surgery), although lowering of the blood pressure helps prevent rupture and may permit longer survival.

FURTHER READING

Banning AP, Rutley MST, Musumeci F, Fraser AG. Acute dissection of the thoracic aorta. *Br Med J* 1995; 310: 72.

Cigarroa JE, Isselbacher EM, De Sanctis RW, Eagle KA. Diagnostic imaging in evaluation of suspected aortic dissection—old standards and new directions. *N Engl J Med* 1993; 328: 35.

DeSanctis RW, Doroghazi RM, Austen WG, Buckley MJ. Aortic dissection. *N Engl J Med* 1987; 317: 1060.

Ernst CB. Abdominal aortic aneurysm. *N Engl J Med* 1993; 328: 1167.

Vlahaker GJ, Warren RL. Traumatic rupture of the aorta. *N Engl J Med* 1995; 332: 389.

CHAPTER 14

Pulmonary Embolism and Pulmonary Heart Disease

CONTENTS

SUMMARY

Acute pulmonary embolism is usually a complication of deep venous thrombosis involving the iliofemoral veins. Its severity is determined by the extent of pulmonary vascular obstruction and only when this exceeds 50% *(massive embolism)* does pulmonary resistance rise sufficiently to cause right ventricular failure (RVF). *Minor embolism* is often clinically silent, occasionally causing pleurisy and haemoptysis. Massive embolism presents with abrupt onset dyspnoea and chest pain associated with tachypnoea, tachycardia and a loud P2; shock and sudden death are not uncommon. Diagnosis is difficult and the ECG and chest X-ray (CXR) are often unhelpful. Arterial gas analysis shows hypoxaemia, hypocapnia and respiratory alkalosis in massive embolism, but definitive diagnosis requires demonstration of ventilation–perfusion mismatch on pulmonary scintigraphy. Treatment is with heparin and oxygen. In severe cases thrombolytic therapy is recommended but failure to respond may require pulmonary angiography and emergency embolectomy.

Chronic pulmonary embolism often remains clinically silent until repeated embolic episodes with progressive obliteration of the vascular bed have caused advanced pulmonary hypertension evidenced by a left parasternal systolic thrust and a loud P2, often associated with the early diastolic murmur of pulmonary regurgitation. The development of RVF produces elevation of the jugular venous pulse (JVP), usually associated with functional tricuspid regurgitation, hepatomegaly and peripheral oedema. The ECG shows RV hypertrophy and the CXR an enlarged heart with prominence of the proximal pulmonary arteries and attenuation ('pruning') of the peripheral vessels. Treatment with long-term warfarin is directed at preventing further embolism but prognosis is poor.

Primary pulmonary hypertension is an uncommon disorder, usually affecting young women, in which obliterative pulmonary arteriolar disease of unknown cause results in progressive pulmonary hypertension and RVF. Prognosis is poor and heart–lung transplantation the only effective treatment.

Pulmonary heart disease, also called cor pulmonale, is usually caused by chronic bronchitis and emphysema in which progressive destruction of the pulmonary vascular bed and hypoxic pulmonary arteriolar constriction lead to pulmonary hypertension and RVF. Initially RVF is intermittent, coinciding with winter exacerbations of bronchitis, but eventually it becomes sustained as pulmonary vascular reserve is exhausted. The patient presents with signs of pulmonary hypertension and RVF. Polycythaemia is common, and respiratory function tests and arterial gas analysis confirm the underlying lung disease. Treatment is directed at preventing progression of pulmonary disease by prophylactic antibiotic therapy and stopping smoking. Diuretics correct peripheral oedema but significant improvement in RV function requires sustained reductions in pulmonary vascular resistance: oxygen therapy is helpful and the role of lung transplantation is under investigation.

ACUTE PULMONARY EMBOLISM

Aetiology

In the majority of cases, pulmonary embolism (PE) is caused by thrombus, usually deriving from the iliofemoral veins (deep venous thrombosis) and, less commonly, from the right-sided cardiac chambers. The thrombus migrates through the right side of the heart into the pulmonary arterial bed causing variable obstruction to flow (Fig. 14.1). Non-thrombotic PE is less common but may be caused by air, amniotic fluid and fat.

Deep venous thrombosis

Deep venous thrombosis (DVT) is usually a complication of prolonged immobility in bed, particularly following abdominal and hip surgery. Other risk factors are shown in Table 14.1. About 10% of cases are complicated by PE. This is unlikely if thrombosis is confined to the calf veins but becomes more likely with extension to the iliofemoral veins. Symptoms and signs of DVT are variable and non-diagnostic. Indeed, although swelling of the affected leg sometimes occurs, many

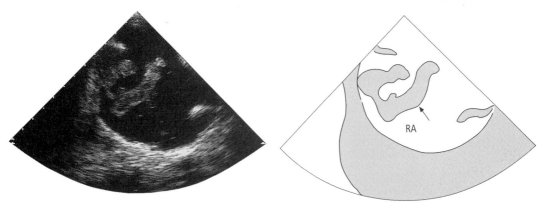

Fig. 14.1 Transoesophageal echocardiogram showing a large serpiginous thrombus (arrowed) in the right atrium (RA) migrating from the iliofemoral veins towards the pulmonary arterial bed. The patient had already experienced one massive pulmonary embolus and later died.

cases are clinically silent. Doppler ultrasound is usually diagnostic but in difficult cases venography provides definitive diagnosis.

Pathophysiology

The severity of PE is largely determined by the extent of pulmonary vascular obstruction; it is classified as *massive* if more than 50% of the major pulmonary arteries are involved, and as *minor* if less extensive. Massive embolism significantly increases pulmonary vascular resistance, causing acute right ventricular failure (RVF). Pulmonary artery systolic pressure, however, does not usually rise above 40 mmHg because the thin-walled right ventricle is unable to generate sufficient pressure to overcome the vascular obstruction. Occasionally, the increase in pulmonary resistance is out of proportion to the extent of vascular obstruction. It has been proposed, therefore, that pulmonary arteriolar constriction caused by ill-defined neurohumoral mechanisms may contribute to the pathophysiology of PE.

Minor PE involving less than 50% of the vascular bed does not compromise right ventricular function because the pulmonary vascular reserve ensures that resistance to flow does not rise significantly. Minor embolism of this type is therefore clinically silent unless it causes pulmonary infarction. This affects only

Table 14.1 Risk factors for deep venous thrombosis.

Immobility—particularly following hip and abdominal surgery
Venous stasis in legs—varicose veins, vena cava compression (e.g. gravid uterus), bony fractures of legs
Heart disease—myocardial infarction, heart failure
Endocrine/metabolic factors—diabetes, obesity, contraceptive pill, postpartum period
Malignant disease—particularly pancreatic and bronchial carcinoma
Miscellaneous—polycythaemia, Behçet's disease

about 10% of cases because the lung is protected by the bronchial arterial supply from the thoracic aorta and also obtains oxygen directly from the alveoli.

Clinical manifestations

These are very variable and usually non-diagnostic. Minor embolism is often asymptomatic but, if it causes pulmonary infarction, pleuritic chest pain with or without haemoptysis may occur.

In massive embolism, patients commonly complain of acute-onset dyspnoea with or without chest pain which is usually retrosternal and not necessarily pleuritic in nature. Cough, haemoptysis, diaphoresis and syncope occur less frequently. The most consistent clinical signs are tachypnoea, tachycardia and accentuation of the pulmonary component of the second heart sound; elevation of the jugular venous pulse (JVP), a third heart sound and cyanosis are more variable. In the most severe cases, the patient is shocked with severe hypotension and other signs of critically impaired cardiac output. Sudden death is not uncommon.

Complications

Non-fatal PE usually resolves without complications. In patients who develop pulmonary infarction, cavitation and secondary infection of the infarct occasionally occurs (Fig. 14.2). In a minority of cases recurrent (often subclinical) thromboembolism results in worsening pulmonary hypertension and RVF (see below).

Diagnosis

The chest X-ray (CXR) is often normal, although loss of lung volume (elevated hemidiaphragm) and regional oligaemia are sometimes seen. A pleural reaction is common and may produce a small effusion although this rarely becomes visible until at least 12–24 hours after the event. When pulmonary infarction occurs, the development of a radiographic density is also a relatively late finding.

The ECG changes are as variable as the clinical features and are rarely diagnostic. Tachycardia may be the only abnormality but, in massive embolism, features of acute right heart strain are sometimes seen. These include P pulmonale, an S wave in lead I and a narrow Q wave in lead III associated with T-wave inversion (S1, Q3, T3). Right bundle branch block and atrial fibrillation may also occur.

Arterial gas analysis is unhelpful in minor embolism but, in more severe cases, hypoxaemia associated with hypocapnia and respiratory alkalosis are characteristic findings.

More useful diagnostic information is provided by the radionuclide lung scan. A normal perfusion scan rules out significant PE. However, the demonstration of perfusion defects is suggestive, particularly when simultaneous ventilation scanning confirms ventilation–perfusion mismatch (see Fig. 3.14).

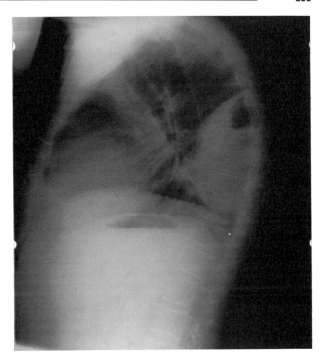

Fig. 14.2 Pulmonary embolism with cavitating infarct. A week after massive pulmonary embolism the lateral chest X-ray showed a posteriorly located infarct with a fluid level indicating cavitation.

Pulmonary arteriography is the definitive method of diagnosis (Fig. 14.3) but is only indicated in patients suspected of having massive PE when surgical embolectomy is under consideration. Arteriography is diagnostic if intraluminal filling defects and vessel cut-offs are seen. Other abnormalities, including regional oligaemia, are less specific.

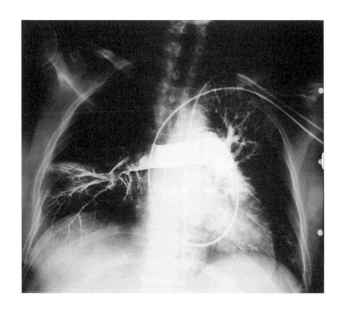

Fig. 14.3 Massive pulmonary embolism—pulmonary arteriogram. There is extensive pulmonary arterial obstruction with opacification limited to the left upper lobe and to a few branches in the right lower zone. Note the intraluminal thrombus which is clearly visible as a filling defect in the right pulmonary artery.

Differential diagnosis

Minor PE must be differentiated from other causes of pleurisy and haemoptysis, particularly pneumonia. The CXR and the results of blood and sputum culture are usually sufficient to confirm infection which usually responds promptly to antibiotics. In difficult cases the radionuclide lung scan is helpful because, in pneumonia, ventilation–perfusion defects are matched, unlike in PE when they are mismatched. Massive PE requires differentiation from myocardial infarction (MI) and other causes of collapse and shock. Typical cardiac pain associated with the diagnostic evolution of ECG and serum enzyme changes is usually sufficient to confirm MI. Hypovolaemic and septic shock can be diagnosed from the clinical context in which they occur. Moreover, in neither condition is the JVP elevated.

Treatment

Prophylaxis

Treatment to prevent DVT in patients at risk (see Table 14.1) significantly reduces the incidence of PE. Thus, prophylactic heparin is recommended in patients with acute MI and also in patients undergoing surgery. Subcutaneous heparin 5000 units 8-hourly is effective and in surgical patients should start preoperatively. Now available is low molecular weight heparin for once daily administration which may be more effective. Other techniques to prevent DVT include electrical stimulation and compression or passive movement of the legs, all of which help prevent venous stasis during bed-rest and surgery.

Minor pulmonary embolism

Initial treatment with oxygen and heparin should be given immediately PE is suspected and should not await the results of diagnostic tests. Heparin prevents extension of thrombosis within the lungs and allows endogenous thrombolysis to proceed uninterrupted; it also guards against recurrent thromboembolism. Following an initial intravenous bolus of 10 000 units, treatment should continue with up to 40 000 units daily in order to keep the partial thromboplastin time at at least twice normal. After 7 days, warfarin should be substituted and continued for 3–6 months. The dose is titrated against the prothrombin time which should be maintained at at least twice to three times normal.

Massive pulmonary embolism

Initial treatment again is with heparin and oxygen. Low-output heart failure requires haemodynamic support with inotropic agents (see page 87). If recovery is delayed, thrombolytic therapy with streptokinase is recommended to hasten resolution of the embolus. Although streptokinase is often given through a catheter positioned in the pulmonary artery, delivery by a peripheral vein is probably equally effective. A loading dose of 600 000 units is followed by an infusion of 100 000 units/hour. In the shocked patient who fails to respond rapidly to these measures, pulmonary arteriography with a view to embolectomy must be considered, though the mortality is high.

Prognosis

In minor PE, spontaneous resolution usually occurs and provided that no further emboli occur the prognosis is good, albeit dependent on the underlying disorder. In massive PE, sudden death is common. In those patients who survive the acute episode, however, complete resolution of the embolus can be expected, following which prognosis is usually good, depending again on the underlying disorder.

Non-thrombotic pulmonary embolism

Air embolism

Major air embolism into the venous circulation is rare. Relatively large volumes (in excess of 50–100 ml) delivered rapidly are required to cause significant haemodynamic disturbance. Air usually gains access through indwelling venous sheaths which do not have haemostatic valves although, occasionally, faulty intravenous infusion equipment is responsible. In the most severe cases, shock or cardiac arrest occurs; nevertheless vigorous resuscitation may permit absorption of the air into the bloodstream following which recovery is possible.

Fat embolism

This is seen following extensive accidental or surgical bony injury. Marrow fat gains access to the venous circulation and embolizes to the lungs. Presentation is usually after a latent period of 12–36 hours and is due not only to pulmonary vascular obstruction by globules of fat but also to local toxic vasculitis caused by free fatty acid release. Mental confusion and severe cardiopulmonary embarrassment occur and mortality is high.

Amniotic fluid embolism

This may complicate both normal and Caesarean deliveries. Significant quantities of amniotic fluid leaking into the venous circulation cause massive PE which is often abruptly fatal. In those patients who survive the acute episode, the subsequent course is complicated by disseminated intravascular coagulation because of the thromboplastic properties of amniotic fluid. Mortality is high.

CHRONIC PULMONARY EMBOLISM

Repeated, often subclinical, episodes of pulmonary thromboembolism may lead to

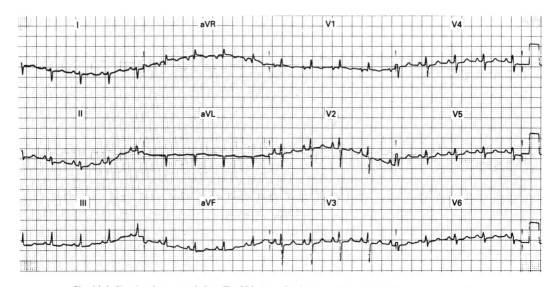

Fig. 14.4 Chronic pulmonary embolism. The ECG shows P pulmonale, right axis deviation and a dominant R wave in lead V1 associated with T-wave inversion. These are typical features of pulmonary hypertension.

progressive obliteration of the pulmonary vascular tree. This is a chronic process associated with a slowly rising pulmonary vascular resistance which provides time for the development of compensatory right ventricular hypertrophy. Pulmonary hypertension is always severe, and RVF eventually supervenes (see page 83).

The patient presents with shortness of breath, sometimes episodic over several months (reflecting repeated embolic episodes), but more commonly progressive without any clear history to suggest PE. Signs of right-sided failure, often with fluid retention, are invariable.

The ECG usually shows evidence of RV hypertrophy with right axis deviation and prominent R waves in leads V1–V3, which may be associated with T-wave inversion (Fig. 14.4). The CXR shows cardiac enlargement and considerable dilatation of the proximal pulmonary arteries, although the peripheral lung fields often appear oligaemic (peripheral 'pruning', Fig. 14.5). Nevertheless, these changes are non-specific and occur in other conditions associated with pulmonary hypertension.

By the time the patient presents, the pulmonary vascular disease is usually irreversible and treatment must be directed at preventing further embolic events. Lifelong anticoagulation with warfarin is essential and, in some cases, surgical procedures are undertaken to prevent further embolism from the iliofemoral veins. Ligation or plication of the inferior vena cava has been widely used but the beneficial effects are usually only temporary because, as large venous collaterals open up, thromboembolism continues. More recently, intraluminal filters (introduced into the inferior vena cava by the percutaneous transvenous route) have been used which filter the blood and remove small emboli without impeding flow. Whether this improves prognosis is uncertain, however, and few patients survive more than 5 years from the time of diagnosis.

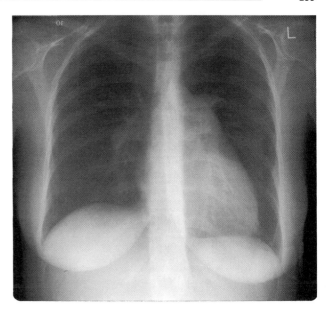

Fig. 14.5 Chronic pulmonary embolism. The chest X-ray shows enlargement of the proximal pulmonary arteries and oligaemic lung fields.

PRIMARY PULMONARY HYPERTENSION

Primary pulmonary hypertension is an uncommon condition, usually affecting young women. It is characterized pathologically by muscular hypertrophy and intimal hyperplasia of the small pulmonary arteries, often associated with intravascular thrombosis. The cause is, by definition, unknown although a link with oestrogens is suggested by its association with female sex and the rapid deterioration that occurs in pregnancy and also, rarely, with use of the contraceptive pill. Pulmonary hypertension is unremitting and progressive, resulting in severe hypertrophy of the right ventricle, which eventually dilates and fails. Exertional dyspnoea and fatigue are the predominant symptoms, although up to 50% of patients also complain of exertional chest discomfort. Physical signs are those of severe pulmonary hypertension and include a left parasternal systolic thrust (due to RV hypertrophy) and accentuation of the pulmonary component of the second heart sound, sometimes associated with the early diastolic murmur of pulmonary regurgitation. The ECG and CXR show changes consistent with right ventricular hypertrophy, pulmonary hypertension and pulmonary vascular obstruction, similar to those seen in chronic PE and other causes of pulmonary hypertension (see above). It is essential, therefore, that other potentially treatable conditions, particularly chronic PE, are excluded before the diagnosis of primary pulmonary hypertension is made.

Anticoagulation is recommended in all patients based on the small-vessel pulmonary thrombosis that can be demonstrated pathologically. Other treatments widely used include vasodilators (particularly high-dose nifedipine), most of which have been shown to lower pulmonary artery pressure when given acutely. However, there is little evidence that drugs of this type are of long-term benefit. Ambulatory infusions of prostacyclin (a potent pulmonary vasodilator with additional antithrombotic effects) have been associated with clinical improvement in patients with severe disease awaiting transplantation. Heart–lung transplantation is at present the only treatment of potential long-term value, indicated in severely incapacitated patients with end-stage disease.

The prognosis is poor—most patients die within 10 years of diagnosis. In many cases death is sudden, presumably due to ventricular arrhythmias; the remainder die of progressive RVF.

PULMONARY HEART DISEASE

Pulmonary heart disease—also called cor pulmonale—is diagnosed when right ventricular hypertrophy and dilatation result from disease of the lungs or pulmonary circulation. Because the basic problem resides in the lungs (or less commonly in the mechanisms of respiratory control), prevention of progressive right heart failure can be achieved only by correction of the pulmonary disorder.

Aetiology (Table 14.2)

Chronic obstructive pulmonary disease caused by bronchitis and emphysema is responsible for the large majority of cases of pulmonary heart disease. Destruction of the pulmonary vascular bed as a result of alveolar damage and interstitial fibrosis increases the pulmonary vascular resistance. Air trapping and hypoxia exacerbate the process, by capillary compression and stimulation of bronchial arteriolar constriction, respectively. These factors combine to produce pulmonary hypertension which overloads the right ventricle, leading eventually to heart failure.

Pulmonary parenchymal disease due to fibrotic, infective or granulomatous disorders (e.g. pneumoconiosis, bronchiectasis, sarcoidosis) is not often so severe

Table 14.2 Causes of pulmonary heart disease.

Obstructive airways disease
Bronchitis
Emphysema
Asthma

Parenchymal lung disease
Sarcoidosis
Pneumoconiosis
Bronchiectasis

Neuromuscular and chest wall diseases
Poliomyelitis
Kyphoscoliosis

Impaired respiratory drive
Pickwickian syndrome

Pulmonary vascular disease
Primary pulmonary hypertension
Chronic pulmonary embolism

as to cause significant pulmonary hypertension. Obliterative pulmonary vascular disease (e.g. chronic PE), on the other hand, almost invariably leads to pulmonary hypertension and right heart failure.

In certain neuromuscular and chest-wall disorders, hypoxaemia due to inadequate pulmonary ventilation stimulates pulmonary arteriolar constriction. Increments in pulmonary vascular resistance may be sufficient to cause right heart failure. Impaired respiratory drive—sometimes seen in severe obesity (Pickwickian syndrome)—causes pulmonary heart disease by a similar mechanism.

Pathophysiology

Pulmonary heart disease is always the result of chronic (sustained or episodic) pulmonary hypertension. The increase in pulmonary vascular resistance which characterizes pulmonary hypertension is caused either by destructive or obliterative disease of the vascular bed or by pulmonary arteriolar constriction, or both.

The vascular reserve of the pulmonary circulation is considerable. Thus, a three-fold increase in cardiac output during exercise causes only a small increase in pulmonary artery pressure; even after pneumonectomy, increments in pulmonary artery pressure during exercise remain small. Therefore, pulmonary disease must be extensive before anatomical reductions in vascular reserve are sufficient to cause pulmonary hypertension. The effects of alveolar hypoxia—a potent stimulus for pulmonary arteriolar constriction—exacerbate anatomical reductions in pulmonary vascular reserve. Indeed, in patients with neuromuscular disorders or diminished respiratory drive, alveolar hypoxia is the primary mechanism.

The interaction between anatomical reductions in pulmonary vascular reserve and hypoxia is important. In patients with chronic bronchitis and emphysema, for example, pulmonary hypertension is usually episodic, coinciding with infective exacerbations of the lung disease. The exacerbations produce alveolar hypoxia which triggers pulmonary vasoconstriction unmasking the underlying reduction in pulmonary vascular reserve. Similarly, in other parenchymal lung disorders, superimposed infection is often the trigger for episodes of pulmonary hypertension and right heart failure. Only when the pulmonary vascular reserve is completely exhausted by the destructive effects of the underlying disease, do pulmonary hypertension and right heart failure become sustained. The pattern is often different, however, in obliterative pulmonary vascular disease caused by chronic PE. In this there is an unremitting increase in pulmonary artery pressure, associated with worsening right ventricular hypertrophy as the pulmonary vascular bed becomes progressively obliterated.

An additional factor in the development of pulmonary hypertension is polycythaemia which occurs in response to chronic hypoxia. The increase in red-cell mass increases blood viscosity and pulmonary resistance; nevertheless, only when the haematocrit exceeds 60% does the disadvantage of increased viscosity exceed the benefit of increased oxygen-carrying capacity.

Pulmonary heart disease exerts its major effects on the right ventricle, which hypertrophies in response to the chronic increase in afterload leading eventually to ventricular dilatation and contractile failure. Nevertheless, abnormalities of left ventricular (LV) function may also exist, although the cause is not always clear. Occult ischaemia—due to the effects of hypoxaemia and coronary artery disease—may be important in certain cases, while in other hypertrophy and bulging of the interventricular septum interfere with LV filling, particularly when RV hypertrophy and dilatation are severe.

Clinical manifestations

The typical patient is a middle-aged or elderly man with a long history of winter bronchitis caused by cigarette smoking. Clinical manifestations are those of the underlying respiratory disorder associated with pulmonary hypertension and right heart failure. Common complaints are dyspnoea, fatigue, abdominal discomfort (caused by hepatic congestion) and peripheral oedema. The patient is often centrally cyanosed—particularly during exacerbations of obstructive pulmonary disease—and may be jaundiced or clubbed. Carbon dioxide retention produces a bounding pulse (due to peripheral vasodilatation) and, in severe cases, tremor and clouding of consciousness may occur.

Signs of pulmonary hypertension are usually prominent. These include a left parasternal systolic thrust due to RV hypertrophy and a loud pulmonary component of the second heart sound, sometimes associated with the early diastolic murmur of pulmonary regurgitation. Nevertheless, hyperinflation of the lungs may make palpation of the RV impulse difficult and may also muffle the heart sounds. The development of frank RVF produces elevation of the JVP, hepatomegaly and peripheral oedema. Functional tricuspid regurgitation is almost invariable in advanced cases.

Complications

Complications of pulmonary heart disease are the same as occur in other cases of right heart failure. They include cardiac arrhythmias, particularly AF, and deep venous and intracardiac thrombosis which predispose to PE. In end-stage disease, progressive renal and hepatic failure usually occur.

Diagnosis

Polycythaemia is commonly present, but the haematocrit rarely rises above 65%. In obstructive pulmonary disease arterial gas analysis shows hypoxaemia and hypercapnia with partially compensated respiratory acidosis. Respiratory function tests confirm an obstructive defect, although in other causes of pulmonary heart disease a restrictive defect may be more prominent. The ECG shows signs suggestive of right ventricular hypertrophy, including: dominant R waves in leads V1 and V2 (see Fig. 2.12); P pulmonale; and right axis deviation, sometimes associated with right bundle branch block (Fig. 14.6). The CXR shows an

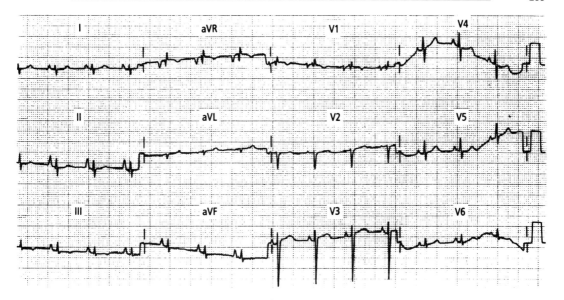

Fig. 14.6 Pulmonary heart disease—12-lead ECG. Note P pulmonale, right axis deviation and the dominant R wave in lead V1 associated with T-wave inversion. The ECG is in all respects similar to that of chronic pulmonary embolism (see Fig. 14.4) and other causes of pulmonary hypertension.

enlarged heart and, on the lateral film, obliteration of the retrosternal space indicates dilatation of the right ventricle. The proximal pulmonary arteries are prominent and, in advanced pulmonary hypertension, attenuation ('pruning') of the peripheral vessels may be present. The echocardiogram confirms dilatation of the right-sided cardiac chambers.

Differential diagnosis

Pulmonary heart disease must be differentiated from other causes of right heart failure including LVF, mitral valve disease, cardiomyopathy, pulmonary and tricuspid valve disease and constrictive pericarditis. In these conditions, however, signs of pulmonary hypertension, if present, are rarely as marked as those that characterize pulmonary heart disease. Indeed, only in mitral stenosis is the severity of pulmonary hypertension sometimes comparable. The echocardiogram, however, is diagnostic of mitral stenosis; it also identifies right-sided valvular disease and LV impairment in patients with congestive heart failure and cardio-myopathy.

Treatment

Treatment is directed towards the underlying pulmonary disease as well as RVF.

Pulmonary disease

In patients with pulmonary heart disease caused by chronic bronchitis and emphysema, presentation is usually with an acute exacerbation which precipitates RVF. Treatment with antibiotics, bronchodilators, inhaled oxygen and physiotherapy is directed at resolving the exacerbation and lowering pulmonary artery pressure in order to correct RVF. Prophylaxis is by prompt antibiotic therapy at the first sign of a chest infection and encouragement to stop cigarette smoking.

Measures directed at controlling progressive disease in other causes of pulmonary hypertension include: antibiotics and physiotherapy in bronchiectasis; steroid therapy in asthma and advanced pulmonary sarcoidosis; anticoagulant therapy in chronic PE; and weight reduction in severe obesity.

Right ventricular failure

Diuretic therapy is usually effective for controlling peripheral oedema and visceral congestion. Moreover, by reducing RV volume, diuretics may correct functional tricuspid regurgitation and increase cardiac output. Generally speaking, however, significant improvements in RV function can be achieved only by inotropic stimulation or reductions in afterload. Inotropic therapy (e.g. intravenous dobutamine) is certainly of value in acute exacerbations of RVF associated with severe low-output states. In chronic RVF, however, there are no orally active inotropic agents of value for long-term outpatient management, although digoxin plays an important role in patients with AF.

Afterload reduction in pulmonary heart disease requires effective pulmonary arteriolar dilatation. Drugs such as hydralazine and calcium antagonists reduce pulmonary vascular resistance and improve cardiac output acutely. In some patients, significant symptomatic improvement occurs but, in the majority, sustained benefit during long-term therapy is difficult to demonstrate. Continuous oxygen therapy is of greater value for afterload reduction in pulmonary heart disease. For domiciliary management, oxygen is conveniently delivered by nasal catheters at a flow rate of 2 l/minute. If an arterial oxygen tension of at least 8 kPa (60 mmHg) can be achieved and sustained for 15 hours/day, pulmonary vascular resistance will usually fall. The improvement is often sustained and has been associated with a significant mortality reduction in patients with advanced pulmonary heart disease.

Oxygen therapy also provides the most effective means of reducing haematocrit. The associated reduction in blood viscosity lowers pulmonary vascular resistance and improves RV function. In patients for whom continuous oxygen therapy is inappropriate (advanced age, continued cigarette smoking), polycythaemia can be treated by regular venesection, which is only necessary, however, for haematocrit values above 65% because, at this level, the effect on pulmonary vascular resistance and the risk of intravascular thrombosis become excessive.

The role of lung transplantation for correcting pulmonary hypertension in end-stage pulmonary heart disease is now receiving attention, but at present the long-term result is not satisfactory.

Prognosis

In pulmonary heart disease, prognosis is poor once RVF develops. Following the first episode of RVF in patients with chronic bronchitis, survival beyond 5 years is unusual.

FURTHER READING

Anonymous. Surgery for pulmonary emboli? *Lancet* 1989; i: 198.

Bishop A, Oldershaw P. Thromboembolism in primary pulmonary hypertension. *Br Med J* 1996; 313: 1418.

Goldhaber SZ, Meyerovitz MF, Markis JE *et al.* Thrombolytic therapy of acute pulmonary embolism: current status and future potential. *J Am Coll Cardiol* 1987;10 (suppl B): 96.

Hirsh J. The optimal duration of anticoagulant therapy for venous thrombosis. *N Engl J Med* 1995; 332: 1710.

Moser KM, Auger WR, Fedullo PF. Chronic major vessel thromboembolic pulmonary hypertension. *Circulation* 1990; 81: 1735.

Peacock A. Pulmonary hypertension due to chronic hypoxia. *Br Med J* 1990; 300: 763.

Uren NG, Oakley CM. The treatment of primary pulmonary hypertension. *Br Heart J* 1991; 66: 119.

Verstraete M. The diagnosis and treatment of deep-vein thrombosis. *N Engl J Med* 1993; 329: 1418.

Weinmann EE, Salzman EW. Deep-vein thrombosis. *N Engl J Med* 1994; 331: 1630.

CHAPTER 15

Paediatric Cardiology

CONTENTS

SUMMARY

About 8 of every 1000 liveborn infants have congenital heart defects. These range from trivial to lethal abnormalities. The major attrition is in infancy, and the emphasis in contemporary paediatric cardiology is in this age-group. Echocardiography has facilitated diagnosis of structural heart disease prenatally and in infancy and early childhood, whereas cardiac catheterization has had an increasing therapeutic role with the development of various catheter-directed interventional techniques. Most structural heart abnormalities are relatively simple abnormalities, such as ventricular septal defect. Sequential segmental analysis of cardiac structures provides the framework for the description of complex congenital heart malformations. With the decline in the incidence of acute rheumatic heart disease, Kawasaki disease has become the most common acquired heart abnormality in childhood in many developed countries. The success of infant surgery for previously lethal congenital heart defects has resulted in a new population with surgically modified congenital heart disease whose numbers will continue to grow.

INTRODUCTION

Cardiac abnormalities are more common than congenital defects of any other system. About 8 in every 1000 liveborn infants have congenital heart defects. Natural history data from the presurgical era are difficult to interpret because of uncertainties about case ascertainment. However, there is a high attrition rate among symptomatic infants, with survival after presentation in infancy of approximately 60%, 30% and 20% at 1 month, 1 year and 5 years of age, respectively (Fig. 15.1). Expressed differently, of all cardiac deaths occurring before adult life, 50% will have occurred by 1 month and 80% by 1 year of age (Fig. 15.2). As a result, clinical paediatric cardiology has had an increasing emphasis on neonatal and infant practice, and has evolved from being an adjunct of adult cardiology to becoming a speciality in its own right.

Embryology

Two endothelial tubes run in the belly of the developing embryo and fuse in the neck region to form the single heart tube. Venous inflow and arterial outflow are at the caudal and cephalic ends of the heart tube, respectively. During the fourth week of gestation, complex looping of the heart tube occurs. The four-chamber arrangement of the heart requires separation and septation of the atrial and ventricular components of the heart tube, and division of the arterial segment into aorta and pulmonary artery. This occurs during the fifth and sixth weeks of gestation and is the process most prone to aberrant development. By the end of the eighth week, the structural arrangement of the heart is complete.

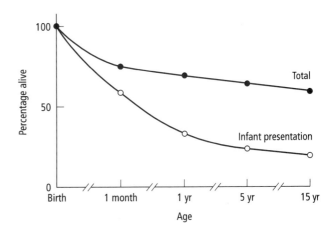

Fig. 15.1 Natural history of congenital heart disease. (After Hoffman, 1987.)

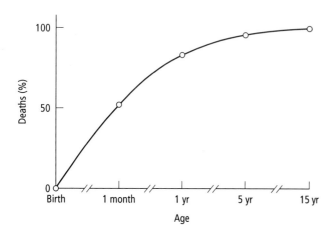

Fig. 15.2 Natural history of age at death in childhood from congenital heart disease. (After Hoffman, 1987.)

Aetiology

The aetiology of congenital heart disease is complex and cannot be identified in most individual cases at present, so that these occur sporadically and are unexpected. Demonstrable chromosome defects probably account for about 10% of cases of heart abnormalities in liveborn infants, and a greater proportion of fetuses with heart malformations who die *in utero*. About 40% of infants born with Down's syndrome (trisomy 21) have heart defects, most often atrioventricular septal defect. Heart defects are even more common in trisomy 18 (Edwards' syndrome) and trisomy 13 (Patau's syndrome), but most liveborns with these conditions die in early infancy because of multiple malformations. Turner's syndrome, characterized by the presence of a single sex chromosome (45X), has associated coarctation of the aorta and/or aortic valve stenosis in about 10% of affected individuals. There has been increasing detection of small chromosome deletions and duplications. The best example relevant to congenital heart disease is chromosome 22q11 deletion which is associated with conotruncal abnormalities such as tetralogy of Fallot or interrupted aortic arch. However, several families with recurrent conotruncal abnormalities do not have this deletion. This suggests that increasingly sophisticated diagnostic techniques will almost certainly disclose other subtle chromosome abnormalities in future.

Single-gene defects account for a few cases of congenital heart disease. Many of these have associated recognizable patterns of malformation and are termed syndromes. Examples involving the heart include autosomal dominant inheritance in Marfan's syndrome, where cystic medial necrosis of the aortic wall may lead to dilatation of the aorta and aortic regurgitation; and Noonan's syndrome which is associated with pulmonary valve stenosis and hypertrophic cardiomyopathy. Isolated hypertrophic cardiomyopathy has autosomal dominant inheritance in some families: a number of specific gene abnormalities have been identified in different families. Some complex forms of congenital heart disease are more common in communities where consanguinity occurs, suggesting that an autosomal recessive pattern of inheritance may be important.

Specific teratogenetic factors may also contribute to abnormal cardiac development. Intrauterine rubella infection, high maternal alcohol intake, poorly controlled maternal diabetes and maternal anticonvulsant or lithium therapy have all been associated with an increased incidence of congenital heart disease. The presence of maternal anti-Ro antibodies is associated with fetal heart block, which is the result of immune-mediated damage to the developing cardiac conduction tissue whether there is symptomatic maternal connective tissue disease or not. In many of the cases of teratogenetic influence, there may be additional polygenic predisposition in the fetus.

Terminology

The nomenclature used to describe congenital heart defects can be confusing. Most patients with congenital heart disease have relatively simple lesions. However, the description of complex heart defects is facilitated by the use of sequential segmental analysis: this requires description of the atrial, ventricular and arterial segments of the heart, and the connections between them.

The structure of the atrial appendage is the most reliable feature allowing the morphological right atrium to be distinguished from the morphological left atrium. In the morphological right atrium, the appendage is a triangular structure with a broad base and a blunt apex, whereas the morphological left atrium has a narrow tubular appendage. Most hearts have usual atrial arrangement (situs solitus) in which the morphological right atrium is to the right and the morphological left atrium to the left; in mirror-image atrial arrangement (situs inversus), the other thoracoabdominal organs usually share the mirror image arrangement. When both atrial appendages are of the same morphology, atrial isomerism exists. There is usually coexisting isomerism of the bronchi, but variability in abdominal organ anatomy (Fig. 15.3).

The ventricular mass almost always contains two ventricles. Coarse apical trabeculations and tricuspid valve cords attaching to the septal surface characterize the morphological right ventricle, whereas the morphological left ventricle has fine apical trabeculations. The atrioventricular connection may be biventricular or univentricular. In biventricular atrioventricular connections, each atrium is connected to a separate ventricle: this connection is usually concordant, with morphological right atrium connected to morphological right ventricle, and morphological left atrium connected to morphological left ventricle; but is discordant when morphological right atrium is connected to morphological left ventricle, and morphological left atrium is connected to morphological right ventricle. When there is atrial isomerism, biventricular atrioventricular connections are ambiguous (Fig. 15.4). A univentricular atrioventricular connection exists when a ventricle has a double inlet (Fig. 15.5) or when either the right- or left-sided atrioventricular connection is absent (Fig. 15.6). A dominant morphological left ventricle with a rudimentary right ventricle is usual when there is a univentricular atrioventricular connection but other arrangements occur. In double-inlet atrioventricular connection

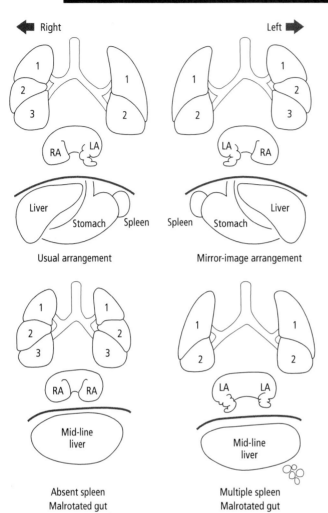

Right ◀   Left ▶

Usual arrangement   Mirror-image arrangement

Absent spleen   Multiple spleen
Malrotated gut   Malrotated gut
Right isomerism   Left isomerism

Fig. 15.3 The possible variations in atrial arrangement with associated bronchial and abdominal organ anatomy. Adapted with permission from original figure by Professor R H Anderson.

there may be two atrioventricular valves or a single common valve (Fig. 15.7).

The arteries at the ventriculoarterial junction are identified by their branching patterns. When two arterial trunks are present, the ventriculoarterial connection is usually concordant, with aorta arising from left ventricle and pulmonary artery from right ventricle, but may be discordant where aorta arises from morphological right ventricle and pulmonary artery arises from morphological left ventricle (Figs 15.5 and 15.8), or double outlet where both great arteries arise from one ventricle, almost always the morphological right ventricle. When an artery overrides the trabecular part of the ventricular septum in the presence of a ventricular septal defect, it is assigned to whichever ventricle it overrides by more than 50% (Fig. 15.9). When only a single artery is connected to the ventricular mass, it may be a common trunk giving rise to coronary, pulmonary and systemic arteries, or a solitary trunk in the absence of central intrapericardial pulmonary arteries (Fig. 15.10).

Concordant atrioventricular connexion

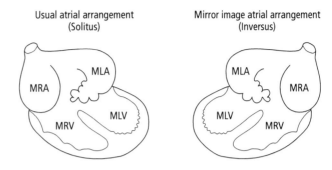

Usual atrial arrangement
(Solitus)

Mirror image atrial arrangement
(Inversus)

Discordant atrioventricular connexion

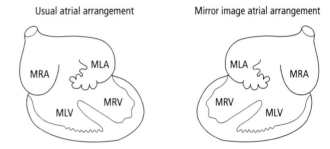

Usual atrial arrangement

Mirror image atrial arrangement

Ambiguous atrioventricular connexion

Right atrial isomerism

Left atrial isomerism

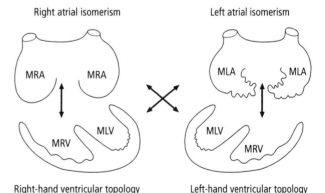

Right-hand ventricular topology

Left-hand ventricular topology

Fig. 15.4 The types of biventricular atrioventricular connection. Reproduced with permission from Anderson R H *et al. Paediatric Cardiology*. Edinburgh: Churchill Livingstone, 1987. MLA, morphological left atruim; MLV, morphological left ventricle; MRA, morphological right atruim, MRV, morphological right ventricle.

An abnormal position of the heart in the chest should be described separately. For example, 'dextrocardia' is an imprecise term which means merely that the heart is located predominantly in the right rather than the left chest. Possible explanations would include displacement of an otherwise normal heart as might be seen in left-sided diaphragmatic hernia or hypoplasia of the right lung; mirror-image atrial arrangement with normal cardiac connections but an otherwise normal heart, which is sometimes associated with airway ciliary dysfunction; or many forms of congenital heart disease of varying complexity where the abnormalities of cardiac connections and associated cardiac malformations are more important than the position of the heart.

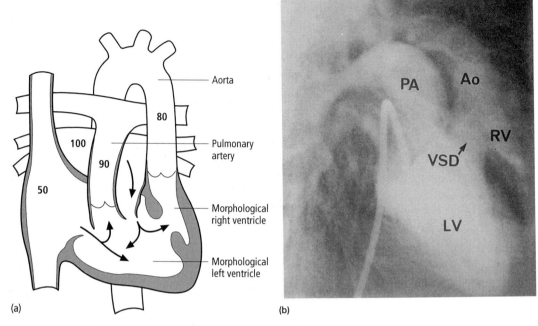

(a)   (b)

Fig. 15.5 (a) Double-inlet left ventricle with ventriculoarterial discordance. Arrows indicate direction and magnitude of flow and numbers are representative percentage oxygen saturations. (b) Left ventricular angiogram in right oblique projection demonstrating the same anatomy. VSD, ventricular septal defect.

Prenatal diagnosis

Structural heart abnormalities can be diagnosed by transabdominal fetal echocardiography from about 16–18 weeks' gestation. When a previous child has been affected, the recurrence risk for congenital heart disease is generally in the order of 2–3%. When a parent is affected, recurrence risk for congenital

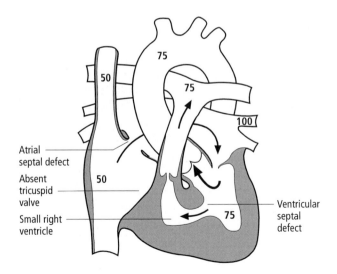

Fig. 15.6 Absent right atrioventricular connection (tricuspid atresia) with ventriculoarterial concordance. Arrows indicate direction and magnitude of flow and numbers are representative percentage oxygen saturations.

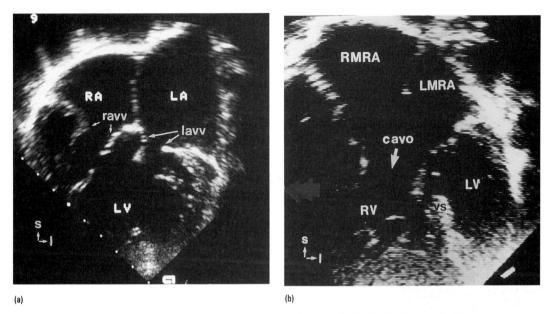

(a)   (b)

Fig. 15.7 (a) Double-inlet left ventricle with two atrioventricular valves. (b) Double-inlet right ventricle via a common atrioventricular orifice in a patient with right atrial isomerism. cavo, common atrioventricular orifice; l, left; lav, left atrioventricular valve; LMRA, left-sided morphological right atrium; ravv, right atrioventricular valve; RMRA, right-sided morphological right atrium; s, superior; vs, ventricular septum.

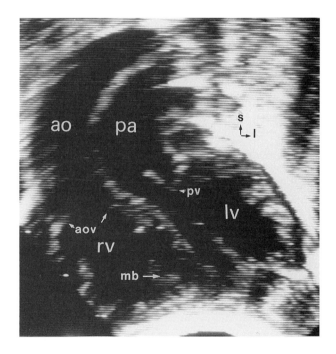

Fig. 15.8 Ventriculoarterial discordance in an infant with simple transposition of the great arteries. aov, aortic valve; mb moderator band; pv, pulmonary valve.

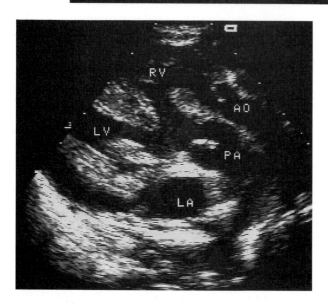

Fig. 15.9 Double-outlet right ventricle with subpulmonary ventricular septal defect. The pulmonary artery overrides the ventricular septum, but slightly more than 50% is committed to right ventricle. There is also a pericardial effusion.

heart disease may be 5–10%, although relatively few data are available. An increasing number of congenital heart defects are now detected prenatally because a heart abnormality is suspected on routine ultrasound scanning. This has led to the advocacy of mid-trimester population screening for congenital heart defects and other lesions at 18–20 weeks' gestation. A transverse section of the fetal thorax demonstrates the four-chamber view of the fetal heart (Fig. 15.11). Recognition of abnormalities from this single view of the heart would potentially allow detection of about one-third of cases of congenital heart disease currently seen in infancy, although those detected would include the most severe structural cardiac abnormalities (Fig. 15.12). Effective screening may be possible

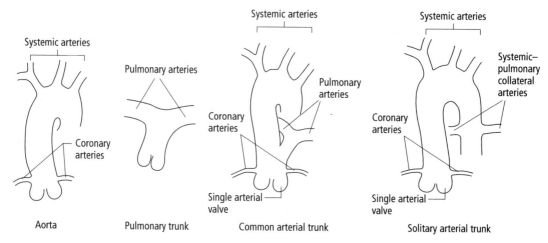

Fig. 15.10 The different types of great arteries. Reproduced with permission from Anderson R H *et al. Paediatric Cardiology*. Edinburgh: Churchill Livingstone, 1987.

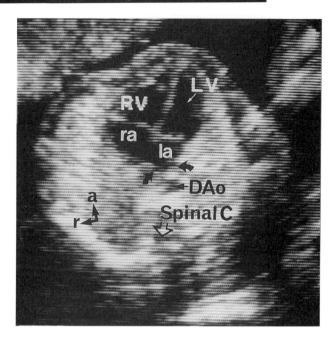

Fig. 15.11 Fetal four-chamber echocardiographic view obtained from a transverse section through the fetal thorax. DAo, descending aorta; Spinal C, spinal canal. The curved black arrows indicate pulmonary veins entering left atrium.

with intensive training of ultrasonographers, but this is difficult to achieve and sustain on a wide basis.

An increasing role for fetal echocardiography is assessment of fetal cardiac performance, which may assist in the management of complicated pregnancies. Detection and treatment of fetal supraventricular tachycardia has also been facilitated. Supraventricular tachycardia is an important reversible cause of fetal heart failure (Fig. 15.13), and can be effectively controlled in most cases by

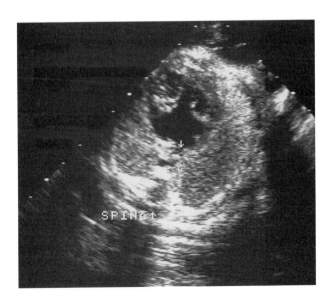

Fig. 15.12 Transverse thoracic echocardiographic section in a fetus with right atrial isomerism, common atrium, double-inlet left ventricle via a common atrioventricular valve.

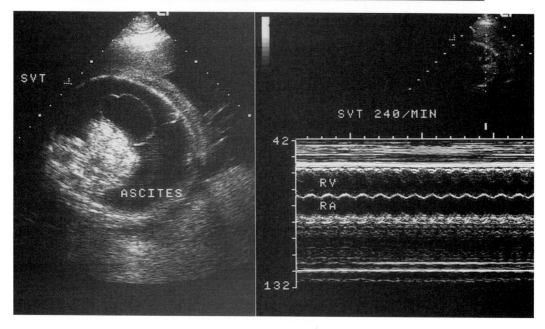

Fig. 15.13 Severe fetal hydrops (left) secondary to heart failure because of sustained atrioventricular re-entry tachycardia which is demonstrated by the M-mode recording of fetal heart rate (right). There is 1 : 1 atrioventricular relationship in tachycardia.

antiarrhythmic drug therapy delivered to the mother or, occasionally, directly to the fetus.

Circulatory changes at birth

In utero, the widely patent arterial duct means that both right ventricle and left ventricle perfuse the systemic circulation in parallel (Fig. 15.14). Gas exchange takes place at the placenta, so that the most-oxygen-saturated blood returns to the fetal inferior caval vein via the umbilical vein. The Eustachian valve in the right atrium preferentially directs this more-oxygenated blood through the oval foramen to the left side of the heart, and thence it is pumped preferentially to the developing fetal brain. Blood from the superior caval vein streams preferentially via the tricuspid valve and right ventricle to the pulmonary trunk. Most of right ventricular stroke volume flows into the low-resistance systemic circulation via the arterial duct. Fetal survival is not usually compromised by congenital heart defects so long as at least one ventricle can perfuse the systemic and placental circulation. At birth, the lungs inflate and take over the role of gas exchange. Clamping of the umbilical cord deprives the systemic circulation of the low-resistance placental circuit. Systemic resistance rises and right-to-left shunting through the oval foramen and the arterial duct falls abruptly. Pulmonary blood flow increases substantially, facilitated by the reduction in pulmonary vascular resistance that coincides with inflation of the lungs and subsequent remodelling of pulmonary arteriolar structure. The delivery of oxygen-saturated blood into

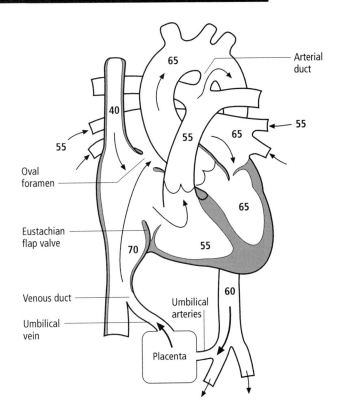

Fig. 15.14 The fetal circulation. In this and Figs 15.15–15.20 and 15.22 arrows indicate direction and magnitude of flow and numbers are representative percentage oxygen saturations.

the aorta and the effects of local prostaglandins stimulate constriction of the arterial duct. Closure of the arterial duct is usually complete within 24 hours of birth in term infants. The flap valve of the oval foramen allows functional closure of the interatrial communication.

Haemodynamic consequences of congenital heart defects

Postnatal presentation of congenital heart disease is largely dependent on the adequacy, and balance between, pulmonary and systemic blood flow. Structural heart defects can be classified on this basis. Such a physiological classification has advantages in that details of the anatomy of specific heart abnormalities are often complex, and categorization by diagnosis alone can be confusing. For example, tetralogy of Fallot may give rise to a range of pulmonary blood flow, from excessive to critically low, depending on the severity of right ventricular outflow tract obstruction.

Systemic to pulmonary shunts

This category includes the most common structural heart lesions such as ventricular septal defect, atrial septal defect and persistent arterial duct (Figs 15.15–15.17). The magnitude of the left-to-right shunt is dependent on the

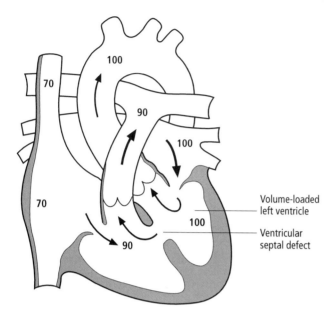

Fig. 15.15 Ventricular septal defect.

relative impedances of the systemic and pulmonary vascular beds, and the size of the intra- or extracardiac communication(s). Pulmonary blood flow will normally increase progressively during the early weeks of life as pulmonary vascular resistance falls. Infants with large left-to-right shunts will be acyanotic, tachypnoeic, typically poor feeders and prone to respiratory tract infections, and will usually fail to thrive.

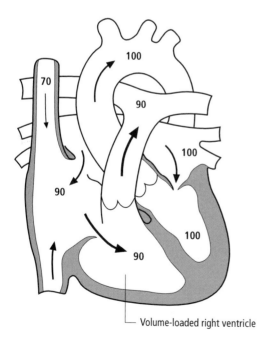

Fig. 15.16 Secundum atrial septal defect.

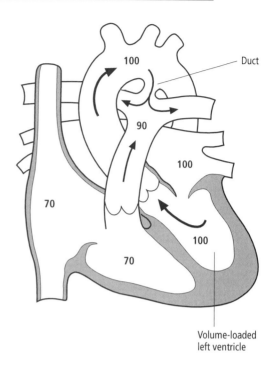

100

Duct

90

100

70

100

70

Volume-loaded
left ventricle

Fig. 15.17 Persistent arterial duct.

Excessive pulmonary blood flow, especially in association with high pulmonary artery perfusion pressure such as occurs with a large ventricular septal defect or large arterial duct, will result in medial hypertrophy of the walls of the pulmonary arterioles, and subsequently intimal proliferation may occur. This progressive alteration in the morphology of the pulmonary arteriolar vasculature increases pulmonary vascular resistance. When this exceeds systemic vascular resistance, shunt reversal will occur at the site of the intracardiac or extracardiac communication, resulting in cyanosis. This is the Eisenmenger syndrome. The rate at which pulmonary vascular obstructive disease develops varies greatly according to the structural cardiac abnormality and individual susceptibility, but may become irreversible within the first 2 years of life. Consequently, if corrective surgery is possible, this should be undertaken early, usually in infancy. In very rare individuals, there may be progression in pulmonary vascular obstructive disease despite appropriate surgical correction of the structural cardiac abnormality in infancy.

Intracardiac mixing

In many structural heart defects oxygenated pulmonary venous blood and deoxygenated systemic venous blood mix at venous, cardiac or great artery level. Patients may be cyanosed as a result. This will be most obvious when there is inadequate pulmonary blood flow or when intracardiac streaming allows relatively little mixing between the pulmonary and systemic circulations.

Inadequate pulmonary blood flow may occur when there is obstruction to

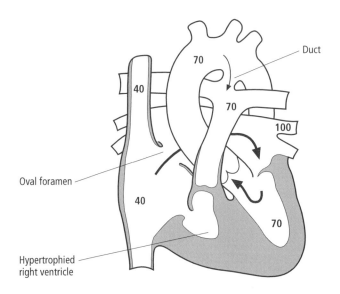

Fig. 15.18 Neonatal severe pulmonary stenosis or atresia with duct-dependent pulmonary blood flow: intact ventricular septum.

pulmonary blood flow, for example in severe pulmonary valve stenosis with right atrial-to-left atrial flow at the oval foramen (Fig. 15.18), or in tetralogy of Fallot with severe right ventricular outflow tract obstruction (Fig. 15.19) so that right ventricular stroke volume is predominantly ejected into the systemic circulation via the subaortic ventricular septal defect (Plate 15.1, opposite p. 244). In such cases, pulmonary blood flow may be dependent on continued patency of the arterial duct, which can be maintained in the short term postnatally by intravenous infusion of prostaglandin E. Neonates with these abnormalities will be cyanosed but not unduly tachypnoeic, unless hypoxia has resulted in metabolic acidosis.

Inadequate mixing between the pulmonary and systemic circulations is characteristic of simple transposition of the great arteries (Fig. 15.20), when

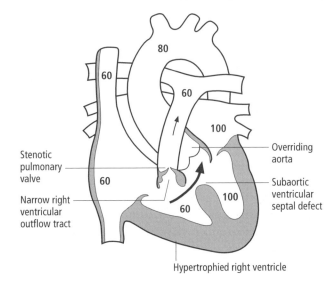

Fig. 15.19 Tetralogy of Fallot.

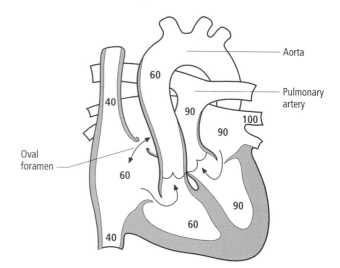

Aorta

Pulmonary artery

Oval foramen

Fig. 15.20 Simple transposition of the great arteries.

actual pulmonary blood flow may be normal or high, but the level of cyanosis profound. The effective pulmonary blood flow in this situation is that proportion of total pulmonary blood flow which reaches the systemic circulation. Balloon atrial septostomy, whereby the interatrial communication at the oval foramen is enlarged by tearing the atrial septum by pulling an inflated balloon catheter through it, is the emergency neonatal treatment to facilitate mixing of systemic and pulmonary venous blood at atrial level (Fig. 15.21). In other mixing situations, total pulmonary blood flow may be high, and there may be sufficient effective pulmonary blood flow that systemic arterial blood contains a sufficiently large proportion of oxygenated blood, so that cyanosis is not discernible clinically. Traditionally, it is said that more than 5 g/dl of deoxygenated haemoglobin in systemic arterial blood is required for central cyanosis to be clinically evident.

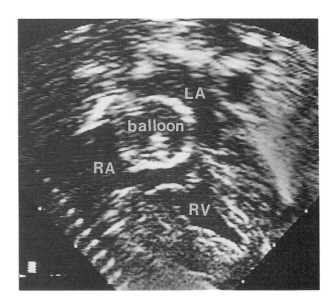

Fig. 15.21 Balloon atrial septostomy. The inflated balloon is pulled rapidly from left atrium to right atrium to enlarge the communication at the oval foramen.

Transcutaneous measurement of oxygen saturation by pulse oximetry has simplified the clinical assessment of systemic oxygen desaturation considerably, and also the differentiation of oxygen desaturation of cardiac cause, compared to the much more common pulmonary origin in neonates. By far the most common cause of cyanosis in a newborn infant is pulmonary venous oxygen desaturation. This can usually be readily corrected by providing an increased fraction of inspired oxygen. The other main pulmonary origin for neonatal cyanosis occurs when the pulmonary vascular resistance does not reduce normally in the period immediately after birth. Cyanosis will occur because of right atrial-to-left atrial flow at the oval foramen, sometimes together with flow from the pulmonary trunk into the descending aorta via the arterial duct. This is persistent pulmonary hypertension of the newborn which has some characteristics of a persisting fetal circulation. Treatment is directed to any underlying cause, such as infection, and to reduction of pulmonary vascular resistance.

Compromised systemic blood flow

Presentation of lesions such as hypoplastic left heart syndrome (Fig. 15.22), critical aortic stenosis or severe coarctation of the aorta, is characterized by inadequate systemic blood flow. Typically, these infants present on the second or third day of life, as the duct constricts, with cool peripheries, weak or absent arterial pulses (femoral pulses in the case of isolated coarctation of the aorta) and hepatomegaly. Dyspnoea and tachypnoea occur because of progressive metabolic acidosis secondary to hypoxia, but also because pulmonary venous congestion, increased pulmonary blood flow, or both, may accompany these lesions. Emergency treatment will include intravenous infusion of prostaglandin E to maintain ductal patency, as adequate systemic blood flow is likely to be dependent on continuing pulmonary artery-to-aorta flow via the duct. Inadequate systemic

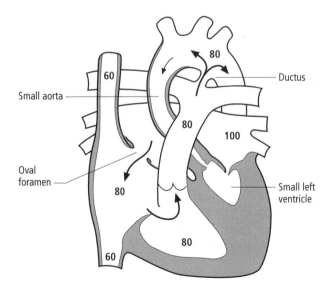

Fig. 15.22 Hypoplastic left heart syndrome.

blood flow may become manifest less acutely beyond the neonatal period because of lesions such as dilated cardiomyopathy, acute viral myocarditis, incessant tachyarrhythmia or left ventricular infarction secondary to anomalous origin of the left coronary artery from the pulmonary trunk.

INVESTIGATION

Echocardiography

Analysis of structural heart disease in infants and children is ideally suited to two-dimensional and Doppler echocardiography. Infinite imaging planes are available for displaying anatomy which is frequently complex. In comparison with cardiac structures in adults, those in infants and children are close to the body surface, which means that higher frequency ultrasound, which has poorer tissue penetration but provides better image resolution, can be used. Doppler signals of better quality can also be obtained more easily in infants and children because of the shorter distances involved. The technique is non-invasive, painless and safe; these considerations are important in all patients but especially so in neonates and infants who are haemodynamically unstable. Echocardiographic studies can be performed at a patient's bedside, serial studies are easy to conduct and the technique is affordable in comparison with other forms of imaging and haemodynamic measurement. While the standard echocardiographic planes familiar to adult cardiologists are employed, there are several important differences. The best acoustic window in children is usually subcostal, and more diagnostic information is obtained from this site than from any other. In order that a three-dimensional description of cardiac structure can be obtained from a series of two-dimensional images, the scan head is moved in sweeps from each transducer position so that the real-time image conveys information about the relationship of adjacent structures which may not be apparent from photographs of single frames. The operator must correlate the real-time images with the movement of the transducer head and scanning plane to describe the anatomy. The superimposition of spatially orientated colour-flow Doppler information on the anatomical image provides an eye-catching demonstration of abnormal flow patterns which are so common in congenital heart defects. Interrogation of the selected site of disturbed flow can be undertaken by conventional spectral Doppler analysis. This allows haemodynamic assessment of many abnormalities. The simplified Bernoulli equation (pressure difference in mmHg = $4 \times$ (peak-flow velocity in m/s)^2) allows estimation of peak instantaneous pressure gradient across a stenotic valve, or of right ventricular systolic pressure from the peak-flow velocity of a tricuspid regurgitant or ventricular septal defect jet (Plate 15.2, opposite p. 244), but is not applicable to all flow disturbances encountered in congenital cardiac malformations.

Transoesophageal echocardiography has been increasingly applied in the assessment of congenital heart disease. In particular, the availability of smaller transoesophageal echocardiography probes in recent years has facilitated the use of this technique for intraoperative and early postoperative investigation in infants and young children at a time when access for conventional echocardiography examination is impaired by surgical dressings and chest drains. The other main indication for transoesophageal echocardiography is assessment of congenital heart disease in adolescent and adult patients (Plate 15.3, opposite p. 244). This will often be during late postoperative follow-up. Another indication may be simultaneous use of transoesophageal echocardiography to assist in selected interventional cardiac catheterization procedures.

The presentation format of echocardiographic images can be confusing. Early two-dimensional echocardiography machines did not include the ability to inverse the sector image, and the part of the heart closest to the transducer was always at the top of the screen. Consequently, it was necessary to present the heart in an upside-down format when imaged from a subcostal or apical position. This is not necessarily a disadvantage with conventional cardiac anatomy, but it may make the analysis of complex structural abnormalities more difficult. Electronic inversion of the sector means that views from subcostal and apical locations can be presented in an anatomical format. This undoubtedly makes echocardiography of complex congenital heart defects an easier skill to acquire. Similarly, electronic inversion of the sector image during transoesophageal echocardiography, when views are obtained from a transgastric position, or longitudinal or multiplane views are obtained from the oesophagus, means easier correlation with conventional echocardiographic images is achieved. Echocardiographic images in this chapter are orientated accordingly.

Cardiac catheterization

Diagnostic, as opposed to therapeutic, cardiac catheterization and angiography are now rarely necessary in infants and small children, provided high-quality echocardiographic images and Doppler signals are obtained in a sedated or cooperative subject. Continuing indications for diagnostic cardiac catheterization include the angiographic assessment of sources of multifocal pulmonary blood flow (Fig. 15.23), and of peripheral pulmonary vasculature, and detailed haemodynamic measurement when this is required, such as when a Fontan-type operation is being considered (see below). Instead, cardiac catheterization has now assumed a dominantly therapeutic role.

The first interventional catheter technique in congenital heart disease was balloon atrial septostomy, which was described in the 1960s. This involves enlarging the interatrial communication at the oval foramen by tearing the adjacent tissue by the rapid passage of a catheter-mounted balloon (Fig. 15.21). It was not until the 1980s that a wide range of interventional procedures in congenital heart disease were developed. This occurred in parallel with advances in technology which were stimulated mainly by applications in the management of coronary artery or peripheral vascular disease. Indications for balloon dilatation include important pulmonary valve stenosis at any age (Fig. 15.24), recurrent postoperative coarctation of the aorta (Fig. 15.25), palliation of congenital

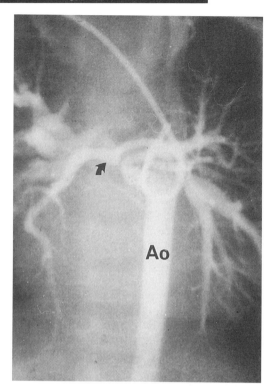

Fig. 15.23 Descending aorta angiogram in a patient who has tetralogy of Fallot with pulmonary atresia and multifocal pulmonary blood supply via collateral arteries from the descending aorta. Hypoplastic central pulmonary arteries (arrow) are opacified.

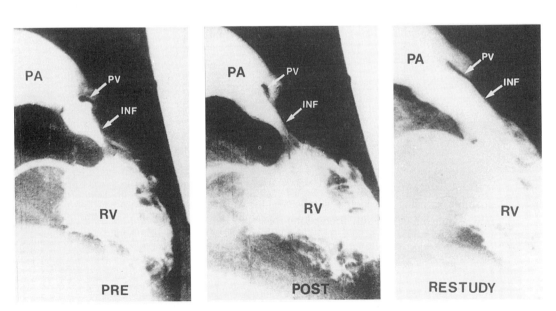

Fig. 15.24 Lateral right ventricular angiographic views. (Pre) Before balloon dilatation there is severe right ventricular hypertrophy, and doming of thickened pulmonary valve leaflets. There is additional obstruction at infundibular level. (Post) Immediately after balloon dilatation the pulmonary valve has been disrupted, although there is persisting infundibular narrowing. (Restudy) Six months later the infundibular narrowing has resolved because of regression of right ventricular hypertrophy. INF, infundibulum.

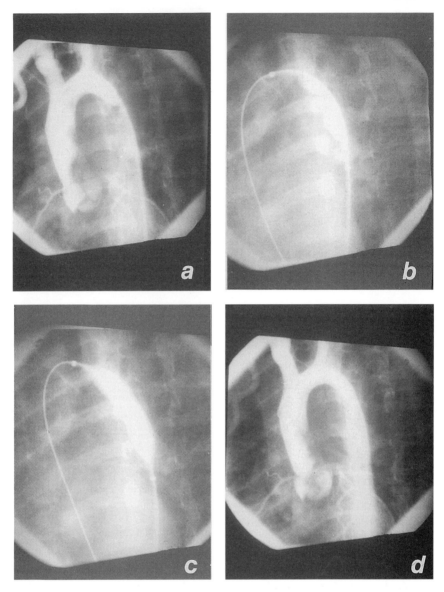

Fig. 15.25 (a) Left anterior oblique angiographic view of the aortic arch in an infant with recurrent obstruction following neonatal subclavian flap repair for coarctation of the aorta. (b) Indentation at the site of obstruction in the partly inflated balloon. (c) Full balloon inflation. (d) Following dilatation there has been good relief of obstruction.

aortic valve stenosis in childhood, and baffle stenosis following atrial repair for transposition of the great arteries. Transcatheter occlusion of a patent arterial duct is frequently undertaken, although the advantage over the surgical alternative of duct ligation, which is safe and effective, is less clear-cut. Device occlusion of a muscular ventricular septal defect is sometimes indicated if the location of the defect makes surgical access difficult. Controversial or experimental indica-

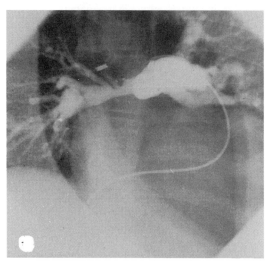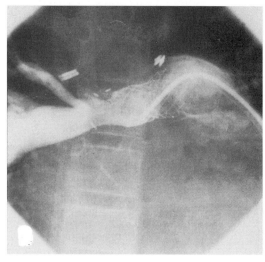

(a)   (b)

Fig. 15.26 (a) Proximal right pulmonary artery stenosis following previous surgical repair of tetralogy of Fallot with pulmonary atresia. (b) Palliation by stent enlargement (higher magnification).

tions for therapeutic cardiac catheterization include balloon dilatation of neonatal aortic valve stenosis, dilatation of unoperated coarctation of the aorta, and device occlusion of some secundum atrial septal defects. Deployment of metallic stents to enlarge pulmonary arterial stenoses or right ventricular outflow tract obstruction is usually undertaken following previous surgery (Fig. 15.26), and is a good example of the collaboration and cooperation between cardiologist and surgeon which is essential for optimal management of many forms of complex congenital heart disease.

The child with an asymptomatic murmur

Assessment of an asymptomatic heart murmur in infants and children can be difficult. A systolic murmur or a venous hum will be present in many infants and children under good examination conditions (72% of 12 000 school-age children in one study). In contrast, the incidence of significant structural heart disease is less than 1%. An innocent systolic murmur is usually a relatively soft, short, systolic ejection murmur heard at the left sternal border. The cause of innocent systolic murmurs is controversial. Postulated mechanisms include increased left ventricular outflow tract velocities into a slightly small ascending aorta, high left ventricular or right ventricular outflow tract flow velocities with normal aortic size, or vibration of intracardiac structures such as fibrous intracavity left ventricular bands (Plate 15.4, opposite p. 244). A venous hum is a soft continuous murmur heard over the base of the heart which is related to flow in the superior caval vein and its main tributaries. This can usually be abolished by changes in head posture or gentle pressure over the jugular veins at the base of the neck. Description of a heart murmur as innocent should be a clinical diagnosis. Occasionally, when there is doubt, echocardiography may be indicated. However, it should be remembered that Doppler colour-flow mapping is a very sensitive technique for detecting flow disturbance, and may demonstrate trivial abnormality such as a small muscular ventricular septal defect or tiny patent arterial duct in hearts which would previously have been considered completely normal. The flow disturbance detected may not necessarily be the source of the murmur.

SPECIFIC MALFORMATIONS

The more common congenital heart abnormalities are described below in the order of frequency in which they occur in liveborn infants. It must be remembered that the abnormalities described may coexist: for example, coarctation of the aorta often has an associated ventricular septal defect.

Ventricular septal defect

In the normal heart, the right ventricle wraps around the anterior aspect of the left ventricle, so that the ventricular septum is a complicated curved structure. As might be expected, ventricular septal morphology varies considerably with different structural abnormalities. In atrioventricular discordance, for example, the ventricles are usually side by side so that the ventricular septum has a more or less sagittal orientation. The normal ventricular septum has a small membranous and a much larger muscular portion. The membranous septum is continuous with the central fibrous body which is the area of fibrous continuity between the tricuspid, aortic and mitral valves. The septal leaflet of the tricuspid valve attaches to the membranous septum, dividing it into atrioventricular and ventricular components above and below this line of attachment, respectively (Fig. 15.27). The importance of the membranous septum is that the majority of ventricular septal defects abut this area so that part of their margin is composed of fibrous tissue (Fig. 15.28). Recognition that such a defect is perimembranous allows identification of the region of the penetrating bundle of cardiac conducting tissue in the posteroinferior margin of the defect which must not be damaged during surgical closure of the hole if heart block is to be avoided. A minority of ventricular septal defects have entirely muscular margins (Fig. 15.29), or are roofed by the aortic and pulmonary valves which are in fibrous continuity and are then termed doubly committed subarterial (Fig. 15.30). This latter abnormality is much more common in Oriental populations than in Caucasians.

Most small perimembranous and trabecular ventricular septal defects become spontaneously smaller and often close. Large defects result in a large left-to-right shunt and pulmonary hypertension (Fig. 15.15). Infants with large defects are tachypnoeic, prone to respiratory infection and have poor weight gain. The precordial impulse is overactive. The systolic murmur of flow through a ventri-

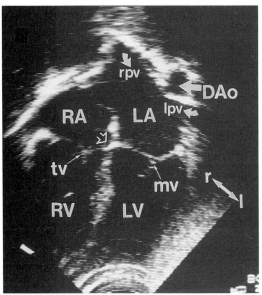
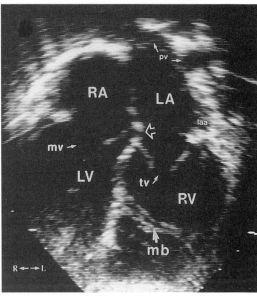

(a)   (b)

Fig. 15.27 Apical four-chamber echocardiographic views (a) in a normal heart and (b) in atrioventricular discordance. The atrioventricular septum is indicated by the open arrows. laa, left atrial appendage; lpv, left pulmonary vein; mb, moderator band; mv, mitral valve; rpv, right pulmonary vein; tv, tricuspid valve.

cular septal defect flow is dependent on the degree of restriction between left ventricle and right ventricle: generally, the more restrictive the defect the louder the systolic murmur. An apical diastolic murmur because of increased left ventricular inflow velocity is usually present if pulmonary to systemic flow ratio is more than about 2 : 1. The chest X-ray shows cardiomegaly with pulmonary plethora, and the ECG will demonstrate biventricular hypertrophy. Surgical closure of a high-flow ventricular septal defect in infancy is often indicated, unless the morphology of the defect suggests that there is a good chance of spontaneous reduction in size. Indications for later surgical closure include persisting high pulmonary blood flow, complications such as aortic valve prolapse (Fig. 15.30), or the development of left ventricular or right ventricular outflow tract obstruction which may be predicted to develop in ventricular septal defects of particular morphology (Fig. 15.31). Surgical mortality for closure of an isolated ventricular septal defect should be extremely low, in the order of 1%, and a successful operation is essentially curative, although it is usually advised that antibiotic prophylaxis against infective endocarditis at times of predictable bacteraemia should continue indefinitely.

Persistent arterial duct

Failure of the arterial duct to close completely after birth results in a systemic-to-

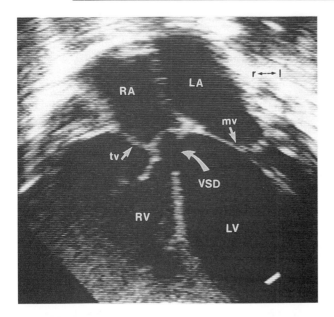

Fig. 15.28 Large perimembraneous ventricular septal defect (VSD). Note the enlargement of the left ventricle.

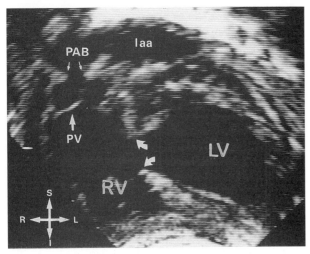

Fig. 15.29 Subcostal echocardiographic view demonstrating large muscular ventricular septal defect (curved arrows). Palliative banding of the pulmonary trunk has been performed. Iaa, Left atrial appendage; PAB, pulmonary artery band; PV, pulmonary valve.

pulmonary shunt once pulmonary vascular resistance has diminished (Fig. 15.17). Failure of ductal closure occurs most often in infants born prematurely, who may require surgical clipping or ligation of the duct because of dependence on mechanical ventilation in the neonatal period. In older infants and children, a patent arterial duct may cause relatively few symptoms unless the left-to-right shunt is large. Clinical features when there is at least a moderate-sized shunt include wide pulse pressure because of the diastolic run-off of systemic blood through the duct, and a continuous murmur over the base of the heart. Chest X-ray will show cardiomegaly with pulmonary plethora, and the ECG will demonstrate dominant left ventricular voltages. There is no question that inter-

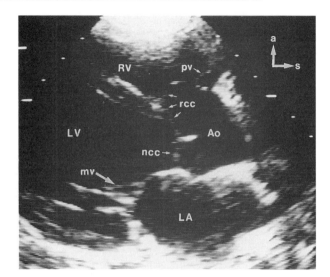

Fig. 15.30 Parasternal long axis view in a patient with a doubly committed subarterial ventricular septal defect into which the right coronary cusp of the aortic valve has prolapsed. The ventricular septal defect is roofed by the aortic and pulmonary valves which are in fibrous continuity. ncc, non-coronary cusp; rcc, right coronary cusp.

vention is indicated for a duct with more than a modest left-to-right shunt (Fig. 15.32). Transcatheter occlusion with stainless steel coils or other devices is usually the preferred approach (Plate 15.5, opposite p. 244) although large ducts may still require surgical ligation. Occlusion of even a very small arterial duct with a negligible left-to-right shunt is widely advocated as a form of prophylaxis against endarteritis, but there is little contemporary evidence to support this approach.

Atrial septal defect

A secundum atrial septal defect is a hole at the oval foramen which occurs when the flap valve fails to close the interatrial communication after birth, and is by far

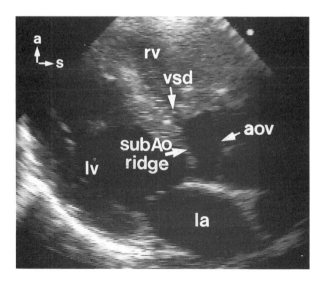

Fig. 15.31 Fixed subaortic stenosis which has developed in a patient with a ventricular septal defect (vsd) where there is malalignment between the trabecular and outlet portions of the ventricular septum.

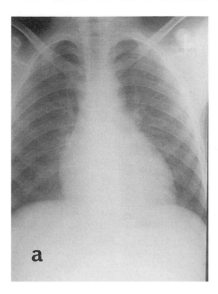
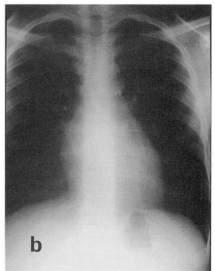

Fig. 15.32 (a) Chest X-ray showing cardiomegaly and pulmonary plethora in a boy with a patent arterial duct. (b) Reduction in heart size after transcatheter double umbrella device occlusion of the duct.

the most common form of atrial septal defect (Plate 15.6, opposite p. 244). The so-called primum atrial septal defect is actually an abnormality of development of the atrioventricular septum and is a form of atrioventricular septal defect, which is considered separately below. An isolated secundum atrial septal defect rarely causes overt symptoms in infancy, although high pulmonary blood flow may result in susceptibility to respiratory infection and reduced effort tolerance in early childhood (Fig. 15.16). Physical findings include an ejection systolic murmur best heard at the left sternal border and fixed splitting of the second heart sound. The systolic murmur arises from the right ventricular outflow tract, because of increased right ventricular stroke volume, and there may sometimes also be an audible mid-diastolic murmur because of increased velocity of right ventricular filling. Pulmonary valve closure is slightly delayed compared to aortic valve closure, even in expiration, because of the left-to-right shunt at atrial level and the increase in right ventricular stroke volume, and accounts for the fixed splitting of the second heart sound. Chest X-ray shows variable degrees of cardiac enlargement, with prominence of the pulmonary trunk, and pulmonary plethora. The ECG shows right axis deviation and incomplete right bundle branch block. Natural history data indicate a risk of supraventricular arrhythmias in young adult life with the potential for later right heart failure, so that secundum atrial septal defects with significant left-to-right shunts are usually closed in pre-school life even in minimally symptomatic children. Surgical mortality should be virtually zero. The symptomatic improvement which occurs following surgery is often striking, and unexpected by parents who may have considered their child to be asymptomatic preoperatively.

A much less common form of interatrial communication is the so-called sinus venosus atrial septal defect. In this situation, the superior caval vein overrides the

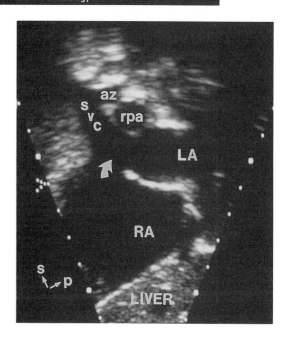

Fig. 15.33 Parasagittal subcostal echo view demonstrating a sinus venosus 'atrial septal defect' (curved arrow). az, azygous vein; rpa, right pulmonary artery; svc, superior vena cava.

atrial septum (Fig. 15.33) and the interatrial communication is actually beyond the confines of the true interatrial septum. One or more right pulmonary veins drain to the superior caval vein or right atrium in this situation. The main clinical importance of this abnormality is that it may easily be overlooked on echocardiography unless specifically sought. Surgical correction in childhood is usually indicated.

Pulmonary valve stenosis

Severe pulmonary valve stenosis presents with cyanosis in the newborn period because of right atrial-to-left atrial flow, and pulmonary blood flow may be dependent on continued patency of the arterial duct, which can be maintained in the short term by intravenous infusion of prostaglandin E (Fig. 15.18). Less severe pulmonary valve stenosis generally presents with an asymptomatic ejection systolic murmur at the left sternal border, which is preceded by an ejection click, and may be accompanied by a systolic thrill. In children, the chest X-ray may demonstrate prominence of the pulmonary trunk because of post-stenotic dilatation. The ECG demonstrates right ventricular hypertrophy. The severity of right ventricular outflow tract obstruction may increase quite rapidly during infancy, but the natural history of the condition is that mild pulmonary valve stenosis (systolic pressure gradient < 40 mmHg) seems not to increase in severity beyond the age of 5 years. Percutaneous balloon dilatation of the pulmonary valve is the treatment of choice (Fig. 15.24). Intervention in the newborn period is required for critical pulmonary valve stenosis. Infants and children with pulmonary stenosis of moderate severity will be asymptomatic, but balloon dilatation is advised when the Doppler-estimated right ventricle–pulmonary artery systolic pressure drop exceeds 40–50 mmHg.

At the most severe end of the spectrum of this abnormality, pulmonary valve stenosis may have progressed in utero to complete obstruction of the right ventricular outflow tract. Retrograde flow via the arterial duct to the pulmonary arteries in fetal life can be observed. Pulmonary blood flow following birth remains dependent on continued patency of the arterial duct (Fig. 15.18). This condition is called pulmonary atresia and intact ventricular septum, and preferred initial management is decompression of the right ventricle, usually together with placement of a systemic-to-pulmonary artery shunt. The long-term prognosis depends most on how much useful function can be recruited from the severely hypertrophied and small-cavity right ventricle.

Abnormalities of left heart development

Abnormalities of left heart development range in severity from a functionally normal but anatomically bicuspid aortic valve, which may occur in close to 1% of the 'normal' population, to a combination of left heart obstructive lesions in series, which in its most severe form is hypoplastic left heart syndrome (Fig. 15.22). As this group of abnormalities are related, they will be considered together.

Coarctation

Coarctation of the aorta is the most common form of aortic arch obstruction, and

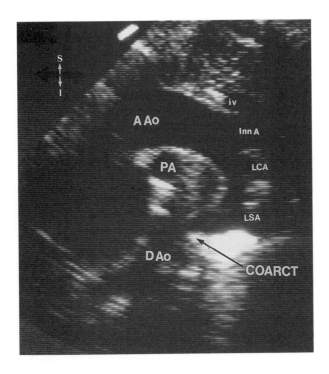

Fig. 15.34 Coarctation of the aorta. Inn A, innominate artery; iv, innominate vein; LCA, left carotid artery; LSA, left subclavian artery.

usually presents in the newborn period. There is localized narrowing of the aorta beyond the origin of the left subclavian artery (Fig. 15.34), immediately proximal to the site of ductal entry to the descending aorta. This may be an isolated abnormality, but often there is associated hypoplasia of the aortic arch, and intracardiac abnormalities of varying complexity (Fig. 15.35). In severe coarctation, lower body perfusion is dependent on flow to the descending aorta via the arterial duct, so that prostaglandin E infusion to maintain ductal patency is first-line treatment, just as it is when there is duct-dependent pulmonary blood flow. Urgent surgical repair of the arch obstruction is required. Less commonly, milder forms of coarctation of the aorta are detected in later infancy or childhood because of the detection of diminished or absent femoral pulses, often with associated upper limb hypertension. Percutaneous balloon dilatation has been advocated as primary treatment, but the consensus view is that surgical repair is preferred for native coarctation. Conversely, balloon dilatation provides effective management for recurrent or persistent postoperative coarctation (Fig. 15.25). Interruption of the aortic arch occurs when a portion of the aorta, most commonly the segment between the origins of the left common carotid artery and left subclavian artery, is missing. An associated ventricular septal defect is almost invariable. Urgent neonatal surgical repair is required.

Aortic stenosis

Similarly, severely compromised systemic blood flow which is dependent on flow via the arterial duct may occur in severe aortic valve stenosis. In neonatal critical

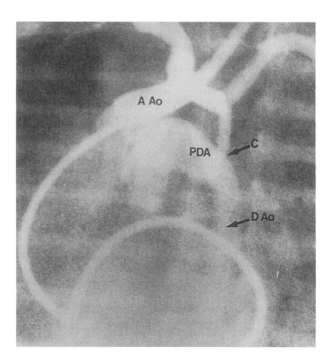

Fig. 15.35 Neonatal coarctation of the aorta with hypoplasia of the aortic arch and double outlet right ventricle. c, coarctation.

aortic valve stenosis, the valve is typically thick and dysplastic, and often unicommissural. Either surgical aortic valvotomy on cardiopulmonary bypass or percutaneous balloon dilatation of the aortic valve may be acceptable initial management: early survival depends most on the adequacy of left ventricular cavity size and myocardial performance. Less severe aortic valve stenosis is usually detected because of an asymptomatic ejection systolic murmur, preceded by an ejection click which is often best heard at the lower left sternal border, and accompanied by a suprasternal thrill. In contrast to adult practice, arterial pulse volume and ECG features of left ventricular hypertrophy are often not very helpful in the clinical assessment of the severity of aortic valve stenosis in children. Congenitally stenotic aortic valves presenting in childhood are usually bicuspid, with a raphe representing the rudimentary undeveloped commissure, and variable degrees of fusion of the other two commissures. Percutaneous balloon dilatation of the aortic valve with the aim of splitting the fused commissures is the preferred technique for initial intervention in childhood. A usually accepted indication for intervention in childhood aortic stenosis is a Doppler-derived peak instantaneous pressure gradient > 70 mmHg, but each case requires individual assessment. Further intervention will be needed in due course in most patients. It is likely that aortic valve replacement will be required ultimately.

Subaortic stenosis

Fixed subaortic stenosis occurs when fibromuscular tissue develops in the left ventricular outflow tract and obstructs flow. Subaortic stenosis is rarely seen in infancy, but typically develops and becomes more severely obstructive as childhood progresses (Fig. 15.31). Like aortic valve stenosis in childhood, presentation is usually because of an asymptomatic ejection systolic murmur with a suprasternal thrill, but without an ejection click. Echocardiographic studies have suggested that subaortic stenosis may be caused by localized tissue proliferation in response to flow disturbance in the left ventricular outflow tract. The progressive development of increasingly severe left ventricular outflow tract obstruction and aortic valve regurgitation are the main concerns. Fixed lesions causing important obstruction require surgical resection; the management of mild to moderate obstruction is controversial, but requires as a minimum careful serial echocardiographic assessment to detect progression.

Left ventricular inflow obstruction

Congenital mitral valve stenosis is rare, but is almost always the result of chordal and papillary muscle malformations, and associated with other cardiac abnormalities. Surgical revision of the mitral valve in this situation is difficult. Supravalvular mitral stenosis occurs when a closely adherent 'membrane' develops on the left atrial aspect of the mitral valve. It is crucial to recognize this abnormality, as it is possible to peel the membrane away from the underlying valve during surgery. There are often coexisting abnormalities of the mitral valve

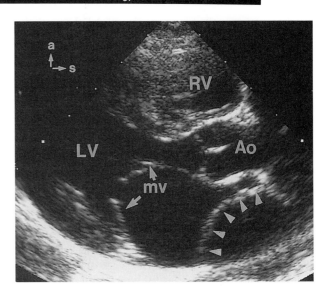

Fig. 15.36 Cor triatriatum. A fibrous shelf (arrowheads) divides the left atrium, causing obstruction to pulmonary venous return.

attachments, and other cardiac malformations, however. Cor triatriatum describes a fibrous shelf which divides the left atrium and may cause severe obstruction to left ventricular filling (Fig. 15.36). It is rare, but recognition is important because it is a potentially lethal malformation which is readily amenable to corrective surgery.

Hypoplastic left heart

Hypoplastic left heart syndrome exists when the left heart structures are insufficiently developed to support the systemic circulation (Fig. 15.22), even after relief of specific obstructive lesions such as aortic valve stenosis or coarctation of the aorta. The left ventricular cavity is usually small by 18–20 weeks' gestation, and this leads to prenatal diagnosis in many cases. Systemic blood flow is duct dependent postnatally. Therapeutic options are difficult: staged surgical palliation with a view to establishing a Fontan type of circulation (see below) is available, but surgical morbidity and mortality over at least three operations remain high, with an uncertain long-term outlook. Neonatal heart transplantation is a theoretical option which has been confounded by a shortfall of donor organs.

Tetralogy of Fallot

The essential abnormality in tetralogy of Fallot is anterior and cephalad deviation of the outlet portion of the ventricular septum. This results in a malalignment ventricular septal defect in which the aorta overrides the trabecular portion of the septum, and right ventricular outflow tract obstruction at subpulmonary level (Fig. 15.19, Plate 15.1). The right ventricular outflow tract obstruction is of variable severity at birth but tends to progress. When this is mild, there is a pure left-to-right shunt in early life so that patients are not cyanosed and may even have features of high pulmonary blood flow. Conversely, if right ventricular outflow tract obstruction is severe at birth, pulmonary blood flow may be duct dependent and urgent surgery is required. In most infants, a variable degree of cyanosis and an ejection systolic murmur at the left sternal border is usual. Hypercyanotic spells occur if there is transient critical reduction in pulmonary blood flow. Onset is usually in infancy; episodes often occur after feeding, with irritability and increased cyanosis followed by fairly abrupt quietening and sleeping with pallor and hypotonia. Flexing the infant's knees against the chest increases systemic vascular resistance and is a useful first-aid manoeuvre. This is analogous to the squatting posture which children with unoperated tetralogy of Fallot often adopt in order to maximize pulmonary blood flow. Chest X-ray shows a boot-shaped heart because right ventricular hypertrophy causes tilting up of the cardiac apex, and pulmonary artery hypoplasia results in a concave aspect to the cardiac silhouette in the region of the right ventricular outflow tract (Fig. 15.37). The ECG will confirm right ventricular hypertrophy. A palliative systemic-to-pulmonary shunt operation may be appropriate in a neonate with low pulmonary blood flow. Beyond the neonatal period, primary intracardiac repair is usually performed towards the end of infancy, unless symptoms indicate earlier intervention.

If right ventricular outflow tract obstruction is sufficiently severe to cause complete obstruction to right ventricular outflow, tetralogy of Fallot with pulmonary atresia exists. If there are reasonably sized central pulmonary arteries, pulmonary blood flow will be duct dependent (Plate 15.7, opposite p. 244). In more severe forms, the central pulmonary arteries may be extremely hypoplastic or even absent. In this situation, pulmonary blood supply is via collateral arteries

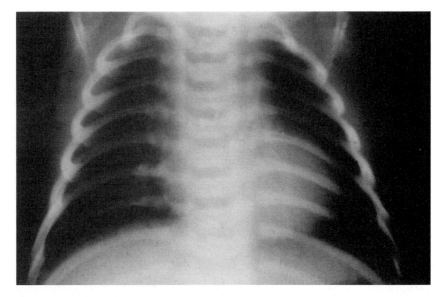

Fig. 15.37 Chest X-ray in an infant with tetralogy of Fallot.

which usually arise from the descending aorta (Fig. 15.23). Complex surgical reconstruction of pulmonary arterial blood supply can be undertaken in these patients, but it can be difficult to decide optimal management.

Atrioventricular septal defect

The atrioventricular septum may be thought of as the region where the atrial septum and ventricular septum 'overlap', and it effectively separates the left ventricle from the right atrium in the normal heart (Fig. 15.27). An atrioventricular septal defect, which is the same as an 'atrioventricular canal', occurs when there is failure of normal development of the atrioventricular septum. There is interatrial communication which can be below the true atrial septum, although the atrial septum is almost always deficient as well, atrioventricular valve morphology is altered and there is frequently an interventricular communication immediately below the atrioventricular valve leaflets (Plate 15.8, opposite p. 244). When the atrioventricular valve tissue is firmly tethered to the ventricular septum, there is no ventricular component to the defect and the isolated atrial communication is sometimes referred to as an ostium primum atrial septal defect (Fig. 15.38). The ECG has a characteristic superior frontal plane axis in atrioventricular septal defect.

Approximately 50% of infants with atrioventricular septal defect have Down's syndrome. Presentation depends on the details of cardiac morphology. If there is a large ventricular communication and regurgitant common atrioventricular valve (Plate 15.8), heart failure will occur in early infancy. Surgical repair of atrioventricular septal defects with a ventricular communication is indicated within the first 6 months of life.

When the left-to-right shunt is confined to atrial level (Fig. 15.38), presenta-

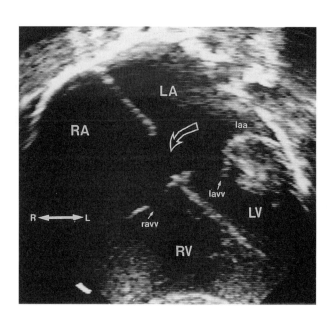

Fig. 15.38 Atrioventricular septal defect in which the atrioventricular valve is partitioned, and firmly tethered to the ventricular septum, so that left-to-right shunting is confined to atrial level (curved arrow). This is an ostium primum atrial septal defect.

tion is similar to a secundum atrial septal defect. Down's syndrome is much less common in this situation. The ECG should allow clinical differentiation from other forms of left-to-right shunting at atrial level. Surgical repair will normally be required, but there is less urgency.

Transposition of the great arteries

Simple transposition of the great arteries (ventriculoarterial discordance) is the most common cause of cyanotic congenital heart disease in newborns (Figs 15.8 and 15.20). Cyanosis in a newborn infant who otherwise has no abnormal physical findings, with normal ECG and chest X-ray, is the usual presentation, but severe hypoxia resulting in acidaemia may develop rapidly if there is inadequate mixing of blood between the systemic and pulmonary circulations. The main sites of communication between these circulations are the arterial duct and the oval foramen, although mixing can also occur at ventricular level if a ventricular septal defect is present. Emergency treatment consists of prostaglandin E infusion to maintain ductal patency prior to enlargement of the interatrial communication by balloon atrial septostomy (Fig. 15.21). For 20 years, until the mid-1980s, surgical treatment consisted of physiological repair at atrial level, so that systemic venous blood was channelled to the left ventricle, and pulmonary venous blood redirected to the right ventricle (Mustard or Senning operation). This operation has worked in the medium term, but there are inherent abnormalities of intracardiac venous flow and the systemic ventricle is a morphological right ventricle which is not ideally designed for this role. Consequently, concern about suboptimal long-term results with atrial level repair has led to the adoption of arterial switch repair (Fig. 15.39). This is nearly always performed in the neonatal period. Relocation of the coronary arteries is required as part of an arterial switch procedure, and it is the variation in coronary artery anatomy which is the main risk factor for surgical mortality. However, mortality after an arterial switch operation for simple transposition of the great arteries or transposition with ventricular septal defect is now less than 5% in leading centres, and medium-term follow-up results are excellent. Concern remains, however, about the long-term impact on coronary perfusion of neonatal coronary artery relocation.

Double-outlet right ventricle

Double-outlet right ventricle describes a heterogeneous group of hearts in which both aorta and pulmonary trunk arise entirely or predominantly from the morphological right ventricle. It is not a particularly helpful category in the sense that presentation and management will be determined by the details of cardiac morphology in any individual case. The relationship of the great arteries to each other and to the ventricular septal defect, and the nature of any outflow obstruction present, are especially important. For example, a heart with tetralogy of Fallot in which more than 50% of the aorta arises from the right ventricle (Fig. 15.40), and a heart with transposition of the great arteries with a subpulmo-

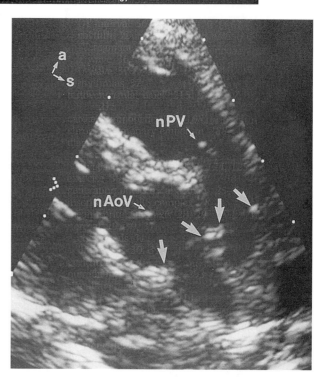

Fig. 15.39 Oblique long axis view in an infant after arterial switch operation for transposition of the great arteries. The large arrows indicate suture lines in the neoaorta and neopulmonary trunk. nAoV, neoaortic valve; nPV, neopulmonary valve.

nary ventricular septal defect where more than 50% of the pulmonary trunk arises from the right ventricle (Fig. 15.9), are both forms of double-outlet right ventricle, but require entirely different management. In most cases of double-outlet right ventricle, it is possible surgically to commit a ventricle to each of the great arteries and to perform a biventricular repair.

Anomalous pulmonary venous connection

Anomalous pulmonary venous connection is the connection of pulmonary veins to sites other than the left atrium. When all pulmonary veins are involved, there is total anomalous pulmonary venous connection (TAPVC). When only some pulmonary veins are connected abnormally, there is partial anomalous pulmonary venous connection. In TAPVC, pulmonary veins drain to a confluence posterior to the left atrium, and then drain to right atrium via a supracardiac (more than 50% of cases), cardiac, or infracardiac connection (Fig. 15.41). Presentation is highly variable, with a spectrum which ranges from a moribund newborn to an asymptomatic child. The variation depends mainly on whether the abnormal venous channel is obstructed or not. Obstruction is most likely with infradiaphragmatic drainage when pulmonary venous flow is via the portal venous system and hepatic sinusoids (Fig. 15.41b). Results of surgical repair are excellent except for the rare cases where there is narrowing of pulmonary veins within the lung parenchyma.

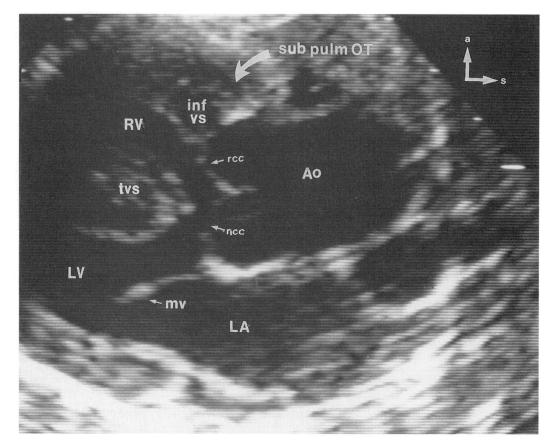

Fig. 15.40 Parasternal long axis view in a patient with tetralogy of Fallot. Anterior deviation of the infundibular (outlet) ventricular septum results in a subaortic ventricular septal defect, and narrowing of the subpulmonary right ventricular outflow tract. More than 50% of the aorta is committed to the right ventricle so, strictly speaking, this is double-outlet right ventricle. inf vs, infundibular septum; mv, mitral valve; ncc, non-coronary cusp; rcc, right coronary cusp; subpulm OT, subpulmonary outflow tract; tvs, trabecular ventricular septum.

Univentricular atrioventricular connection

This describes the group of hearts in which the atria are connected to a single ventricle (see terminology above). There is almost always a second, rudimentary ventricle present but, in physiological terms, the heart has one effective ventricle. The most common examples are tricuspid atresia (absent right atrioventricular connection) (Fig. 15.6) and double-inlet left ventricle (Fig. 15.5). Abnormalities of this sort have been increasingly recognized prenatally (Fig. 15.12). Presentation in early infancy depends mostly on the ventriculoarterial connection: in tricuspid atresia, for example, about two-thirds have ventriculoarterial concordance (Fig. 15.6), and have obstruction to pulmonary blood flow of varying degree, but often severe enough to require a palliative neonatal systemic-to-pulmonary shunt; conversely, about one-third of patients have ventriculoarterial discordance and typically have high pulmonary blood flow, often in association with

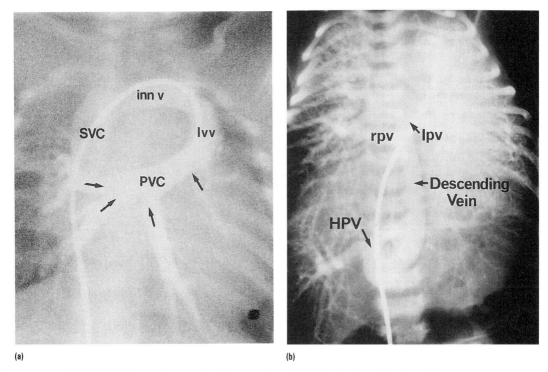

Fig. 15.41 Angiograms demonstrating (a) supracardiac and (b) infracardiac forms of total anomalous pulmonary venous connection. In contemporary practice, preoperative diagnosis in infancy is by echocardiography. HPV, hepatic portal vein; inn v; innominate vein; lpv, left pulmonary vein; lvv, left vertical vein; PVC, pulmonary venous confluence; rpv, right pulmonary vein; svc, superior vena cava.

aortic arch obstruction, and require a completely different approach to surgical management.

The aim of surgical treatment in any heart with one effective ventricle is to achieve a Fontan type of circulation. The 'only' ventricle powers a circulation in which the systemic venous return is surgically redirected to the pulmonary arteries. This is usually achieved by performing total cavopulmonary connection (Fig. 15.42). Prerequisites for this type of circulation to be effective are low pulmonary vascular resistance, good ventricular function and absence of atrioventricular valve regurgitation.

Atrial isomerism

Atrial morphology is best identified by the characteristics of the atrial appendages. When both atria are of right atrial morphology right atrial isomerism exists, whereas left atrial isomerism occurs when both atria are of left atrial morphology (Fig. 15.3). The complex cardiac malformations usually associated with, atrial isomerism determine presentation, management and outcome. There are frequently abnormalities of systemic and pulmonary veins, of the atrioventricular

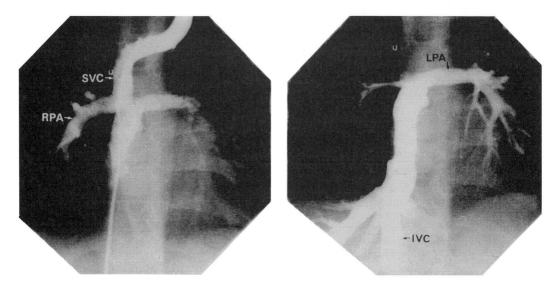

Fig. 15.42 Total cavopulmonary connection. In this patient superior vena caval (SVC) blood flows preferentially to right pulmonary artery (RPA), and inferior vena caval (IVC) blood is routed preferentially to left pulmonary artery (LPA) via an intracardiac tunnel.

junction which is often a univentricular connection via a common valve (Figs 15.7 and 15.12), and of the ventriculoarterial connection and great arteries.

Congenitally corrected transposition

Sometimes called 'double discordance', this abnormality occurs when there is atrioventricular and ventriculoarterial discordance. If there are no associated malformations, the circulation is physiologically normal, and occasionally congenitally corrected transposition may be an incidental finding in late adult life. However, the majority of patients have associated lesions, particularly ventricular septal defect and left ventricular outflow tract obstruction (subpulmonary stenosis). Regurgitation of the systemic atrioventricular valve, which is a morphological tricuspid valve, and heart block, which can occur spontaneously or postoperatively because of the tortuous anterior course of the atrioventricular conduction tissue, are the other main problems encountered (Plate 15.3). The nature and timing of surgical intervention in these patients requires detailed consideration in any individual case. A non-surgical approach is appropriate in some. In others, a total cavopulmonary connection (Fig. 15.42) may be definitive surgery preferable to attempting biventricular repair if the latter is likely to be compromised by a small morphological right ventricular cavity with a regurgitant atrioventricular valve and the need for an extracardiac valved conduit. In others, a 'double switch' procedure which involves redirection of systemic venous return as well as an arterial switch may be appropriate.

Tricuspid regurgitation

Tricuspid regurgitation is among the most common cardiac abnormalities detected prenatally and occurs because of fetal right ventricular failure, developmental abnormality of the tricuspid valve, or both. Most severely affected fetuses die *in utero* or immediately after delivery, so that important isolated tricuspid regurgitation is uncommon in postnatal practice.

Ebstein's anomaly of the tricuspid valve occurs when cleavage of the septal and inferior tricuspid valve leaflets from the right ventricular endocardium is incomplete, so that these leaflets are plastered against the endocardial surface (Fig. 15.43). There are frequently abnormal chordal and papillary muscle attachments of the anterosuperior leaflet. Severe tricuspid regurgitation may occur, with right-to-left shunting at atrial level resulting in cyanosis. The prognosis is extremely variable and correlates broadly with the severity of the structural abnormality. Accessory atrioventricular conduction pathways are common, so that the most common presentation in older children and young adults is atrioventricular re-entry tachycardia. Some cases of Ebstein's anomaly of the tricuspid valve have been associated with maternal lithium therapy.

Mitral or aortic regurgitation

Mitral regurgitation is often a consequence of left ventricular cavity enlargement as occurs in dilated cardiomyopathy. Isolated mitral regurgitation is rare, but may be caused by mitral valve prolapse (Fig. 15.44), chordal rupture or an

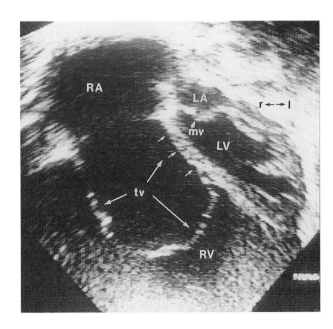

Fig. 15.43 Ebstein's anomaly of the tricuspid valve (tv). The septal leaflet of the tricuspid valve is adherent to the septal surface (small arrows) so that its functional septal attachment is displaced into the right ventricle.

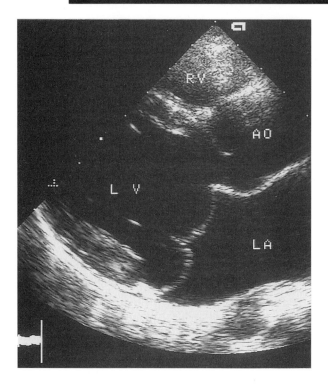

Fig. 15.44 Mitral valve prolapse and dilatation of the aortic root in Marfan's syndrome.

isolated cleft in the anterior mitral valve leaflet. The importance of the latter is that surgical repair of the mitral valve is extremely effective.

Isolated congenital aortic regurgitation is rare, but aortic regurgitation may occur in association with aortic stenosis; or because of aortic valve prolapse into a perimembranous or doubly committed ventricular septal defect (Fig. 15.30); or when the aortic root is dilated as occurs in Marfan's syndrome (Fig. 15.44) and other connective tissue disease. Infective endocarditis is an important cause of both mitral regurgitation and aortic regurgitation. If aortic root abscess is detected on echocardiography, this is an indication for urgent homograft aortic root replacement.

Common arterial trunk

Failure of separation of the pulmonary trunk from the ascending aorta during embryogenesis is the cause of common arterial trunk (truncus arteriosus). There is a single arterial outlet from the heart, the truncal valve usually overrides the trabecular septum, and the pulmonary arteries arise from the proximal part of the common trunk (Fig. 15.10). The truncal valve is often dysplastic and may be both stenotic and regurgitant (Plate 15.9, opposite p. 244), and the aortic arch is interrupted in about 20% of cases. Young infants present with features of high pulmonary blood flow. Surgical repair in early infancy is indicated. Reoperation will be needed in due course to replace the extracardiac right ventricle-to-pulmonary artery valved conduit which is required as part of the surgical repair.

Absent pulmonary valve syndrome

Rudimentary pulmonary valve tissue and very large central pulmonary arteries, often with an associated subaortic ventricular septal defect, are the hallmarks of this condition. Congenital absence of the arterial duct and consequent exposure of the central pulmonary arteries to ventricular ejection without the decompression that the arterial duct provides in prenatal life might explain aetiology in some cases. The main problem is airway obstruction, either because of compression of the adjacent bronchi by the large central pulmonary arteries, or because of intrinsic airway abnormality. The minority of neonates with severe respiratory failure have a poor outlook but results after cardiac surgical repair are good in the remaining patients. This condition is one of the group of so-called conotruncal abnormalities, which includes tetralogy of Fallot, common arterial trunk and interrupted aortic arch. These malformations may be familial.

Vascular rings

Rare abnormalities of the great arteries in the superior mediastinum may compress the trachea and oesophagus. This possibility should be considered in any infant or child with stridor, especially if this is becoming increasingly severe, rather than gradually improving, as tends to occur with intrinsic airway abnormality. There are several possible anatomical variants, but by far the most common type of vascular ring is a double aortic arch: the ascending aorta gives rise to one arch which passes to the right and another which passes to the left of the trachea and oesophagus before merging posteriorly to form the descending aorta (Fig. 15.45). The central mediastinal structures are compressed within this

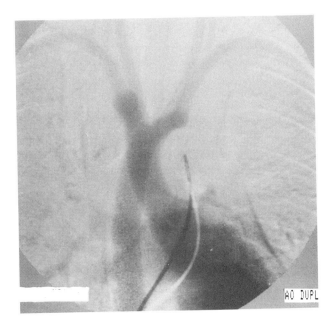

Fig. 15.45 Double aortic arch. The two arches compress the central mediastinal structure. Unusually, in this patient the descending aorta is right sided.

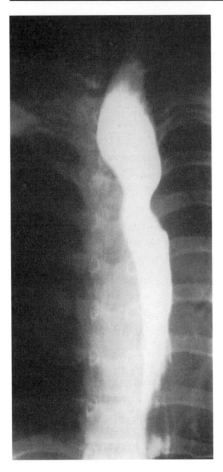

Fig. 15.46 Barium swallow showing extrinsic oesophageal compression from a double aortic arch.

vascular vice. Barium swallow demonstrates fixed extrinsic oesophageal compression (Fig. 15.46). Echocardiography can confirm the diagnosis and delineate the vascular anatomy. Surgical division of the constricting ring is curative.

Aortopulmonary window

This is a large and usually non-restrictive communication between the proximal ascending aorta and proximal pulmonary trunk (Fig. 15.47). As a result, there is high pulmonary blood flow with pulmonary hypertension in early infancy. About 50% of cases have a ventricular septal defect or other associated cardiac malformations. Management is surgical.

ACQUIRED HEART ABNORMALITIES

Cardiomyopathy

Strictly, cardiomyopathy describes myocardial dysfunction of unknown cause. Left ventricular cavity dilatation and impaired myocardial performance in infants

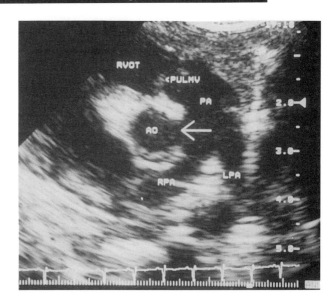

Fig. 15.47 Aortopulmonary window (arrow). PULMV, pulmonary valve; RVOT, right ventricular outflow tract.

and children is usually idiopathic. Occasionally, however, evidence for preceding enterovirus infection causing myocarditis or, rarely, an inborn error of metabolism may be detected. There is also increasing evidence that a proportion of cases considered to be idiopathic may have a familial basis. In any infant who presents with a dilated and poorly functioning left ventricle, it is crucial to exclude anomalous origin of the left coronary artery from the pulmonary trunk (Plate 15.10, opposite p. 244), or incessant tachyarrhythmia, as both of these conditions are treatable. In anomalous origin of the left coronary artery from the pulmonary trunk, the ECG will usually show features of anterolateral myocardial infarction. Left ventricular function may recover following surgical reimplantation of the anomalous coronary artery to the aorta. Incessant or prolonged tachycardia may not be immediately apparent, as sinus tachycardia rates in a sick infant may easily exceed 200 beats/minute. In older children or young adults, a problem apparent with increasing frequency is heart failure occurring late after treatment for childhood malignancy with cardiotoxic anthracycline drugs such as adriamycin. Principles of treatment of heart failure in childhood are similar to those in adults.

Hypertrophic cardiomyopathy (Fig. 15.48) is not often diagnosed in young children, partly because the condition may not necessarily be manifest in the first decade of life. Diagnosis may be made in an asymptomatic child because of family screening following diagnosis of an index case. However, at least 50% of children diagnosed to have hypertrophic cardiomyopathy have no identifiable family history or involvement of other family members, and most likely represent a new mutation for the condition. Several abnormal gene loci involving regulation of myocardial contractile proteins have been identified in different families. This genetic heterogeneity presumably contributes to the wide variation in morphological severity and prognosis in hypertrophic cardiomyopathy. However, myo-

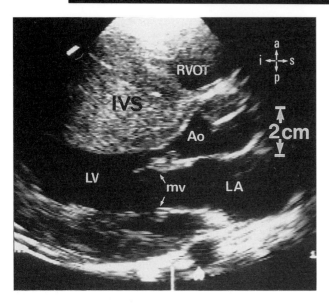

Fig. 15.48 Hypertrophic cardiomyopathy with severe asymmetrical septal hypertrophy. RVOT, right ventricular outflow tract; IVS, interventricular septum.

cardial hypertrophy in infancy is more likely to be caused by metabolic disease than hypertrophic cardiomyopathy, because of conditions such as excess insulin production, glycogen storage disease or respiratory chain defects. Noonan's syndrome may cause hypertrophic cardiomyopathy as well as pulmonary valve dysplasia.

Kawasaki disease

Kawasaki disease is a systemic vasculitis of unknown aetiology. Presenting features include fever, skin rash, erythema of tongue and pharynx, conjunctivitis, lymphadenopathy, swollen hands/feet and, later, desquamation of skin at the extremities. Epidemiological evidence suggests exposure to an infectious agent in susceptible individuals. The condition was first described in 1967 in Japan, and it has replaced rheumatic heart disease as the leading cause of acquired heart disease in most developed countries. It may be a genuinely 'new' disorder, but it seems more likely that the ability to diagnose coronary artery aneurysms by echocardiography is the main reason for the increasing number of cases identified. About 80% of patients are aged < 4 years and the annual incidence in Japanese people, 90/100 000 children aged < 5 years, is much higher than the incidence in Europeans. About 20% of patients with Kawasaki disease develop coronary artery aneurysms detectable with echocardiography. Treatment includes intravenous infusion of gamma-globulin as early in the course of the disease as possible, and aspirin which is initially given in anti-inflammatory doses, then as an antiplatelet agent (3–5 mg/kg daily). Antiplatelet treatment is usually discontinued after about 6–8 weeks if no coronary artery abnormalities are detected, but should be continued indefinitely in the presence of coronary artery abnormalities. Symptomatic acute myocardial ischaemia is rare consider-

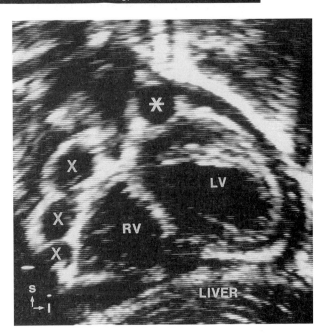

Fig. 15.49 Kawasaki disease. Subcostal view. Three large aneurysms involving the proximal right coronary artery (X) and one involving the proximal left coronary artery (*) are evident. There is also a small pericardial effusion.

ing the gross coronary artery morphological changes which are sometimes seen (Fig. 15.49), but both acute myocardial infarction and sudden death do occur occasionally. Anticoagulation with warfarin should be considered in the presence of large coronary artery aneurysms, and thrombolysis may be indicated when intraluminal thrombus is detected. Late follow-up data are lacking regarding the outlook for children with coronary artery abnormalities. There is anecdotal evidence that a few young adults investigated for myocardial ischaemia have coronary artery morphology consistent with previous undiagnosed Kawasaki disease in early childhood.

Rheumatic heart disease

On a global basis, acute rheumatic fever and rheumatic heart disease are the most common heart abnormalities in childhood. With a few geographical exceptions, acute rheumatic fever is now very rarely seen in developed countries. Improved living standards are probably the most important reason for this reduction in incidence, but widespread use of penicillin in the past 50 years and reduced streptococcal virulence are other factors. Acute rheumatic fever is the result of an immune-mediated process which follows infection with group A streptococci in susceptible individuals. The usual main clinical features include arthritis, carditis and chorea in a school-age child who has evidence of recent streptococcal infection. Arthritis and carditis occur usually 2–6 weeks after streptococcal infection whereas chorea occurs several months later. Not all features are likely to be manifest in an individual. The arthritis may be fleeting, involving middle-sized joints. Pancarditis occurs with valvulitis, myocarditis and pericarditis. Echocardiographic demonstration of impaired myocardial function and colour Doppler detection of valvar regurgitation, especially mitral regurgitation, enhances diagnosis. Acute heart failure may be the consequence. Treatment of the acute episode is with rest and aspirin in anti-inflammatory doses (blood salicylate levels should be monitored); alternatively, steroid therapy may be required. This should be continued until inflammatory markers such as erythrocyte sedimentation rate (ESR) have subsided. Heart failure, if present, requires conventional treatment. Penicillin should be given acutely, and as prophylaxis against recurrent episodes of acute rheumatic fever at least until adult life. The main long-term consequences are mitral and aortic valve disease, especially mitral valve stenosis.

HEART AND HEART–LUNG TRANSPLANTATION

Heart or heart–lung transplantation is theoretically an attractive therapeutic option for infants and children with complex congenital heart defects. However, the development of neonatal heart transplantation has been greatly restricted by an insuperable shortfall of donor organs, and this remains a problem in later infancy and childhood as well. There are technical problems in transplanting patients with complex abnormalities of pulmonary and systemic venous drainage, and the likelihood of multiple previous operations in children with complex heart disease, and the presence of acquired collateral arteries in cyanotic patients, makes perioperative bleeding a major problem. As a result, the early postoperative mortality for children undergoing heart transplantation for congenital heart disease is higher than for children with cardiomyopathy, although the medium-term survival rate thereafter is similar (Fig. 15.50). Immunosuppressive therapy needs close surveillance indefinitely. There are late concerns such as coronary artery occlusive disease in heart transplant recipients. Obliterative bronchiolitis developing in lung recipients is the main reason why medium-term survival after heart transplantation remains considerably better than after heart–lung transplantation (Fig. 15.50). Nevertheless, quality of life is considerably enhanced in most recipients after heart or heart–lung transplantation. Xeno-

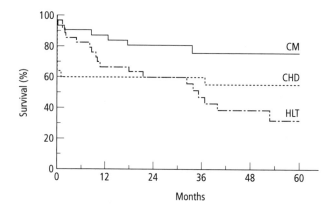

Fig. 15.50 Great Ormond Street Hospital survival data after heart transplantation for cardiomyopathy (CM) or congenital heart disease (CHD), or after heart and lung transplantation (HLT). The main indication for HLT has been cystic fibrosis.

transplantation is a potentially exciting development which may possibly improve the problem of donor organ shortage in the future.

ARRHYTHMIAS

This subject is covered in detail elsewhere, and only a few points especially pertinent to paediatric practice will be highlighted. Fetal supraventricular tachyarrhythmia is an important treatable cause of intrauterine heart failure (Fig. 15.13). It must be remembered that the tachycardia may be intermittent. In neonates and infants, by far the most common mechanism of tachycardia is atrioventricular re-entry via an accessory pathway which is usually concealed. There is a bimodal incidence of atrioventricular re-entry tachycardia, with a large peak in early infancy and a second peak around the end of the first decade of life. Facial immersion in ice-cold water is effective in terminating episodes of tachycardia in neonates and young infants. Children often learn to perform vagal stimulation such as a Valsalva manoeuvre to abort episodes of tachycardia. Adenosine as an intravenous bolus (usual dose 0.2 mg/kg) is effective in terminating episodes of tachycardia. When there are recurrent episodes, flecainide is the most effective prophylactic treatment. Serum levels should be monitored. The natural history of tachyarrhythmias in children should be considered before definitive intervention such as transcatheter ablation of an accessory pathway is undertaken. This procedure is rarely indicated in infants or toddlers. The second most common mechanism for supraventricular tachycardia in the fetus or infant is atrial flutter. The natural history is favourable. Atrial flutter may occur late postoperatively in patients where there has been extensive atrial surgery, such as atrial repair for transposition of the great arteries or Fontan-type surgery. Rare but important forms of supraventricular tachycardia in infants and young children are atrial ectopic tachycardia and paroxysmal reciprocating junctional tachycardia. Both of these may be incessant, and present with features that may be confused with dilated cardiomyopathy. Atrial fibrillation is almost never seen in infants and young children, and atrioventricular nodal re-entry tachycardia is rare. Cardiac structure is usually normal in infants with supraventricular tachycardia, but atrioventricular accessory pathways are more common in Ebstein's anomaly of the tricuspid valve (Fig. 15.43) and hearts with atrioventricular discordance (Plate 15.3).

Junctional ectopic tachycardia (His bundle tachycardia) is common after operations for congenital heart disease. Strictly speaking, this is a type of ventricular tachycardia, and is the most clinically important arrhythmia in this setting, as the combination of rapid ventricular rate and atrioventricular dissociation is potentially lethal. The increased diagnosis in recent years probably reflects both an expanded surgical repertoire and failure of accurate diagnosis in an earlier era. This arrhythmia arises because of an ectopic focus with increased automaticity high in the ventricular septum in the region of the bundle of His. There is usually atrioventricular dissociation, in which the ventricular rate is faster than the atrial rate, although retrograde ventriculoatrial conduction

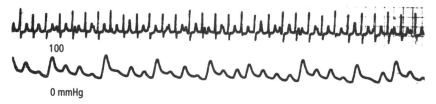

100

0 mmHg

Fig. 15.51 His bundle tachycardia showing narrow QRS complexes, atrioventricular dissociation and marked beat-to-beat variation in arterial blood pressure.

occasionally occurs. The atrioventricular dissociation may be apparent from the beat-to-beat variation in the continuously monitored arterial blood pressure tracing (Fig. 15.51), and the diagnosis is often confirmed by recording the atrial electrogram from an atrial pacing wire (Fig. 15.52). Our current preference for management of this arrhythmia is to use moderate systemic hypothermia (core temperature 33–34°C) to reduce the rate of the ectopic focus. Full ventilatory support and neuromuscular blockade must be used simultaneously. Further benefit may be obtained by amiodarone intravenous infusion, and by atrial pacing when the ectopic focus tachycardia rate has been reduced sufficiently to allow capture at a slightly faster rate than the tachycardia rate. This management approach is essentially supportive while spontaneous resolution of the His bundle tachycardia is awaited.

Other forms of ventricular tachycardia are rare in children. Paroxysmal ventricular tachycardia may occur in long QT syndrome, where there is prolongation of ventricular repolarization. This may have a familial basis, and both dominant and recessive forms of inheritance have been described. However, most new cases do not have a family history, nor is the condition detectable in asymptomatic family members. A problem with family screening is that individuals susceptible to ventricular tachycardia will not necessarily have a QT interval which is prolonged beyond the normal range on the surface ECG. Myocardial tumours, typically rhabdomyomas which are often associated with tuberous sclerosis (Fig. 15.53), sometimes provide the substrate for ventricular tachycardia

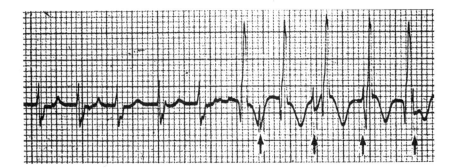

Fig. 15.52 Electrogram recorded from atrial epicardial pacing wire (right) showing His bundle tachycardia in a patient in whom the standard electrocardiogram lead II (left) was not diagnostic. The arrows indicate atrial depolarization.

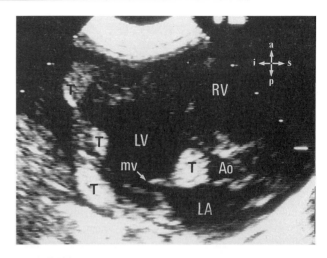

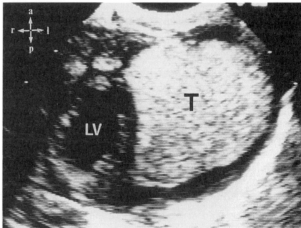

Fig. 15.53 Long axis (top) and short axis (below) echocardiographic views in a neonate with multiple myocardial tumours (T) who presented with ventricular tachycardia.

in infants and children. Ventricular tachycardia has also been a problem during late follow-up after surgical repair of tetralogy of Fallot, although the incidence of this complication seems to have been very much reduced by performing cardiac surgical repair at a younger age.

Congenital heart block is usually the consequence of transplacental transfer of maternal anti-Ro autoantibodies. In the absence of symptoms, indications for pacemaker insertion are not clear-cut. However, pacing would normally be undertaken if there is a mean daytime ventricular heart rate of less than about 50 beats/minute, if the junctional escape focus fails to track the atrial rate during activity, or if there is evidence of instability of the junctional escape focus such as prolonged pauses. Postoperative heart block has become less common with better knowledge of the surgical anatomy of cardiac conduction tissue in congenital heart defects. Heart block after intracardiac surgery is often transient, but persisting heart block 2 weeks after operation is a generally accepted indication for pacemaker insertion. Spontaneous heart block occurs frequently in hearts with atrioventricular discordance (Plate 15.3).

GROWING UP WITH CONGENITAL HEART DISEASE

The development of infant cardiac surgery and interventional catheterization techniques over the past 30 years has resulted in survival beyond infancy and early childhood of the majority of children born with conditions which were previously lethal. This has resulted in a new population of adolescents and young adults with surgically modified congenital heart malformations (Fig. 15.54). Often these patients are not 'cured' and have continuing special needs. Some nominally corrective surgical procedures will have an inevitable requirement for late reintervention, such as prosthetic valve replacement in childhood, or procedures including insertion of an extracardiac valved conduit. An apparently corrective surgical procedure may have residual abnormality: with long-term follow-up after repair of tetralogy of Fallot, for example, it is becoming clear that late survivors may sometimes benefit from homograft valve insertion to the pulmonary position. Other procedures in childhood, such as balloon or surgical aortic valvotomy, are palliative with an almost certain requirement for further surgery. Alternatively, there may have been no indication to repair some congenital abnormalities in childhood, but later surgical intervention is required, as might occur with aortic dilatation in Marfan's syndrome. Late postoperative complications might not have been known or anticipated at the time of childhood surgery, such as recurrence of subaortic stenosis, or venous pathway obstruction developing late after atrial level repair using the Mustard or Senning operation for transposition of the great arteries. Infective endocarditis is a lifelong possibility in most patients with congenital heart malformations. Arrhythmias may complicate late follow-up after tetralogy of Fallot, atrial repair for transposition of the great arteries or Fontan-type surgery in particular, and may occur as part of the natural history of Ebstein's anomaly of the tricuspid valve or atrioventricular discordance, even without surgery. All of these patients may also require specialized advice or management with regard to choice of career, fitness to drive or participate in sport, life insurance, genetic counselling, contraception, pregnancy and coexisting medical problems. Delivery of the optimal care for this increasing population of adults with congenital heart defects is a major challenge.

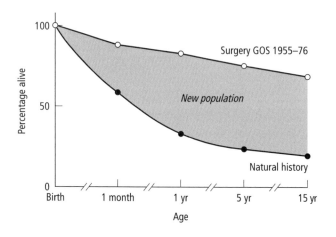

Fig. 15.54 Natural history data for infants presenting with congenital heart disease in the presurgical era, compared to survival after infant cardiac surgery in the early surgical era. There is a new population of young adults with surgically modified congenital heart disease. (After Macartney *et al.*, 1980; Hoffman, 1987.)

FURTHER READING

Anderson RH, Macartney FJ, Shinebourne EA, Tynan M (eds). *Paediatric Cardiology*. Edinburgh: Churchill Livingstone, 1987.

Rees PG, Tunstill A, Pope T, Kinnear D, Rees S. *Heart Children. A Practical Hhandbook for Parents*. Camberley: Heartline Association, 2nd edn. 1992.

Stark J, de Leval M (eds). *Surgery for Congenital Heart Defects*, 2nd edn. Philadelphia: W B Saunders, 1994.

Wren C, Campbell RWF (eds). *Paediatric Cardiac Arrhythmias*. Oxford: Oxford University Press, 1996.

CHAPTER 16

Pregnancy, Systemic Disorders, Neoplastic Disease and the Heart

CONTENTS

SUMMARY

Pregnancy is associated with increased plasma volume, vasodilatation, hyper-dynamic circulation and variable compression of the heart by the uterine fundus. These changes often produce flow murmurs, added heart sounds, peripheral oedema and minor ECG and chest X-ray abnormalities, any of which may give rise to a spurious impression of heart disease. When organic heart disease does occur it is mitral stenosis and cardiomyopathy that are most hazardous because of the risk of life-threatening pulmonary oedema in the third trimester. Echocardiography is the safest and most reliable diagnostic technique.

Endocrine disorders. Diabetes and thyroid disease are the most important endocrine disorders affecting the heart. Diabetes is a major risk factor for atherosclerosis and is commonly associated with premature coronary and peripheral vascular disease. Cardiomyopathy may also occur. The effects of thyrotoxicosis on the heart, including tachycardia and arrhythmias (particularly atrial fibrillation), largely resemble those of sympathetic overstimulation and respond to beta-blockers. Hypothyroidism causes bradycardia and pericardial effusion and, in longstanding disease, may result in cardiac dilatation and congestive failure.

Connective tissue disorders. These are associated with vasculitis that may affect almost any part of the heart. Pericarditis is the most common cardiac manifestation of rheumatoid arthritis and systemic lupus erythematosus, while aortic root disease leading to aortic regurgitation is the characteristic lesion in ankylosing spondylitis and Marfan's syndrome.

Infiltrative disorders such as amyloidosis and haemochromatosis are important causes of cardiomyopathy, but in sarcoidosis granulomatous destruction of conducting tissue with varying degrees of AV block is a more frequent mode of presentation.

Infective disease is usually viral, causing pericarditis or myocarditis. Bacterial infection is a more common cause of endocarditis, although tuberculous pericarditis remains an important problem in many parts of the world. Chronic trypanosomiasis is a major cause of cardiomyopathy and conducting tissue disease in Central and South America.

Neoplastic disease affecting the heart is usually metastatic from lung or breast and, when clinically evident, presents with pericardial effusion and tamponade. Of the primary cardiac tumours, the histologically benign left atrial myxoma is the most common. Typically it is pedunculated and attached to the interatrial septum, causing variable obstruction to mitral flow during diastole. Symptoms and signs are similar to mitral stenosis but the echocardiogram permits reliable differential diagnosis. Primary malignant tumours are rare and are nearly all sarcomas; death early in the clinical course is invariable.

PREGNANCY

Circulatory changes

During pregnancy, plasma volume and cardiac output increase to meet the requirements of the uterus. By the third trimester, plasma volume may be increased by 40–50%. Plasma volume expansion is associated with a fall in colloid osmotic pressure which predisposes to oedema even in the absence of pre-eclampsia. Oedema is usually mild and tends to affect the lower limbs due to compression of the pelvic veins by the uterus. Elevated venous pressure is also an important factor in the development of varicose veins and haemorrhoids which are common in pregnancy. Following delivery, there is a sharp drop in plasma volume due to blood loss associated with shedding of the placenta. Thereafter, plasma volume and cardiac output decline more gradually, returning to pre-pregnancy levels after about 6 weeks.

Clinical manifestations

The skin is warm and often flushed due to peripheral vasodilatation. The heart rate is increased and the pulse has a collapsing quality. During the third trimester the pregnant uterus may cause upward displacement of the diaphragm. This compresses the heart so that the apex beat becomes palpable in the fourth intercostal space in the anterior axillary line. Auscultation during this period commonly reveals an 'innocent' ejection murmur at the base of the heart and a third heart sound—both manifestations of the hyperdynamic circulation.

The ECG and chest X-ray are usually normal but, late in pregnancy, may show changes reflecting cardiac compression. These include a degree of left axis deviation and apparent radiological cardiac enlargement. Atrial and ventricular ectopic beats are frequently found.

Heart disease in pregnancy

Flow murmurs, added heart sounds, peripheral oedema and minor ECG and chest X-ray abnormalities often give rise to a spurious impression of heart disease in the pregnant woman. In such cases, the echocardiogram provides a safe and useful means of ruling out valvular and myocardial disorders.

Coronary artery disease is unusual in premenopausal women but valvular and myocardial disease are seen more often. Presentation is typically during the third trimester, or at the time of delivery, when increments in plasma volume and cardiac output are at their peak. Mitral stenosis in particular is poorly tolerated and there is a considerable risk of acute pulmonary oedema. It is best treated by valvotomy before the onset of labour but, if valvular calcification or regurgitation contraindicate this procedure, medical management is preferable. Beta-blockers are particularly helpful in mitral stenosis because, by slowing the heart rate, they improve ventricular filling. Aortic and right-sided valvular disorders are better tolerated during pregnancy and definitive surgical treatment can usually be delayed until after delivery. In women with valvular disease antibiotic prophylaxis against endocarditis (intravenous gentamicin and amoxycillin) is unnecessary for normal vaginal deliveries but is recommended for instrumented deliveries and for all women with prosthetic valves or a history of previous endocarditis. Generally speaking, if valve replacement is required in pregnancy (or in women who wish to become pregnant at a future date) a porcine xenograft should be chosen (see page 187) since this avoids the need for anticoagulation, which poses special problems during pregnancy due to the teratogenic effects of warfarin and the risk of uterine bleeding. The usual recommendation for women needing anticoagulation during pregnancy is for treatment with heparin, although the need for parenteral administration throughout the 9-month period makes the management difficult.

Women with cardiomyopathy usually tolerate pregnancy well, although in severe cases there is always a risk of pulmonary oedema during the third trimester or at delivery. Dilated cardiomyopathy presenting within 3 months before or after labour has been named peripartum cardiomyopathy. This appears to be a specific entity related to pregnancy and is particularly common in women of West African origin. Nevertheless, it remains unclear whether peripartum cardiomyopathy represents the direct effects of pregnancy on a previously normal heart or merely a deterioration in a pre-existing cardiomyopathy. Peripartum cardiomyopathy can present with life-threatening pulmonary oedema in the peripartum period demanding urgent Caesarean section and, although variable (sometimes complete) clinical recovery usually occurs following delivery, the risk of recurrent decompensation in future pregnancies is considerable.

ENDOCRINE DISEASE

Thyroid disease

Cardiovascular manifestations of thyrotoxicosis include palpitation, dyspnoea, tachycardia, systolic hypertension and a third heart sound. Arrhythmias are common, particularly atrial fibrillation, which may be the only sign of thyrotoxicosis in the elderly patient. Tachycardia and arrhythmias exacerbate angina in patients with coronary artery disease and may lead to heart failure. It is noteworthy that the effects of thyrotoxicosis on the cardiovascular system largely resemble those of sympathetic overstimulation, and beta-blockers (propranolol 40–80 mg three times daily) provide the most effective treatment pending definitive measures to reduce secretion of thyroid hormone.

Hypothyroidism has a direct effect on myocardial structure and function which leads ultimately to cardiac dilatation and congestive failure. Bradycardia, hypotension and pericardial effusion are common findings. The hypercholesterolaemia associated with hypothyroidism may predispose to coronary artery disease. The ECG shows low-voltage QRS complexes which often persist despite removal of pericardial fluid. Following thyroid replacement therapy, reversal of cardiovascular abnormalities nearly always occurs. Nevertheless, treatment must be given cautiously—particularly in the elderly and those known to have underlying organic heart disease—because abrupt myocardial stimulation by thyroid hormone may precipitate acute ischaemia or cardiac arrhythmias. Thus, initial therapy is with very low doses of thyroid hormone which are gradually increased over a period of weeks.

Diabetes

Diabetes is a major risk factor for atherosclerotic arterial disease affecting the coronary, cerebral or peripheral circulations. The relative risk of coronary heart disease increases at least two-fold among diabetic women. Diabetics are more likely to sustain an acute myocardial infarction then non-diabetics, and, in these patients, diabetes is a major predictor of morbidity and mortality. The distribution of disease differs from that of non-diabetic patients in that the small distal arteries in the coronary circulation and the legs tend to be involved, often to the same extent as the proximal arteries. This increases the technical difficulties of vascular bypass surgery and angioplasty procedures.

The sensory supply of the heart runs with the autonomic innervation, and silent ischaemia (see page 109) is therefore common in patients with diabetic neuropathy. Painless MI is common for the same reason but, in other respects, MI is usually more severe than in the non-diabetic patient and the incidence of all complications (including arrhythmias, heart failure and death) is higher. Catecholamine release exacerbates the diabetic state and adequate metabolic control in the coronary care unit demands regular administration of short-acting insulin even in patients usually controlled with oral hypoglycaemic agents.

Diabetes may cause cardiomyopathy which is unrelated to atherosclerotic coronary artery disease. The precise cause is uncertain, but some studies of myocardial histology have provided evidence of microvascular obliterative disease. Treatment is the same as for dilated cardiomyopathy (see page 152).

Acromegaly

Cardiac enlargement is almost invariable in acromegaly and is due principally to the effects of growth hormone on the myocardium, although hypertension, which affects up to 50% of patients, contributes to this. Premature coronary artery disease is common in acromegaly, not only because of hypertension but also because of abnormal lipid and carbohydrate metabolism.

Adrenal disease

In Cushing's disease, hypertension and abnormalities of lipid and carbohydrate metabolism commonly lead to accelerated atherosclerosis. MI is a common cause of death in untreated cases. Primary hyperaldosteronism (Conn's syndrome) is associated with hypertension and hypokalaemia which predispose to myocardial disease, coronary artery disease and arrhythmias. The only important cardiovascular manifestation of Addison's disease is hypotension, which may cause postural dizziness or syncope. Hyperkalaemia is rarely so severe as to disturb cardiac rhythm.

Catecholamine-secreting tumours of the adrenal medulla (phaeochromocytoma) are an important cause of secondary hypertension. The tumours are usually benign but may occur bilaterally or in extra-adrenal locations. Hypertension caused by phaeochromocytoma is characteristically labile due to episodic release of catecholamines. Arrhythmias are not uncommon and in severe cases diffuse myocardial dysfunction leads to heart failure and death. Myocardial disease is due in part to the effects of hypertension, but has also been attributed to the direct action of catecholamines which may cause focal myocardial necrosis.

Carcinoid syndrome

Carcinoid tumours in the appendix and other parts of small bowel secrete kinin peptides and serotonin, which are largely inactivated in the liver. Following metastasis to the liver, however, the systemic circulation is no longer protected from these toxic substances which are responsible for the characteristic clinical manifestations of carcinoid syndrome. These include diarrhoea, bronchospasm, flushing attacks and telangiectasia. Cardiac manifestations are the result of toxic damage to the tricuspid and pulmonary valves; variable stenosis or regurgitation often develops (see Fig. 9.13). Left-sided valvular disease is rare but is occasionally seen in patients with pulmonary metastases.

NUTRITIONAL DISEASE

Obesity

The excess mortality in severe obesity is largely related to cardiovascular disease. Hypertension is common (see page 258) and associated metabolic abnormalities include diabetes and hyperlipidaemia, all of which are major risk factors for atherosclerosis and predispose to MI and stroke. Obesity is also associated with increased plasma volume and myocardial mass. In advanced disease plasma volume overload and myocardial hypertrophy lead to congestive heart failure. In certain cases, chronic hypoventilation (Pickwickian syndrome) produces pulmonary hypertension and cor pulmonale (see page 291).

Malnutrition

Although anorexia nervosa is associated with reduced myocardial mass and hypotension there is no demonstrable impairment of left ventricular (LV) contractile function However, in advanced protein–calorie malnutrition (e.g. marasmus, kwashiorkor), cardiac atrophy and interstitial oedema commonly lead to LV dysfunction and there is a major risk of acute pulmonary oedema during rehydration of these patients.

Beriberi caused by thiamine deficiency is the only hypovitaminosis associated with heart disease, and occurs in parts of the world where polished rice is the staple carbohydrate source. Reductions in systemic vascular resistance (due probably to autonomic neuropathy) produce a chronically elevated cardiac output which may lead to high-output failure (see page 76). Physical signs are those of a hyperkinetic circulation and include the third heart sound and an ejection systolic murmur.

CONNECTIVE TISSUE DISEASE

Rheumatoid arthritis

Fibrinous pericarditis commonly occurs in rheumatoid disease and is a well-recognized cause of pericardial effusion and tamponade. In patients with widespread subcutaneous rheumatoid nodules, myocardial and valvular nodules also occur. These are granulomatous lesions but they rarely affect myocardial or valvular function. Coronary arteritis can often be demonstrated in post-mortem studies but this rarely causes myocardial ischaemia or infarction.

Systemic lupus erythematosus

The diffuse vasculitis characterizing this condition nearly always involves the heart; however, cardiac disease is rarely prominent. Pericarditis is the most common lesion and may produce effusion and tamponade. Myocarditis is sub-clinical in most cases and, although congestive heart failure occurs, it is usually the result of hypertension secondary to renal disease. Inflammatory endocarditis, originally described by Libman and Sacks, may affect any of the heart valves and consists of extrusions of degenerative tissue on the valve surfaces which, though large (up to 4 mm), rarely cause significant valvular dysfunction.

Polyarteritis nodosa

Vasculitis affecting the pericardial and coronary vessels may lead to pericarditis and MI, though the latter is rare. Myocardial disease and congestive failure are usually the result of hypertension secondary to renal disease.

Ankylosing spondylitis

Though diffuse carditis with pericardial, myocardial and endocardial involvement may occur in ankylosing spondylitis, aortic regurgitation is the most characteristic cardiac manifestation. This is partly the result of valve scarring but dilatation of the aorta due to destruction of elastic tissue is the major cause.

Marfan's syndrome

This is a generalized connective tissue disorder with an autosomal dominant mode of inheritance; about 15% of cases occur sporadically. Phenotypic expression is variable and many of the 'classical' manifestations (particularly long limbs, mobile joints and high-arched palate) do not provide a very reliable diagnostic guide. Much more specific for Marfan's are lens dislocation and aortic root dilatation. Mitral valve prolapse occurs commonly, but potentially lethal cardiovascular complications result from cystic medial necrosis of the aorta which may lead to aortic root dilatation or aortic regurgitation (Fig. 16.1). Death is usually the result of aortic dissection, aneurysmal rupture or severe aortic regurgitation with left ventricular failure (LVF). There is now clear evidence that prophylactic treatment with beta-blockers can protect against these lethal complications. Echocardiographic examination of the aortic root at yearly intervals is essential in patients with Marfan's syndrome. Evidence of progressive aortic dilatation provides indication for surgical replacement of the aortic root before lethal complications occur.

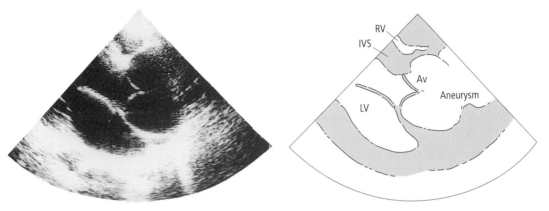

Fig. 16.1 Marfan's syndrome—two-dimensional echocardiogram (long axis view). There is a large aneurysm of the aortic root involving the sinuses of Valsalva.

Scleroderma

Cardiac involvement is common but usually silent, affecting up to 50% of cases. Myocardial fibrosis may present as dilated (or occasionally restrictive) heart-muscle disease while pericarditis sometimes results in significant effusion and tamponade. Lung disease in scleroderma causes pulmonary hypertension and may lead to severe right-sided heart failure.

INFILTRATIVE DISEASE

Amyloidosis

In this condition extracellular deposits of the fibrous protein amyloid occur in various sites of the body. Almost any organ may be involved. When amyloidosis is secondary to chronic infection (e.g. tuberculosis) or inflammation (e.g. rheumatoid arthritis), cardiac involvement is unusual. In primary amyloidosis, however, heart failure is the most common cause of death. Myocardial deposits of amyloid may cause contractile dysfunction leading to cardiac dilatation and congestive failure, but more commonly causing the defect is one of diastolic relaxation and the syndrome resembles restrictive cardiomyopathy (see page 158). Cardiac enlargement may not be prominent but echocardiography demonstrates variable ventricular hypertrophy and, in the most severe cases, characteristic myocardial stippling is seen. Nevertheless, definitive diagnosis is only possible by endomyocardial biopsy. There is no treatment that influences the progression of cardiac amyloidosis.

Haemochromatosis

This is a genetic disorder characterized by excessive intestinal absorption of iron leading to parenchymal deposition of iron in multiple organs, particularly the liver, pancreas, pituitary and heart. Clinical manifestations are rare before the age of 20 and an identical syndrome may result from iron overload secondary to liver disease and multiple blood transfusions. Myocardial deposition of iron leads to fibrosis and contractile dysfunction resulting in cardiomyopathy (often with a significant restrictive component) and congestive failure: definitive diagnosis of cardiac involvement requires endomyocardial biopsy. Regular phlebotomy provides the best means of treating iron overload but chelating agents such as desferrioxamine may also be used. Nevertheless, once congestive heart failure is established, it is always progressive.

Sarcoidosis

This is a multisystem granulomatous disorder of unknown aetiology. Pulmonary sarcoidosis may lead to progressive fibrosis and cor pulmonale which is the most common cardiac manifestation. Although primary cardiac involvement can be demonstrated in up to 25% of post-mortem cases, clinical sarcoid heart disease occurs in less than 5%. Granulomatous destruction of the conducting tissues may cause atrioventricular (AV) block which is the most frequent clinical manifestation of cardiac sarcoidosis. Atrial and ventricular arrhythmias also occur. In patients with extensive granulomatous disease of the ventricular myocardium, congestive heart failure may develop. Sudden death due to heart block or arrhythmias is not uncommon in patients with cardiac sarcoidosis.

NEUROLOGICAL DISEASE

Muscular dystrophy

Sinus tachycardia and ECG abnormalities are common in Duchenne's muscular dystrophy, although the mechanisms are uncertain. Myocardial contractile dysfunction occasionally leads to heart failure but severe cardiac dilatation is unusual.

Dystrophia myotonica

Clinical manifestations of cardiac involvement occur in over 50% of cases. Most common are conduction disturbances, including all degrees of AV block and bundle branch block. Sinus bradycardia and atrial and ventricular arrhythmias also occur.

Friedreich's ataxia

Up to 50% of patients have symptomatic myocardial disease and nearly all patients have ECG abnormalities. Hypertrophic cardiomyopathy is the most common cardiac disorder and is often responsible for death.

Guillain–Barré syndrome

Despite mechanical ventilation, Guillain–Barré syndrome remains fatal in up to 20% of cases: a proportion of these deaths are sudden, and may be attributed to cardiac arrhythmias. Both brady- and tachyarrhythmias occur, and ECG monitoring is recommended, particularly in severe cases.

INFECTIVE DISEASE

Infective endocarditis, viral myocarditis and pericarditis have been previously discussed (see Chapters 6–8) and will not be considered further in this section.

Tuberculosis

In many parts of the world tuberculosis remains a common cause of pericarditis tamponade and constriction although it is seen less often in developed countries (Fig. 16.2). Myocardial involvement is very rare but may lead to AV block, ventricular aneurysm, arrhythmias or heart failure.

Syphilis

Cardiovascular syphilis is now rarely seen due to effective treatment in the early stages of the disease. Spirochaetal invasion of the aortic media occurs soon after the initial infection and is usually localized in the ascending aorta. Medial necrosis, fibrosis and calcification lead to aortic dilatation after a latent period of

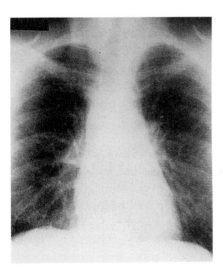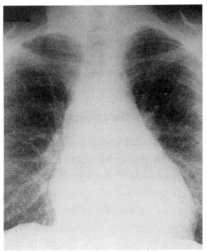

Fig. 16.2 Tuberculous pericardial effusion. The chest X-ray on the left shows hilar lymphadenopathy. Cervical lymph node biopsy 3 weeks later confirmed tuberculosis. Meanwhile a repeat chest X-ray had shown considerable cardiac enlargement due to pericardial effusion.

up to 25 years. Aneurysm formation in the ascending aorta is the most common manifestation, and when this involves the aortic valve ring it leads to aortic regurgitation. Ostial stenoses of the coronary arteries also occur. Aneurysmal compression or erosion of adjacent mediastinal or bony structures may produce a variety of symptoms and signs including pain, dysphagia, stridor and hoarseness. Aortic regurgitation commonly leads to LVF, while coronary ostial stenoses are a cause of angina and, less frequently, MI. Death is usually the result of LVF or aneurysmal rupture.

Diphtheria

This is now rarely seen due to effective immunization in infancy. The diphtheria bacillus infects the pharynx and secretes an exotoxin which causes acute myocarditis in 20% of cases, which is the most common cause of death. By the end of the first week of the illness, the heart is dilated with severe contractile dysfunction, and all grades of heart block may occur. Heart failure with pulmonary congestion commonly develops. Treatment is with antitoxin and penicillin; if the patient survives, recovery of normal myocardial function can be expected in most, but not all, cases.

Trypanosomiasis (Chagas' disease)

This disease, caused by the protozoon parasite *Trypanosoma cruzi*, is endemic in Central and South America where it is responsible for about 30% of all deaths. It is transmitted by the reduviid bug. Occasionally, an acute illness develops at the time of the initial infection but in the majority of cases there is a latent period of up to 25 years before chronic Chagas' disease develops. This is characterized by biventricular dilatation and contractile failure with involvement of the conduction tissues. Symptoms and signs are those of congestive heart failure. The ECG usually shows bundle branch block and, in many patients, complete AV block develops. Ventricular arrhythmias are common.

Acquired immunodeficiency syndrome

Cardiac involvement in acquired immunodeficiency syndrome (AIDS) is common but rarely clinically prominent, usually being obscured by the systemic manifestations of the syndrome. Myocarditis is a consequence of opportunistic infection and a variety of organisms have been implicated including *Pneumocystis carinii*, *Mycobacterium tuberculosis* and *Candida albicans*. In most cases it is asymptomatic and diagnosed only at post-mortem, but occasionally it causes severe congestive heart failure and cardiac arrhythmias. Endocarditis is nearly always the non-bacterial thrombotic variety (marantic endocarditis) that is known to be associated with long-term wasting illnesses and malignancies. Embolic complications have occasionally been reported. Pericarditis is usually associated with concomitant myocardial disease and is caused by infiltration with Kaposi's sarcoma or opportunistic infection.

NEOPLASTIC DISORDERS

Primary tumours

Primary cardiac tumours are rare, the histologically benign myxoma accounting for at least half of all cases. Myxomas usually arise in the left atrium but are also found in the other cardiac chambers. Typically the tumour is pedunculated and attached to the interatrial septum, prolapsing into the mitral valve orifice during diastole (Fig. 16.3). This impedes diastolic filling of the left ventricle and produces symptoms similar to those of mitral stenosis (MS). Nevertheless, the dyspnoea is often episodic and provoked by changes in posture which encourage gravitational prolapse of the tumour into the mitral valve. On examination, there is a low-pitched noise in mid-diastole (tumour plop) probably caused by the myxoma striking the LV wall. This may be mistaken for the mid-diastolic murmur of MS. Other symptoms and signs variably present include fever, weight loss and clubbing. The erythrocyte sedimentation rate (ESR) may be raised and systemic thromboembolism is common. Sudden death may occur if the tumour causes unrelieved obstruction of the mitral valve. In the past, left atrial myxoma was usually misdiagnosed as MS but the echocardiogram now permits visualization of the tumour and rules out mitral valve disease. Treatment is by surgical excision of the tumour.

Other benign tumours of the heart (Table 16.1) usually present with heart failure due to intracavity obstruction to flow, and may also cause myocardial contractile dysfunction (particularly if very large) and conduction disturbance. Rhabdomyomas are most commonly seen in infants and, if large, may be a cause of stillbirth. About half of all cases occur in association with tuberous sclerosis.

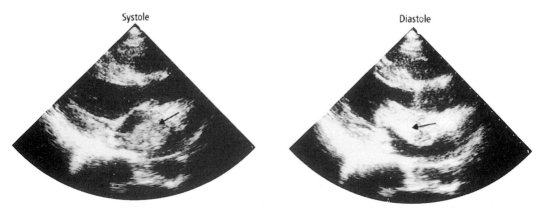

Systole   Diastole

Fig. 16.3 Left atrial myxoma—two-dimensional echocardiogram (long axis view). Note that during diastole the tumour (arrowed) prolapses through the valve obstructing left ventricular filling.

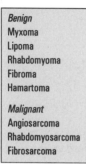

Table 16.1 Classification of primary cardiac tumours.

Benign
Myxoma
Lipoma
Rhabdomyoma
Fibroma
Hamartoma
Malignant
Angiosarcoma
Rhabdomyosarcoma
Fibrosarcoma

Fibromas and hamartomas occur principally in children but lipomas occur in all age groups.

Malignant tumours of the heart are nearly all sarcomas and include angiosarcomas, rhabdomyosarcomas and fibrosarcomas. They usually present in adults and, because they proliferate rapidly, death occurs early in the clinical course (Fig. 16.4).

Metastatic tumours

Metastases account for the majority of cardiac tumours and usually originate from the breast or lung. The pericardium is most commonly affected but any other part of the heart may also be involved. Most cases are clinically silent, but pericardial effusion and tamponade is the most common clinical presentation. Invasion of the conducting tissue may produce heart block, and occasionally extensive myocardial involvement or valvular obstruction leads to heart failure.

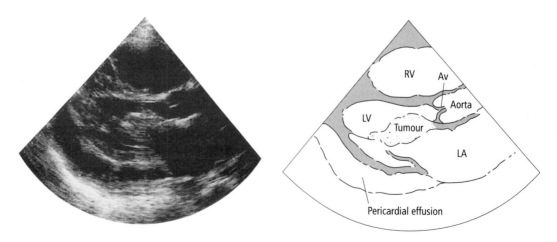

Fig. 16.4 Fibrosarcoma—two-dimensional echocardiogram (long axis view). The large tumour applied to the anterior leaflet of the mitral valve is seen. Pericardial seeding has led to pericardial effusion.

FURTHER READING

Buckley BH, Hutchins GM. Atrial myxoma: a fifty year review. *Am Heart J* 1979; 97: 639.

Doherty NE, Siegel RJ. Cardiovascular manifestations of systemic lupus erythematosus. *Am Heart J* 1985; 110: 1257.

Fleming HA. Sarcoid heart disease. *Br Med J* 1986; 292: 1095.

Francke U, Furthmayr H. Marfan's syndrome and other disorders of fibrillin. *N Engl J Med* 1994; 330: 1385.

Fyke FE, Seward JB, Edwards WD et al. Primary cardiac tumors: experience with 30 consecutive patients since the introduction of two-dimensional echocardiography. *J Am Coll Cardiol* 1985; 5: 1965.

Goldman AP, Kotler MN. Heart disease in scleroderma. *Am Heart J* 1985; 110: 1043.

Gottdiener JS, Hawley RJ, Maron BJ, Bertorini TF, Engle WK. Characteristics of the cardiac hypertrophy in Friedreich's ataxia. *Am Heart J* 1982; 103: 525.

Hayward RP, Emanuel RW, Nabarro JBN. Acromegalic heart disease: influence of treatment of the acromegaly of the heart. *Q J Med* 1987; 237: 41.

Hiromasa S, Ikeda T, Kubota K. Myotonic dystrophy: ambulatory electrocardiogram, electrophysiologic study, and echocardiographic evaluation. *Am Heart J* 1987; 113: 1482.

Homans D. Peripartum cardiomyopathy. *N Engl J Med* 1985; 312: 1432.

Hunsacker RH, Fulkerson PK, Barry FJ, Lewis RO, Leier CV, Unverferth DV. Cardiac function in Duchenne's muscular dystrophy. *Am J Med* 1982; 73: 235.

Jacob AJ, Boon NA. HIV cardiomyopathy: a dark cloud with a silver lining? *Br Heart J* 1991; 66: 1.

Kaul S, Fishbein MC, Siegel RJ. Cardiac manifestations of acquired immune deficiency syndrome: a 1991 update. *Am Heart J* 1991; 122: 535.

Kirk J, Cosh J. The pericarditis of rheumatoid arthritis. *Q J Med* 1969; 38:397.

Oliveira JS. A natural model of intrinsic heart nervous system denervation: Chagas' cardiopathy. *Am Heart J* 1985; 110: 1092.

Roberts WC, Honig HS. The spectrum of cardiovascular disease in the Marfan syndrome: a clinico-morphologic study of 18 necropsy patients and comparison to 151 previously reported patients. *Am Heart J* 1982; 104: 115.

Schrader ML, Hochman JS, Bulkley BH. The heart in polyarteritis nodosa: a clinicopathologic study. *Am Heart J* 1985; 109: 1353.

Stevens MB. Lupus carditis. *N Engl J Med* 1988; 319: 861.

Sullivan JM, Ramanathan KB. Management of medical problems in pregnancy: severe cardiac disease. *N Engl J Med* 1985; 313: 304.

Symons C. Thyroid heart disease. *Br Heart J* 1979; 41: 257.

Zarich SW, Nesto RW. Diabetic cardiomyopathy. *Am Heart J* 1989; 118: 1000.

CHAPTER 17

Surgery and Heart Disease

SUMMARY

Preoperative factors. The perioperative and long-term cardiac risk of non-cardiac surgery is heightened in patients with prior myocardial infarction (MI), angina, congestive heart failure, or diabetes, especially those who are older or have unstable symptoms. If angina is stable the excess risk is trivial and can be reduced further by prophylactic beta-blockers. Recent unstable symptoms, however, provide indication for preoperative angiography and, if necessary, revascularization to protect against perioperative infarction and death. In patients with MI in the previous 6 months, the perioperative risk is particularly high and elective surgical procedures are effectively contraindicated. Heart failure also increases surgical risk and should always be controlled in the preoperative period. Valvular disease requires antibiotic prophylaxis against endocarditis only if the risk of bacteraemia is high (bowel or dental surgery). Anticoagulation with subcutaneous heparin is recommended for all patients prior to surgery to protect against pulmonary embolism.

Perioperative factors. Anaesthetic agents can cause severe hypotension, through direct effects on the myocardium and the autonomic nervous system, leading to coronary hypoperfusion and low-output failure. Risk is particularly high during induction when careful monitoring of blood pressure is essential. The arrhythmogenic properties of anaesthetic agents may also be troublesome and demand continuous ECG monitoring. Myocardial injury may complicate severe hypotension and coronary hypoperfusion, but the risk is particularly high during cardiopulmonary bypass when the incidence of perioperative infarction is related to the duration of the procedure and the adequacy of myocardial protection.

Postoperative factors. Fluid imbalance is the major cause of cardiovascular instability in the postoperative period. Requirements can be monitored with a central venous catheter but, in patients with left ventricular disease, a pulmonary artery (Swan–Ganz) catheter may help by providing an indirect measure of left ventricular filling pressure.

PREOPERATIVE FACTORS

In patients undergoing non-cardiac surgery, a careful preoperative history and examination coupled with a chest X-ray provide a useful estimate of perioperative and long-term cardiac risk. An ECG is also recommended in patients over 65. Patients at greatest risk include those with prior MI, angina, congestive heart failure or diabetes, especially those who are older or have unstable symptoms. The effects of these risk factors are additive: patients with none of them have a 3% risk of perioperative infarction or death during vascular surgery; the risk rises to 15–20% in patients with three or more risk factors.

Coronary artery disease: prior myocardial infarction, angina

Patients with coronary artery disease are at risk of perioperative MI which is an important cause of surgical death. There are three separate components to the heightened surgical risk.

1 Adrenergic stress increasing myocardial oxygen demand and the risk of plaque rupture.

2 Reductions in myocardial oxygen delivery due to hypotension and pulmonary congestion.

3 The hypercoagulable state induced by surgery, predisposing to coronary thrombosis.

In patients who are symptomatically stable (no recent deterioration in angina), however, the risk is remarkably low ($< 2\%$), particularly when surgery is conducted with modern surgical, anaesthetic and postoperative care facilities. Prophylactic beta-blockade reduces the risk still further. Thus, there is no indication for routine preoperative investigation of these patients either by stress testing or by angiography. Patients with recent unstable symptoms, on the other hand, represent a much higher surgical risk and in this group coronary angiography with a view to revascularization is a sensible precaution prior to elective non-cardiac surgery. Perioperative risk is also increased in patients with MI during the previous 6 months in whom there is a 16% risk of recurrent infarction during the perioperative period. For this reason, recent MI should be regarded as a contraindication to elective surgical procedures.

Heart failure

The patient with heart failure is a considerably higher operative risk than the patient with a normal heart, regardless of the cause of heart failure and the nature of the surgical procedure. In major non-cardiac surgery, perioperative mortality rises from 4% in mild heart failure to 67% in severe heart failure. A similar pattern of risk exists in patients undergoing cardiac procedures. Mitral valve replacement, for example, carries a 3% mortality for moderately symptomatic patients but a 17% mortality for the severely symptomatic patient who is dyspnoeic at rest. Thus heart failure should always be controlled before submitting the patient to elective surgical procedures.

Valvular disease

Where possible elective surgery should be avoided in the patient with severe valvular heart disease until after valve replacement. In those patients with less severe lesions undergoing surgery, antibiotic prophylaxis against endocarditis is not necessary unless there is an important risk of bacteraemia, e.g. bowel surgery, dental surgery.

Arrhythmias

Careful control of cardiac arrhythmias is essential before patients are submitted to surgery.

Anticoagulant therapy

Oral anticoagulant therapy (warfarin) should be discontinued at least 3 days before elective surgical procedures because of the risk of bleeding. Subcutaneous heparin (5000 units 8-hourly) can be substituted and continued into the early postoperative period. Indeed heparin is recommended for all surgical procedures to protect against pulmonary embolism, particularly in patients undergoing pelvic or hip surgery. Now available is low molecular weight heparin for once daily administration which may be more effective and is certainly more convenient to use. In the event of bleeding complications, heparin (unlike warfarin) can be rapidly reversed with protamine.

PERIOPERATIVE FACTORS

Heart failure

The cardiovascular properties of anaesthetic agents, mediated through direct effects on the heart and the autonomic nervous system, can have a profound influence on the circulation during surgery. Induction of anaesthesia with thiopentone, for example, can cause myocardial depression and vasodilatation leading to severe hypotension. This is particularly undesirable in patients with coronary artery disease in whom reductions in blood pressure may threaten the perfusion of regionally ischaemic myocardium and lead to MI. Thus, careful monitoring of blood pressure is essential during this critical part of the anaesthetic procedure. Many other anaesthetic agents depress the myocardium and can exacerbate heart failure, although the degree to which this occurs in practice is modified by the extent of simultaneous stimulation of the sympathetic nervous system. Halothane produces little sympathetic stimulation and can cause severe hypotension and myocardial contractile failure in susceptible subjects.

Arrhythmias

Anaesthetic agents also have important arrhythmogenic properties which are heightened by hypoxaemia, electrolyte disorders and acid–base imbalance, all of which may occur during prolonged surgical procedures. Intubation at the start of the anaesthetic procedure elicits a profound vagal response which may cause heart block or asystole.

Myocardial injury

The risk of MI during surgery has already been discussed. Myocardial injury may also occur as a complication of heart surgery. The risk is greatest for open heart procedures when the heart is isolated from the circulation during cardiopulmonary bypass. The incidence of myocardial injury is related to both the duration of the procedure and the adequacy of myocardial protection. Myocardial protection is provided by cooling the heart and, in some cases, by selective perfusion of the coronary arteries with oxygenated blood. In a few cases, however, myocardial injury develops which is not always reversible in the postoperative period. Factors unrelated to the bypass procedure can also contribute to myocardial injury during open heart surgery. These include embolization of air or platelet fragments into the coronary circulation and inadvertent damage to the coronary arteries.

POSTOPERATIVE FACTORS

Fluid balance

Early after major surgical procedures the patient is particularly sensitive to the consequences of fluid imbalance. Under normal circumstances, fluctuations in plasma volume are compensated for by reflex adjustments of venous capacity, such that cardiac filling remains constant within a narrow range. However, these homeostatic responses may be attenuated during the postoperative period due to the effects of anaesthetic and analgesic agents on venous tone. Thus, a relatively minor plasma volume deficit can produce severe reductions in ventricular filling and cardiac output whilst excessive fluid replacement readily causes pulmonary oedema.

Maintenance of haemodynamic stability after major surgery is made easier by measuring ventricular filling pressures. In most patients, fluid requirements can be titrated against right atrial pressure measured with a central venous catheter. The right atrial pressure should be maintained in the normal range, between 5 and 8 mmHg (equivalent to a left atrial pressure of 9–13 mmHg). In the patient with heart failure, however, the relation between the ventricular filling pressures is variable and it is more difficult to predict left atrial pressure from measurements of central venous pressure. In difficult cases, therefore, indirect measurement of left atrial pressure with a Swan–Ganz catheter may be helpful for titration of fluid replacement (see page 67): a pulmonary artery wedge pressure of 15–20 mmHg is optimal because this takes maximal advantage of the Starling effect without producing pulmonary oedema. If cardiac output remain inadequate, despite adjustment of plasma volume, treatment with vasodilators or inotropes is indicated to improve left ventricular performance.

The patient recovering from open heart surgery can present special problems if recovery of myocardial contractile function is delayed. The 'stunned' heart does not always respond to inotropic stimulation and intra-aortic balloon pump therapy may be necessary. This is a useful temporizing measure pending recovery of normal contractile function.

FURTHER READING

Anonymous. Perioperative myocardial ischaemia and non-cardiac surgery. *Lancet* 1991; 337: 1516.

Collins R, Scrimgeour A, Yusuf S, Peto R. Reduction in fatal pulmonary embolism and venous thrombosis by perioperative administration of subcutaneous heparin. Overview of results of randomized trials in general, orthopedic and urologic surgery. *N Engl J Med* 1988; 318: 1162.

Eagle KA, Boucher CA. Cardiac risk of noncardiac surgery. *N Engl J Med* 1989; 321: 1330.

Eagle KA, Froehlich JB. Reducing cardiovascular risk in patients undergoing noncardiac surgery. *N Engl J Med* 1996; 335: 1761.

Goldman L. Assessment of perioperative cardiac risk. *N Engl J Med* 1994; 330: 709.

Mamode M, Cobbe S, Pollock JG. Infarcts after surgery. *Br Med J* 1995; 310: 1215.

Index